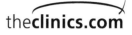

CLINICS IN GERIATRIC MEDICINE

Gastroenterology

GUEST EDITOR
Syed H. Tariq, MD, FACP

November 2007 • Volume 23 • Number 4

SAUNDERS

An Imprint of Elsevier, Inc.
PHILADELPHIA   LONDON   TORONTO   MONTREAL   SYDNEY   TOKYO

W.B. SAUNDERS COMPANY
A Division of Elsevier Inc.

Elsevier, Inc. • 1600 John F. Kennedy Blvd., Suite 1800 • Philadelphia, PA 19103-2899

http://www.theclinics.com

CLINICS IN GERIATRIC MEDICINE
November 2007
Editor: Lisa Richman

Volume 23, Number
ISSN 0749-069
ISBN-13: 978-1-4160-5049-
ISBN-10: 1-4160-5049-

GUEST EDITOR

SYED H. TARIQ, MD, FACP, Associate Professor of Internal Medicine, Department of Internal Medicine, Divisions of Geriatric Medicine, Saint Louis University School of Medicine, St. Louis, Missouri

CONTRIBUTORS

IAN McPHEE CHAPMAN, MBBS, PhD, Associate Professor, Department of Medicine, University of Adelaide, Royal Adelaide Hospital, North Terrace, Adelaide, Australia

SARAH J. CRANE, MD, Senior Associate Consultant, Division of Primary Care Internal Medicine, Mayo Clinic College of Medicine, Rochester, Minnesota

ADRIAN M. DI BISCEGLIE, MD, Acting Chairman, Department of Internal Medicine, Saint Louis University School of Medicine, Saint Louis, Missouri; Professor of Internal Medicine, Division of Gastroenterology and Hepatology, Saint Louis University School of Medicine, Saint Louis, Missouri

BURAK GURSES, MD, Assistant Professor of Medicine, Meharry Medical College, Nashville, Tennessee

MICHAEL HOROWITZ, MBBS, PhD, FRACP, Professor of Medicine, Discipline of Medicine, Royal Adelaide Hospital, North Terrace, Adelaide, South Australia, Australia

OMER JUNAIDI, MD, Clinical Instructor, Department of Internal Medicine, Saint Louis University School of Medicine, Saint Louis, Missouri

PAUL KUO, MBBS, PhD student, Discipline of Medicine, Royal Adelaide Hospital, North Terrace, Adelaide, South Australia, Australia

GEORGE MEKHJIAN, MD, Internal Medicine, St. Anthony's Hospital, Alton, Illinois

JOHN E. MORLEY, MB, BCh, Division of Geriatric Medicine, Saint Louis University, Medical Center, Saint Louis University School of Medicine, St. Louis, Missouri; and GRECC, VA Medical Center, St. Louis, Missouri

NURI OZDEN, MD, Assistant Professor of Medicine, Department of Internal Medicine, Director, Division of Gastroenterology and Hepatology, Meharry Medical College, Nashville, Tennessee

KAVITA PRABHAKAR, MD, MPH, TM, Infectious Diseases and Tropical Medicine Physician, Brookfield, Connecticut

CHRISTOPHER K. RAYNER, MBBS, PhD, FRACP, Senior lecturer, Discipline of Medicine, Royal Adelaide Hospital, North Terrace, Adelaide, South Australia, Australia

HELMUT K. SEITZ, MD, Professor of Medicine and Chief, Department of Medicine & Center of Alcohol Research, Liver Disease and Nutrition, Salem Medical Center, University of Heidelberg, Heidelberg, Germany

FELIX STICKEL, MD, Assistant Professor of Medicine, Institute of Clinical Pharmacology, University of Berne, Berne, Switzerland

PRABHAKAR P. SWAROOP, MD, Assistant Professor of Medicine, Consultant Hepatology, Division of Digestive and Liver Diseases, Department of Internal Medicine, UT Southwestern Medical Center, Dallas, Texas

NICHOLAS J. TALLEY, MD, PhD, Professor of Medicine, Division of Gastroenterology and Hepatology, Chair, Department of Internal Medicine, Mayo Clinic College of Medicine, Jacksonville, Florida

SYED H. TARIQ, MD, FACP, Associate Professor of Internal Medicine, Department of Internal Medicine, Divisions of Geriatric Medicine, Saint Louis University School of Medicine, St. Louis, Missouri

CHANTRI TRINH, MD, Adjunct Assistant Professor, Division of Geriatric Medicine, Department of Internal Medicine, Saint Louis University School of Medicine, St. Louis, Missouri

CONTENTS

Typical and atypical symptoms from acid reflux, dyspepsia, chronic constipation, fecal incontinence, and irritable bowel syndrome are extremely common in adults and remain so in the geriatric population. The presence of these problems may have profound effects on the functional status, independence, and quality of life in the vulnerable older population, making it essential for physicians to inquire actively about them and to be able to recognize atypical presentations when appropriate. This article summarizes the definitions, epidemiology, clinical presentation, and impact of these common problems in the geriatric patient.

Undernutrition is common in the elderly, particularly those in nursing homes and other institutions. It is associated with substantial adverse effects. The age-associated physiologic reduction in appetite and food intake, which has been termed "the anorexia of aging," contributes to the development of pathologic anorexia and undernutrition. This article reviews age-related changes to appetite, food intake, and body composition; undernutrition in the elderly; and the factors contributing to physiologic and pathologic anorexia and undernutrition.

Changes in the physiology of the gastrointestinal tract with aging are less obvious than are seen in other organs, such as the brain.

Nevertheless, physiologic changes play a role in the anorexia of aging, postprandial hypotension, aspiration pneumonia, increased *Clostridium difficile* infections, fecal incontinence, gallstones, and altered drug metabolism.

constipation. Irritable bowel syndrome should be considered in the differential diagnosis of abdominal pain, diarrhea and constipation in older persons.

Diarrhea in the elderly population is one disease that needs special attention in treatment and management, especially in acute- and long-term care residents, because of their multiple comorbidities, immunosenescence, frailty, and poor nutritional status. Close follow-up to ensure adequate hydration and electrolyte replacement and infection control measures to contain outbreaks should be emphasized to caregivers and nursing staff in acute- and long-term care facilities. Although *C difficile* colitis causes significant morbidity and mortality in this population, judicious use of antibiotics is important to decrease the incidence and recurrence of the disease. When the diarrhea is chronic and all stool testings and serologies have been performed, the patient may benefit from endoscopy and colonoscopy for biopsy. Attentive and vigilant nursing staff is crucial in the timely diagnosis and treatment of diarrheal diseases to improve quality of life and reduce mortality.

Fecal incontinence is an underreported and underappreciated problem in older adults. Although fecal incontinence is more common in women than in men, this difference narrows with aging. Risk factors that lead to the development of fecal incontinence include dementia, physical disability, and fecal impaction. Treatment options include medical or conservative therapy for older adults who have mild incontinence, and surgical options can be explored in selected older adults if surgical expertise is available.

Intestinal ischemia is a relatively common disorder in the elderly and, if not treated promptly, still carries a high morbidity and mortality rate. High degree of clinical suspicion is of paramount importance in diagnosis, because there is no specific laboratory test available and physical examination findings may be subtle. Once the diagnosis is made, management relies on early resuscitation, identification, and treatment of the predisposing conditions, along with careful planning of the therapeutic invasive interventions, which altogether may help reduce the mortality and morbidity associated with this condition.

Chronic liver disease and cirrhosis are the tenth leading causes of death in the United States and results in approximately 25,000 deaths annually. As life expectancy in developed countries has increased, so has the number of elderly patients who have liver disease. With an aging population and chronic liver disease becoming an increasingly significant cause of morbidity and mortality, the various causes for hepatitis will need to be evaluated and available treatments considered, even in elderly population. Common causes for hepatitis in elderly individuals include viral, autoimmune, and drug-induced hepatitis, but evidence for treatment of this population is limited. This article reviews the likely causes of hepatitis in elderly individuals and discusses evidence for treating this population.

Although per capita alcohol consumption, and thus the prevalence of alcoholic liver disease, decreases generally with age in Europe and in the United States, recently an increase in alcohol consumption has been reported in individuals over 65 years. Reasons explaining this observation may include an increase in life expectancy or a loss of life partners and, thus, loneliness and depression. Although ethanol metabolism and ethanol distribution change with age, and an elderly person's liver is more susceptible to the toxic effect of ethanol, the spectrum of alcoholic liver diseases and their symptoms and signs is similar to that seen in patients of all ages. However, prognosis of alcoholic liver disease in the elderly is poor. In addition, chronic alcohol consumption may enhance drug associated liver disease and may also act as a cofactor in other liver diseases, such as viral hepatitis and nonalcoholic fatty liver disease.

FORTHCOMING ISSUES

PREVIOUS ISSUES

THE CLINICS ARE NOW AVAILABLE ONLINE!

Access your subscription at:
www.theclinics.com

ELSEVIER
SAUNDERS

Clin Geriatr Med 23 (2007) xi–xiii

CLINICS IN
GERIATRIC
MEDICINE

Preface

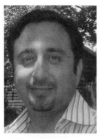

Syed H. Tariq, MD, FACP
Guest Editor

No organ in the body is so misunderstood, so slandered and maltreated as the colon.

—Sir Arthur Hurst, 1935

It is estimated that by the year 2030 there will be 27 million people age 65 years and older. This growing population's livelihood is often complicated by underlying age related changes, polypharmacy, chronic medical conditions, psychosocial stressors resulting from loss of bodily functions (incontinence, inability to walk or live at home), or loss of a spouse or child. Oftentimes, these aliments are further compounded by loss of memory. In older patients with poor cognition it is extremely difficult for the healthcare provider to obtain a good history, and in turn reach the crux of the problem. It is because of this important fact that all older adults should be screened for memory loss using instruments such as the Saint Louis University Mental Status Examination [1]. Older patients should also be screened for depression, along with screening for erectile dysfunction, problems related to appetite, incontinence, as well as other assessments needed to provide a complete comprehensive geriatric evaluation.

In regards to the gastrointestinal (GI) function, aging has a relatively small effect because of the large, efficient reserve of the GI tract. Changes that do occur in the GI tract usually go unnoticed unless severe stress is placed on the gut. In contrast, aging is associated with an increased prevalence of several GI disorders, including those induced by drugs (*eg*, gastrointestinal bleeding caused by nonsteroidal anti-inflammatory drugs),

doi:10.1016/j.cger.2007.09.001
geriatric.theclinics.com

anorexia of aging, development of constipation, diarrhea or fecal incontinence, and postprandial hypotension. In the next few decades, it is expected
that there will be a rise in prevalence of both hepatitis B and C. Therefore,
more in depth research will be necessary to evaluate the treatment of chronic
hepatitis.

One of the most relevant progressions in the geriatric population, that
needs a through evaluation, is the physiologic anorexia of aging that causes
weight loss and possibly cachexia. The first stride is to properly differentiate
physiologic anorexia from pathologic undernutrition. The etiology of anorexia of aging has not been fully defined, but there are some probable
causes, such as decreased sense of smell and taste, reduced palatability of
food, alteration of GI function, age related hormonal changes, and an increase in the level of cytokines [2]. It is also clear that anorexia of aging places older persons at a higher risk of having a severe decrease in food intake,
and is further worsened by special diets [3]. In this population, the magnitude of any problem they face can easily enhance the likelihood of malnutrition. It is therefore important to be familiar with some of the common
causes of geriatric malnutrition, such as poverty, shopping and preparation
of food, limited transport or social support, presence of depression or dementia, alcoholism, and chronic medical conditions, to name a few.

Fecal incontinence is one the most devastating conditions an older person
may face. In the nursing home population alone, fecal incontinence is nearly
50%. Along with urinary incontinence, it makes up one of the leading causes
of nursing home placement. At this time, fecal incontinence is an underreported and undervalued problem in older adults. Although fecal incontinence is more common in women than in men, the difference does begin
to narrow with the increase of age. Some of the risk factors that lead to
the development of fecal incontinence include dementia, physical disability,
and fecal impaction. Treatment options include medical or conservative
therapy. Surgical options may also be explored, based on the availability
of surgical expertise in selected older adults [4].

Constipation is very common in older adults and accounts for increased
physician office visits and hospital admissions. There is no agreement on the
definition of constipation, regarding what patients perceive as constipation
and what physicians traditionally view as constipation. The etiology of constipation is multifactorial, and when left untreated, results in complications,
such as impaction, fecal incontinence, obstruction of the bowel, perforation
of the colon, and even death. Laxative use also increases with age; at times
multiple agents are used to relieve symptoms of constipation. Currently, the
most commonly used laxative is stool softener; however stool softener does
lack efficacy. It appears that osmotic laxatives are effective in older adults
and well tolerated. Psyllium, a bulk laxative, is also effective, and while there
is limited evidence for stimulants, dioctyl sulfosuccinate is also used in the
treatment of constipation. There is a clear need for a large-scale trial to examine an appropriate cost-effective approach to the management of

constipation in older persons, in particular in the nursing home where the problem is of paramount importance [5].

Although the specialty of geriatrics involves many different areas of awareness, this issue of geriatric gastroenterology offers a comprehensive review for some of the most significant concerns that impact the lives of older persons. The authors have done an exemplary job in addressing the most recent information about physiologic changes, disease presentation, and management issues in the ever-growing geriatric population. I hope this issue will serve as a resource for those clinicians who are involved in the care of older persons.

Finally, I would like to thank all the authors who made invaluable contributions to this issue.

Syed H. Tariq, MD, FACP
Saint Louis University School of Medicine
Division of Geriatric Medicine
1402 South Grand Boulevard, M-238
Saint Louis, MO 63104, USA

E-mail address: tariqsh@slu.edu

References

[1] Tariq SH, Tumosa N, Chibnall JT, et al. The Saint Louis University Mental Status (SLUMS) examination for detecting mild cognitive impairment and dementia is more sensitive than Mini Mental Status Examination (MMSE)—A pilot study. Am J Geriatr Psychiatry 2006; 14(11):900–10.

[2] Chapman IM, MacIntosh CG, Morley JE, et al. The anorexia of ageing. Biogerontology 2002; 3(1–2):67–71.

[3] Tariq SH, Karcic E, Thomas DR, et al. Non-concentrated sweets vs. regular diet in the management of type-2 diabetes in nursing homes. Am J of Dietetic Assoc 2001;101:1463–6.

[4] Tariq SH, Morley JE, Prather CM. Health issues in the elderly: fecal incontinence: importance, clinical evaluation and treatment. Am J of Medicine 2003;115(3):217–27.

[5] Tariq SH. Constipation in long-term care. J Am Med Dir Assoc 2007;(8):209–18.

ELSEVIER
SAUNDERS

CLINICS IN
GERIATRIC
MEDICINE

Clin Geriatr Med 23 (2007) 721–734

Chronic Gastrointestinal Symptoms in the Elderly

Sarah J. Crane, MD[a], Nicholas J. Talley, MD, PhD[b],*

[a]Division of Primary Care Internal Medicine, Mayo Clinic College of Medicine,
200 First Street S.W., Rochester, MN 55905, USA
[b]Division of Gastroenterology and Hepatology, Department of Internal Medicine,
Mayo Clinic College of Medicine, 4500 San Pablo Road,
Jacksonville, FL 32224, USA

The population of patients aged 65 years and older is growing rapidly, with an anticipated increase in the United States from 34 million in the year 2000 to 71 million by the year 2030 [1]. Within that age range, there is a tremendous heterogeneity, from the functional young-old, to the more frail old-old, to patients living in long-term care facilities with severe functional impairment and cognitive dysfunction. The oldest-old represent the fastest growing subgroup of this population [2]. Within this changing population, evidence suggests that many gastrointestinal diseases, such as gastroesophageal reflux disease (GERD) and irritable bowel syndrome (IBS), continue to be a lifelong problem for patients extending well into older age. Other problems, such as fecal incontinence and chronic constipation, have an increasing prevalence and impact on quality of life and functional status as patients age.

Common gastrointestinal (GI) complaints may present new challenges for patients and their physicians in geriatric practice. The underlying diagnosis is complicated by the greater prevalence of diseases such as ischemia, pathologic lesions of the upper and lower GI tracts, persisting infections (eg, *Helicobacter pylori*), and acute infectious diseases (eg, *Clostridium difficile* and diverticulitis). In addition, the clinical implications of GI diseases are altered significantly in the older patient who has a decreased physiologic reserve with an increased risk for malnutrition resulting in falls, depression, social isolation, and a deterioration of functional status. Treatment options

* Corresponding author.
E-mail address: talley.nicholas@mayo.edu (N.J. Talley).

0749-0690/07/$ - see front matter © 2007 Elsevier Inc. All rights reserved.
doi:10.1016/j.cger.2007.06.003   *geriatric.theclinics.com*

often are limited by patient comorbidities and the side effects of the medications, which tend to be more pronounced in this population.

This article focuses on the epidemiology, presentation, and impact of five common GI symptom complexes: reflux symptoms, dyspepsia, constipation, fecal incontinence, and IBS. Some of the atypical symptom presentations in the elderly also are highlighted.

Heartburn and reflux symptoms

Definitions

GERD is defined as symptoms or lesions resulting from the reflux of gastric contents into the distal esophagus. Heartburn and acid regurgitation are common; however, the symptom cutoffs that are used to define the disease GERD have varied greatly, resulting in a wide range of prevalence and incidence figures [3]. Defining GERD in the elderly is more challenging because they often present with atypical symptoms that may not be associated with heartburn or reflux. They also may have severe erosive disease with few, if any, symptoms. Thus, a clinical definition of GERD in the elderly may not be an accurate reflection of the spectrum and severity of the disease in this population.

Epidemiology

The prevalence of GERD in the general adult population is estimated to be 10% to 20% based on symptoms that occur at least weekly [4]. By comparison, in a study of 487 Finnish residents aged 65 years or older conducted in 1993, the prevalence of daily GERD symptoms was 8% in men and 15% in women; however, more than half of the respondents reported symptoms at least monthly [5]. The prevalence by age group is summarized in Table 1 and did not differ significantly with increasing age. The investigators noted that the actual prevalence may be significantly higher, given the challenge of identifying the diagnosis [6].

Clinical features

In practice, the diagnosis of symptomatic GERD remains primarily a clinical one based on patient report of symptoms; however, evidence suggests that some elderly patients have significantly altered pain and symptom perception that may affect the manifestation of common GI syndromes, such as GERD [7]. Most older patients who are diagnosed present with typical symptoms of heartburn or acid reflux; however, elder patients with documented GERD by endoscopy also may complain of atypical symptoms, such as chest pain, dysphagia, dyspepsia, hoarseness, postprandial fullness, respiratory symptoms, vomiting, or belching [5,8]. Furthermore, these symptoms may not be associated with the typical heartburn or regurgitation

Table 1
Prevalence (%) of symptoms suggestive of gastroesophageal reflux by age and gender

Age group (y)	Daily	Weekly	Monthly	At least once monthly
Men				
65–69	1.6	19.7	36.1	57.4
70–74	5.4	17.9	30.4	53.7
75–80	15.4	19.2	15.4	50.0
81–84	13.0	15.2	21.7	49.9
85+	9.8	22.0	19.5	51.3
All (age adjusted)	7.7	18.7	26.9	53.5
Women				
65–69	13.6	22.0	44.1	79.7
70–74	16.1	12.5	28.6	57.2
75–79	16.7	21.4	31.0	69.1
80–84	14.6	19.5	24.4	58.5
85+	12.1	6.1	27.3	45.5
All (age adjusted)	14.9	17.9	33.4	66.2

From Raiha I, Impivaara O, Seppala M, et al. Prevalence and characteristics of symptomatic gastroesophageal reflux disease in the elderly. J Am Geriatr Soc 1992;40(12):1210; with permission.

symptoms that are used by clinicians to make this diagnosis. Up to 25% of older patients who have esophagitis may not have typical reflux symptoms [6].

The multiple comorbidities often present in the elderly population also may increase the complexity of the diagnosis, particularly in the setting of atypical symptoms, such as chest pain, cough, or dysphagia, all of which raise concerns about cardiac, respiratory, or neurologic diagnoses. Obtaining a more objective diagnosis by ordering upper endoscopy or pH monitoring may be limited by the presence of many medical complexities, such as end-stage cardiac disease or dementia.

To add to the level of concern, in addition to the atypical presenting symptoms in older patients, there may be decreased sensitivity to the sensation of reflux, even in the setting of more severe esophageal injury [9–11]. In a study of Veterans' Administration patients, 52% of younger patients (<65 years) and 47% of older patients (≥ 66 years) who complained of upper GI symptoms had esophagitis on endoscopy, and both age groups presented with similar symptom severity levels. The most significant difference between the two age groups arose in patients who had Barrett's esophagus. Although both age groups had a similar percentage of patients who had Barrett's esophagus, the older patients who had Barrett's esophagus had significantly lower symptom severity scores than did the younger patients; their symptom scores were more comparable to the asymptomatic controls who were included in the study [9]. In a study of 228 consecutive patients who were referred for endoscopy, Collen and colleagues [10] found that 81% of patients older than age 60 years had significant esophageal mucosal disease as compared with 47% of patients younger than age 60 years. They noted a consistent increase in the prevalence of esophagitis related to patient age by decade. There did not seem to be a significant change in acid output associated with increasing age and, again, symptom scores remained similar to those of younger patients. Additional evidence of decreased reliability of symptom perception in older patients is provided by a study in Italy that found that older patients with symptoms of GERD had more frequent severe grades of esophagitis (21% versus 3.4%) when compared with younger patients and that they had more severe reflux on pH monitoring [11].

In addition to a possible reduction in esophageal sensation with aging, there is increasing evidence that the motility of the esophagus is compromised in older people. Studies have demonstrated an age-related decrease in the pressure of the lower esophageal sphincter as well as decreased peristaltic coordination [12]. This could result in more frequent or severe episodes of esophageal exposure to acid.

Given recent interest in the role of screening endoscopy in the prevention of progression from Barrett's esophagus to esophageal adenocarcinoma, the lack of a strong correlation between the severity of the older patients' symptoms and the likelihood of significant disease is a concern. Esophageal adenocarcinoma is primarily a disease of the elderly, with the average age of diagnosis in the late 60s to early 70s [13]. This is precisely the age at which physiologic changes appear to make the role of endoscopic screening based on symptoms most challenging.

Dyspepsia

Definitions

Dyspepsia is defined primarily as epigastric pain or burning or meal-related discomfort that does not include heartburn [14]. Nonulcer (or functional) dyspepsia refers to the subgroup without structural or biochemical explanation for their symptoms, in contrast to those with endoscopic findings of ulcer disease [15]. These definitions remain unchanged in the geriatric population.

Epidemiology

Prevalence studies of dyspepsia have estimated that approximately 15% of the general adult population suffer from dyspepsia, specifically excluding symptoms suggestive of GERD; most (> 53%) have a normal endoscopy [15,16]. In older patients, the prevalence estimates for dyspepsia range from 9% to 25%, but no study has determined the percentage of patients with endoscopic findings [17]. The concern in the older patient is missing an ulcer or cancer in presenters who have dyspepsia.

Clinical features

As in GERD-related disorders, the presentation of ulcer-related disease in the elderly may be atypical. They may have few symptoms of dyspepsia until the disease is advanced. One study documented that 65% of the time patients older than age 80 years presenting with ulcer-related hemorrhage had no complaint of pain before presentation [18]. In a study comparing older patients who had ulcers to younger patients, just 65% of older patients had abdominal pain before diagnosis as compared with 92% of younger patients [19]. These findings were confirmed in a UK study of 277 prospectively identified patients presenting for endoscopy. Approximately 30% of patients older than 60 years had no complaint of pain, which was significantly different than in younger patients, of whom only 14% had no pain [20]. The most common indications for endoscopy given in patients with no pain but an ulcer on examination were nausea, vomiting, and heartburn; however, the list also included weight loss, belching, dysphagia, anorexia, blood loss, and change in bowel habits.

Increased mortality is associated with upper GI bleeding from ulcers in the elderly [21]. It is likely that the delay in diagnosis caused by a decreased awareness of symptoms or atypical symptoms, in combination with a higher prevalence of risk factors and comorbidities, may account for this finding [21,22]. Studies showed that there is no increase in the risk for endoscopic complications and, that following endoscopy, mortality in older patients is similar to that in younger patients, so that current treatment is adequate and equally effective in all age groups [23]. Therefore, the difference in mortality likely is accounted for primarily by the difference in presentation, not intervention.

The high prevalence of risk factors for peptic ulcer disease in the elderly is well known. Nonsteroidal anti-inflammatory drug (NSAID) use and *H pylori* infection are much more common in the elderly, as are complications resulting from the use of NSAIDs [24,25]. It also is estimated that the routine use of NSAIDs or aspirin leads to a twofold increase in the risk for symptoms involving the upper GI tract [26].

There is little information available regarding the risk factors associated with nonulcer dyspepsia in the geriatric population. Given its prevalence in the adult population, it is a common disorder; however, more research is needed.

Similarly, the impact of dyspepsia on functional status and quality of life in older patients remains largely unexplored. One study documented a significant decrease in mobility and lower limb function in older patients complaining of dyspepsia [27]. It is also known that nonulcer dyspepsia results in a significant decrease in health-related quality of life in the general population [28]; however, these studies have yet to be reproduced in the geriatric population.

Chronic constipation

Definitions

Chronic constipation is an extremely common complaint among older patients; however, what is meant by the term "constipation" may differ significantly between patient and physician. The most commonly accepted medical definition of constipation in the adult population is a stool frequency of less than three times a week [29], but this definition significantly underestimates the perceived prevalence of this complaint among geriatric patients [30]. Older patients are much more likely to complain of constipation when it is associated with the sensation of having to strain to pass stool, rather than based on stool frequency, and they are much more likely to self-medicate, often without consulting their physician. This has resulted in the development of several definitions of constipation in an effort to describe the problem accurately in adults, including the geriatric population.

In patients with constipation who do not have a structural or biochemical explanation, there are two broad groups. Functional constipation has been defined as having any two of the following complaints: straining to defecate, passing hard stools, the sensation of incomplete evacuation, and defecating fewer than three times per week, or—in the absence of symptoms—defecating fewer than two times per week [29,31]. Outlet delay constipation describes a group of patients who experience symptoms because of inappropriate contraction of the external anal sphincter on straining or have another cause of anal obstruction (eg, a large rectocele). Such patients also may complain of a sense of anal blockage and prolonged defecation (greater than 10 minutes) or have a history of self-digitation to assist with bowel movements [29].

A third group of patients who would describe themselves as constipated, but who do not fit the traditional definition, are those who use laxatives on a routine basis, resulting in a regular stool pattern. Because of the self-medication, it is difficult to define the severity of their underlying complaint. Often, these patients are intentionally excluded from studies of prevalence because of these complexities, but it is an important group for their primary care physician to recognize.

Epidemiology

Chronic constipation is an extremely common complaint that increases with age in the geriatric population (Figs. 1 and 2) [29]. Measures of prevalence have been challenged, however, by the role of perception and varying definitions within this older population. Several studies suggested that the actual prevalence of constipation in older patients is similar to that in younger patients, but that they are more likely to consider their defecation too infrequent if it is not daily or if there is significant straining with defecation [29,30]. In one study, the self-reported sensation of constipation increased from 8.4% and 23.0% in men and women, respectively, between the ages of 65 and 69, to 25.7% and 34.1%, respectively, for individuals older than age 84 years [32]. A conservative estimate based on stool frequency resulted in a prevalence of only 4% in patients aged 70 years or older, however

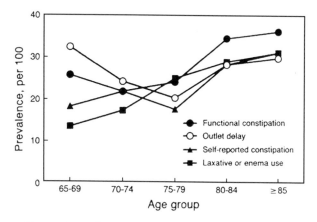

Fig. 1. Age-specific prevalence of symptoms consistent with functional constipation and outlet delay in women. (*From* Talley N, Fleming K, Evans J, et al. Constipation in an elderly community: a study of prevalence and potential risk factors. Am J Gastroenterol 1996;91(1):23; with permission.)

[33]. This demonstrates the important role that factors other than stool frequency play in patient perception of their condition.

The prevalence of functional constipation in community-dwelling patients older than age 65 years was estimated to be 24.4 per 100 [29]. In that same population, when patients with symptoms consistent with outlet delay, self-reported constipation, or laxative use were included, the prevalence increased to 40.1 per 100 [29]. In another study, 52% of men and 65% of women who had an average of one or more stools per day reported

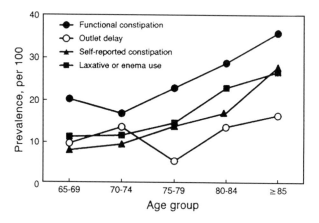

Fig. 2. Age-specific prevalence of symptoms consistent with functional constipation and outlet delay in men. (*From* Talley N, Fleming K, Evans J, et al. Constipation in an elderly community: a study of prevalence and potential risk factors. Am J Gastroenterol 1996;91(1):19–25; with permission.)

themselves as constipated [30]. The sensation of straining to have a stool seemed to explain a self-description of constipation better than did stool frequency [30]. Laxative use is common in the elderly, with estimates demonstrating that 10% to 18% of community-dwelling elders use laxatives on a routine basis [29,34].

The prevalence estimates of constipation that exist for this age group commonly do not include the nursing home patient population; therefore, they likely underestimate the burden of disease in the oldest and most frail patients.

Clinical features

There are many physiologic and iatrogenic conditions that may contribute to the increased prevalence of constipation with age. Inactivity, inadequate hydration, and many medications are risk factors that may contribute to the increased complaint of constipation in older patients. Other risk factors may involve intrinsic changes in the function of the GI tract as well as the medical and functional complexity of the population.

Multiple medications may contribute to constipation, including cardiac medications, antihypertensives, diuretics, pain medications, and iron or calcium supplements. Their use often is unavoidable given the seriousness of the conditions that they are used to treat.

Decreased mobility associated with functional decline may contribute to constipation, particularly in the old-old population and in nursing home patients, and poor dietary intake also is a factor. A decreased sense of thirst, in combination with diuretic medication, and decreased functional independence increase the risk for dehydration in this group, leading to an increased risk for constipation [33].

Pathophysiologic changes also may contribute to the specific symptoms that patients interpret as constipation. For instance, when compared with controls with no complaints of constipation, the elderly group complaining of functional constipation demonstrated a prolonged colonic transit time, particularly in the rectosigmoid region [35]. Pelvic floor dysfunction may contribute to the sensation of anal obstruction.

Other risk factors associated with an increased perception of constipation have included increased use of hypnotics, a feeling of poor health, impaired performance of instrumental activities of daily living [33], anticholinergic medications [32], and an increased number of chronic illnesses [30].

Fecal incontinence

Definition

Fecal incontinence can be a tremendously disabling condition for patients, resulting in great anxiety and fear of public embarrassment. It is defined as the involuntary loss of liquid or solid stool. Severity is categorized by frequency and by the need to wear a pad for protection on a routine basis. Many patients may be continent on a normal basis, but—when challenged by a GI infection—may develop temporary incontinence that subsequently resolves [36]. Incontinence also may be defined as functional. This is a group, often composed of primarily nursing home patients, who, in the setting of decreased mobility, reliance on others for assistance in the performance of activities of daily living, or cognitive dysfunction, are unable to reach a restroom in time to prevent an incontinent episode [36].

Epidemiology

When defined as incontinence more than once a week or the need to wear a pad for protection from stool leakage, the prevalence of fecal incontinence was estimated to be 7.0 per 100 in patients older than 65 years [37]. A more liberal definition of incontinence, defined as loss of control anytime in the last year, resulted in an estimate of 12% [38]. This was almost identical in men and women, 12.4% and 11.6%, respectively, in contradiction to the long-held belief that it is more common in women, a finding that has been confirmed in other studies [39].

The prevalence of fecal incontinence clearly increases with age. When defined as occurring once within the last year, the prevalence increases from 7% in women aged 20 to 29 years to 21% among women aged 80 years or older, with approximately one third of women experiencing onset before age 40 years, an additional third between the ages of 41 and 60 years, and the final third among respondents aged 61 to 80 years [40]. Among most women, the incontinence was infrequent (less than monthly) regardless of age; however, among nursing home residents, between 33% and 66% had severe incontinence, defined as daily [36,41,42].

Clinical features

The clinical conditions associated with fecal incontinence may vary widely, and the cause typically is multifactorial. Sphincter incompetence may be caused by pelvic floor dysfunction; neurologic injury from childbirth; or chronic diseases, such as diabetes mellitus or degenerative spinal disease. Fecal incontinence may be exacerbated by chronic diarrhea, chronic constipation with overflow, or acute infectious events. Factors in this population associated with an increased risk for fecal incontinence in men and women include chronic diarrhea and poor self-perceived health [38]. In men, lower extremity swelling, transient ischemic attacks, depression, living alone, prostate disease, and decreased mobility were additional significant variables. In women, urinary incontinence, increased comorbidities, and a history of hysterectomy were predictive [38]. Forty-two percent of patients suffering from fecal incontinence reported chronic diarrhea, and 17% reported chronic constipation. A large component of fecal incontinence in the older population, however, may not result from primary GI disorders, but from other common geriatric conditions, such as dementia and decreased mobility [36].

Fecal incontinence has significant clinical consequences in this population. One of the most concerning consequences is its effect on patients' quality of life. Among respondents with mild incontinence, only 6% reported a moderate or severe impact on their quality of life, whereas among those with severe symptoms, 82% reported a significant impact. Only 10% of the women included in this survey had visited a physician to discuss their incontinence in the last 12 months [40]. This makes clear the importance of physicians actively inquiring about this common and disabling condition.

Other significant medical consequences of incontinence may include skin breakdown, social isolation resulting in depression, and decreased functional status. Fecal incontinence often may precipitate the decision to move a patient to a more supported environment, such as a long-term care facility, which can have a profound emotional and psychologic effect on the patient and his/her family.

Fecal and urinary incontinence often coexist. For patients older than age 80 years, 39% of men and 27% of women with urinary incontinence also experienced fecal incontinence, demonstrating that it is essential to inquire about both conditions if questions about urinary incontinence are positive [39].

Lower abdominal discomfort and irritable bowel syndrome

Definitions

Many elderly patients report chronic constipation or diarrhea and abdominal discomfort or pain. As in younger patients, older patients with multiple lower GI symptoms may be diagnosed more appropriately as having IBS, although this label may not always be applied. The criteria used to define IBS in the general adult population apply to older patients as well. The Manning criteria include chronic or recurrent abdominal pain with two or three of six additional symptoms, including abdominal pain relieved by defecation, looser or more frequent stools at pain onset, abdominal distension, passage of mucus per rectum, or feelings of incomplete rectal evacuation [7]. The Rome III criteria include two of the three symptoms for at least 3 months, namely abdominal discomfort or pain relieved by defecation, looser or harder stools at pain onset, or altered stool frequency at pain onset [31]. These same definitions should be used to describe the condition in the geriatric population.

Epidemiology

Despite the different definitions of IBS, prevalence studies in older patients provide reasonably consistent results. A systematic review of the studies conducted in the general adult North American population, applying either the Manning or Rome criteria, described a prevalence of 10% to 15% in the adult population [43]. In comparison, a study of 328 Olmsted County, Minnesota residents older than 65 years, using a definition that included positive responses to three of the six symptoms in the Manning criteria, estimated a prevalence of 10.9 per 100 [37]. Another study of 1119 Danish residents estimated a prevalence of 6% to 18% among older patients [17], and a third study out of the United Kingdom found a prevalence of 12% in patients older than 65 years, which was about half that of younger subjects [44]. Presentation after the age of 60 years probably is unusual, because most patients seem to be diagnosed in their 30s and 40s, although better data are needed [45].

Clinical features

IBS in the geriatric population shares many of the same clinical features described in younger patients. It is unclear whether the decrease in prevalence identified in the above studies is explained by physiologic changes associated with aging; however, the elderly seem to have increased rectal sensory thresholds as compared with younger patients with similar degrees of colonic compliance, which may result in a decrease in symptom perception [46].

IBS in the younger population primarily is a clinical diagnosis. In the older population, however, the potential differential diagnosis is wider and more serious, making it arguably more of a diagnosis of exclusion requiring thorough investigation. Because the usual onset of IBS symptoms occurs earlier in life, older patients who present with new symptoms that are suggestive of IBS should be evaluated carefully for the many other diseases that may present similarly: colon cancer, colonic ischemia, inflammatory bowel disease, collagenous or microscopic colitis, diverticulitis, infections (eg, *Clostridium difficile*) after recent antibiotic use, and medication side effects [7].

When a diagnosis of IBS has been made, however, studies performed in elderly community-dwelling patients confirmed that the long-term prognosis was as good as in younger patients. A Danish study that followed patients older than age 70 years for 5 years found that 59% to 79% of patients had resolution of their symptoms at the time of follow up [17]. This may reflect the natural history of this disease, which waxes and wanes with stress, diet, and sleep disturbance [7].

Recognizing how chronic diseases, such as IBS, affect the functional status of patients is one of the key outcomes in geriatric patients and an area of increased investigation. In one study of elderly community-dwelling patients, the presence of chronic GI symptoms, including IBS, frequent abdominal pain, constipation, diarrhea, and fecal incontinence, were associated with lower physical, social, and mental function. IBS, in particular, was associated with significant decreases in all areas of function measured compared with controls with no GI symptoms [47]. This study was cross-sectional, however, and did not address the question of causality. Another study of Danish patients found that older patients with functional status limitations were more likely to suffer from symptoms of IBS or dyspepsia. Furthermore, those patients with IBS were more likely to have experienced a decrease in functional status at reassessment 5 years later. This study points to the concerning predictive role that these symptoms may play in anticipating functional decline [27].

Summary

Many common GI disorders remain clinically relevant throughout the patient's lifespan, but the symptoms and clinical impact often change significantly with aging. Alterations in patient perception, ranging from decreased sensory perception of pain and discomfort associated with significant disease in the upper GI tract to disproportionately increased perception of difficulties with constipation, may explain these observations in part. GI symptoms in the elderly also have a significant impact on important clinical outcomes, such as functional status, quality of life, and the ability to live independently. All of these issues make it essential for a primary care clinician to inquire actively about these symptoms and disorders, to be mindful of the often atypical presentation, and to be respectful of the patient's perspective when considering their clinical impact and importance.

References

[1] United States. Administration on Aging Census Bureau. 2000. Available at: www.aoa.gov/prof/Statistics/statistics.asp. Accessed August 7, 2007.
[2] Census 2000 summary file 1; 1990 census of population, general population characteristics, United States. US Government Census Bureau; 2000.
[3] Dent J, El-Serag H, Wallander M, et al. Epidemiology of gastro-oesophageal reflux disease: a systematic review. Gut 2005;54(5):710–7.
[4] Locke GR, Talley N, Fett S, et al. Prevalence and clinical spectrum of gastroesophageal reflux: a population-based study in Olmsted County, Minnesota. Gastroenterology 1997; 112(5):1448–56.
[5] Raiha I, Impivaara O, Seppala M, et al. Prevalence and characteristics of symptomatic gastroesophageal reflux disease in the elderly. J Am Geriatr Soc 1992;40:1209–11.
[6] Raiha I, Hietanen E, Sourander L. Symptoms of gastro-esophageal reflux disease in elderly people. Age Ageing 1991;5:365–70.
[7] Bennet G, Talley N. Irritable bowel syndrome in the elderly. Best Pract Res Clin Gastroenterol 2002;16(1):63–76.
[8] Malagelada J. Review article: supra-oesophageal manifestations of gastro-oesophageal reflux disease. Aliment Pharmacol Ther 2004;(Suppl 1):43–8.
[9] Triadafilopolous G, Sharma R. Features of symptomatic gastroesophageal reflux disease in elderly patients. Am J Gastroenterol 1997;92:2007–11.
[10] Collen M, Abdulian J, Chen Y. Gastroesophageal reflux disease in the elderly: more severe disease that requires aggressive therapy. Am J Gastroenterol 1995;90:1053–7.

[11] Zhu H, Pace F, Sangaletti O, et al. Features of symptomatic gastroesophageal reflux in elderly patients. Scand J Gastroenterol 1993;28(3):235–8.

[12] Grande L, Lacima G, Ros E, et al. Deterioration of esophageal motility with age: a manometric study of 79 healthy subjects. Am J Gastroenterol 1999;94(7):1795–801.

[13] Crane S, Locke GR, Harmsen W, et al. The changing incidence of esophageal and gastric adenocarcinoma by anatomic sub-site. Aliment Pharmacol Ther 2007;25(4):447–53.

[14] Tack J, Talley N, Camilleri M, et al. Functional gastroduodenal disorders. Gastroenterology 2006;130(5):1466–79.

[15] Locke GR. Nonulcer dyspepsia: what it is and what it is not. Mayo Clin Proc 1999;774(10): 1011–5.

[16] Johnsen R, Bernersen B, Straume B, et al. Prevalence of endoscopic and histological findings in subjects with and without dyspepsia. Br Med J 1991;1991(302):749–52.

[17] Kay L. Prevalence, incidence and prognosis of gastrointestinal symptoms in a random sample of an elderly population. Age Ageing 1994;23(2):146–9.

[18] Wilcox C, Clark W. Features associated with painless peptic ulcer bleeding. Am J Gastroenterol 1997;92(8):1289–92.

[19] Clinch D, Banerjee A, Ostick G. Absence of abdominal pain in elderly patients with peptic ulcer. Age Ageing 1984;13(2):120–3.

[20] Hilton D, Iman N, Burke G, et al. Absence of abdominal pain in older persons with endoscopic ulcers: a prospective study. Am J Gastroenterol 2001;96(2):380–4.

[21] Linder J, Wilcox C. Acid peptic disease in the elderly. Gastroenterol Clin North Am 2001; 30(2):363–76.

[22] Gilinsky N. Peptic ulcer disease in the elderly. Scand J Gastroenterol 1988;146:191–200.

[23] Choudari C, Elton R, Palmer K. Age-related mortality in patients treated endoscopically for bleeding peptic ulcer. Gastrointest Endosc 1995;41(6):557–60.

[24] Greenwald D. Aging, the gastrointestinal tract, and risk of acid-related disease. Am J Gastroenterol 2004;117(5!):8S–13S.

[25] McCarthy D. Acid peptic disease in the elderly. Clin Geriatr Med 1991;7(2):231–54.

[26] Talley N, Evans J, Fleming K, et al. Nonsteroidal antiinflammatory drugs and dyspepsia in the elderly. Dig Dis Sci 1995;40(6):1345–50.

[27] Kay L, Avlund K. Abdominal syndromes and functional ability in the elderly. Aging 1994; 6(6):420–6.

[28] El-Serag H, Talley N. Systematic review: health-related quality of life in functional dyspepsia. Aliment Pharmacol Ther 2003;18:387–93.

[29] Talley N, Fleming K, Evans J, et al. Constipation in an elderly community: a study of prevalence and potential risk factors. Am J Gastroenterol 1996;91(1):19–25.

[30] Whitehead W, Drinkwater D, Cheskin L, et al. Constipation in the elderly living at home. J Am Geriatr Soc 1989;37:423–9.

[31] Longstreth G, Thompson W, Chey W, et al. Functional bowel disorders. Gastroenterology 2006;130:1480–91.

[32] Stewart R, Moore M, Stat M, et al. Correlates of constipation in an ambulatory elderly population. Am J Gastroenterol 1992;87(7):859–64.

[33] Campbell A, Busby W, Horwath C. Factors associated with constipation in a community-based sample of people aged 70 years and over. J Epidemiol Community Health 1993;47: 23–6.

[34] Ruby C, Fillenbaum G, Kuchibhatla M, et al. Laxative use in the community-dwelling elderly. Am J Geriatr Pharmacother 2003;1(1):11–7.

[35] Evans J, Fleming K, Talley N, et al. Relation of colonic transit to functional bowel disease in older people: a population-based study. J Am Geriatr Soc 1998;46:83–7.

[36] Delvaux M. Digestive health in the elderly: faecal incontinence in adults. Aliment Pharmacol Ther 2003;18(Suppl 2):84–9.

[37] Talley N, O'Keefe E, Zinsmeister A, et al. Prevalence of gastrointestinal symptoms in the elderly: a population-based study. Gastroenterology 1992;102:895–901.

[38] Goode P, Burgio K, Halli A, et al. Prevalence and correlates of fecal incontinence in community-dwelling older adults. J Am Geriatr Soc 2005;53:629–35.

[39] Roberts R, Jacobsen S, Reilly W, et al. Prevalence of combined fecal and urinary incontinence: a community-based study. J Am Geriatr Soc 1999;47(7):837–41.

[40] Bharucha A, Zinsmeister A, Locke GR, et al. Prevalence and burden of fecal incontinence: a population-based study in women. Gastroenterology 2005;129:42–9.

[41] Topinkova E, Neuwirth J, Stankova M, et al. Urinary and fecal incontinence in geriatric facilities in the Czech Republic. Cas Lek Cesk 1997;136:573–7.

[42] Denis P, Bercoff E, Bizien M. Prevalence of anal incontinence in adults. Gastroenterol Clin Biol 1992;16:344–50.

[43] Saito Y, Schoenfeld P, Locke GR. The epidemiology of irritable bowel syndrome in North America: a systematic review. Am J Gastroenterol 2002;97(8):1910–5.

[44] Ruigomez A, Wallander M, Joansson S. One year follow-up of newly diagnosed irritable bowel syndrome patients. Aliment Pharmacol Ther 1999;13:1097–102.

[45] O'Keefe E, Talley N. Irritable bowel syndrome in the elderly. Clin Geriatr Med 1991;7(2): 265–86.

[46] Lagier E, Delvaux M, Vellas B, et al. Influence of age on rectal tone and sensitivity to distension in healthy subjects. Neuorogastroenterol Motil 1999;11:101–7.

[47] O'Keefe E, Talley N, Zinsmeister A, et al. Bowel disorders impair functional status and quality of life in the elderly: a population-based study. J Gerontol 1995;50A(4):M184–9.

ELSEVIER
SAUNDERS

CLINICS IN
GERIATRIC
MEDICINE

Clin Geriatr Med 23 (2007) 735–756

The Anorexia of Aging

Ian Mcphee Chapman, MBBS, PhD

Department of Medicine, University of Adelaide, Level 6 Eleanor Harrald Building,
Royal Adelaide Hospital, North Terrace, Adelaide 5000, Australia

Undernutrition is common in the elderly, particularly those in nursing homes and other institutions. It is associated with substantial adverse effects. The age-associated physiologic reduction in appetite and food intake, which has been termed "the anorexia of aging," contributes to the development of pathologic anorexia and undernutrition. This article reviews age-related changes to appetite, food intake, and body composition; undernutrition in the elderly; and the factors contributing to physiologic and pathologic anorexia and undernutrition.

Changes in appetite, food intake, body weight, and body composition with increasing age

Appetite and food intake

On average, people become less hungry and eat less as they get older [1]. Healthy older persons are less hungry and more full before meals, consume smaller meals more slowly, eat fewer snacks between meals, and become more rapidly satiated after eating a standard meal than do younger persons [2,3]. Aging also is associated with consumption of a less varied, more monotonous diet. Average daily energy intake decreases by up to 30% between 20 and 80 years [1]. For example, the 1989 cross-sectional American National Health and Nutrition Examination Survey (NHANES III) study reported a decline in energy intake, between the ages of 20 and 80 years, of 1321 cal/d in men and 629 cal/d in women [4]. A 7-year New Mexico longitudinal study of 156 persons aged 64 to 91 years reported a decrease of 19.3 kcal/d/y in women and 25.1 kcal/d/y in men [5], whereas a Swedish

Supported by a project grant from the National Health and Medical Research Council of Australia.

E-mail address: ian.chapman@adelaide.edu.au

736   CHAPMAN

6-year longitudinal study of 98 people found that between the ages of 70 and
76 years, there was a decrease in energy intake of 610 cal/d in men and
440 cal/d in women [6].

Much of the age-related decrease in energy probably is a response to the
decline in energy expenditure that also occurs as people get older. In many
individuals, however, the decrease in energy intake is greater than the
decrease in energy expenditure, so body weight is lost. This physiologic,
age-related reduction in appetite and energy intake has been termed "the
anorexia of aging" [3].

Body weight

The results of large studies show that, on average, body weight and body
mass index (BMI) increase throughout adult life until about age 50 to
60 years, after which they decline (see Ref. [7]). Although some of the decline
in mean body weight after age 50 to 60 years is due to the premature death
of obese people, there is evidence from longitudinal studies of a decrease in
body weight after about age 60 years. For example, in one prospective
study, community-dwelling American men older than 65 years lost an average of 0.5% of their body weight per year, and 13.1% of the group had
weight loss of 4% per year or more [8].

As a result of this weight loss in older people and the premature death of
obese people at younger ages, the prevalence of overweight and obesity declines after about age 65 years, whereas that of underweight increases. For
example, in the 1997–1998 US National Health Interview Survey of 68,556
adults, more people aged 75 years and older than those aged 45 to 64 years
were "underweight" (BMI < 18.5; 5% versus 1.2%) and substantially less
were "overweight" (BMI > 25; 47.2% versus 63.5%) [9].

A substantial minority of older people have marked weight changes over
time [8,10]. In one study, 17% of home-dwelling people in the United States
older than 65 years lost 5% or more of their initial body weight over 3 years,
whereas 13% gained 5% or more [10]. There is evidence for interactive effects of body weight category and change in body weight on health, particularly adverse effects in already underweight people who lose weight.

Body composition

With normal aging, there is a progressive increase in fat and decrease in
fat-free mass, which is mainly due to loss of skeletal muscle, with loss of up
to 3 kg of lean body mass per decade after age 50 years. Consequently, at
any given weight, older people on average have substantially more body
fat than do young adults, approximately twice as much in 75-year-old
men as in 20-year-old men of the same weight [11]. The increase in body
fat with aging is multifactorial in origin, with decreased physical activity
a major cause, and contributions from reduced growth hormone secretion,

declining sex hormone action, and reduced resting metabolic rate and thermic effect of food. Body fat also is distributed differently in older adults. A greater proportion of body fat in older people is intrahepatic, intramuscular, and intra-abdominal versus subcutaneous [12], changes that are associated with increased insulin resistance. Therefore, they are likely to be associated with adverse metabolic outcomes [13], although it has not been proven.

The causes of age-related skeletal muscle loss are multiple and not fully understood, but probably are similar to those leading to fat gain, including reduced exercise and anabolic hormone action. When excessive, this skeletal muscle loss leads to sarcopenia (from the Greek meaning "poverty of flesh"), which has been defined in various ways (eg, skeletal mass more than two standard deviations below the young adult sex-specific mean) [14]. The prevalence of sarcopenia in older people varies according to the population studied and diagnostic criteria used, but it is on the order of 6% to 15% in people older than 65 years [14]. The reduction of skeletal muscle mass and strength in sarcopenia is so severe that it often is associated with marked functional impairment. The presence of sarcopenia is an independent predictor of poor gait, balance, falls, and fractures. In the NHANES III study, for example, older people who had marked sarcopenia (<5.75 kg skeletal muscle/m^2) were 3.3 times (women) to 4.7 times (men) more likely to have physical disability than were those with low-risk skeletal muscle mass (>6.75 kg/m^2) [15].

Undernutrition in older people

There is no gold standard method for diagnosing undernutrition in older people. Diagnostic methods used are discussed briefly later; however, two of the most important markers of undernutrition and increased risk for morbidity and mortality in older people are low body weight and loss of weight, particularly if unintentional.

"Low" body weight in older people: what is "ideal"?

The relationship between mortality and body weight is a J-shaped curve, with increased mortality at low and high BMIs. For young adults, the BMI associated with the greatest life expectancy is in the range of 20 to 25 kg/m^2 [16,17]. Most evidence suggests that the BMI (and, therefore, body weight) associated with maximum life expectancy increases with age. The lower end of the range increases to about 22 to 23 kg/m^2 and the upper end increases to about 27 to 28 kg/m^2 for people older than 65 years [18–20], with little or no evidence of increased mortality at any BMI for people older than 75 years. At less than 22 to 23 kg/m^2, there is a steady increase in the risk for death, probably particularly at BMI values less than 18.5 kg/m^2 in women and 20.5 kg/m^2 in men [17]. The deleterious effects of being underweight are amplified by increasing age [21].

Weight loss in older people

Body weight tends to decrease after about age 60 years, and a loss of 5% or more of body weight over several years is not uncommon in older people. Numerous studies have shown that weight loss in the elderly is associated with poor outcomes (for review see Ref. [20]). For example, the prospective Cardiovascular Health Study in the United States [10] studied 4714 home-dwelling subjects older than 65 years without known cancer. In the 3 years after study entry, 17% of the subjects lost 5% or more of their initial body weight. This group had significant increases in total (2.09-fold; 95% confidence interval [CI], 1.67–2.62) and risk-adjusted (1.67-fold; 95% CI, 1.29–2.15) mortality during the subsequent 4 years compared with the stable weight group. The increased mortality occurred irrespective of starting weight and apparently irrespective of whether weight was lost intentionally. Similarly, in the Systolic Hypertension in the Elderly Program study [18], subjects who had a weight loss of 1.6 kg/y or more had a 4.9 times greater death rate (95% CI, 3.5–6.8) than those without significant weight change. The association between increased mortality and weight loss was present even in the subjects who were heaviest at baseline (BMI $\geq$ 31) and was independent of baseline weight. Nevertheless, subjects with a low baseline weight (BMI < 23.6 kg/m^2) who lost more than 1.6 kg/y had a mortality of 22.6%, almost 20 times greater than the mortality of those with a baseline BMI of 23.6 to 28 kg/m^2 whose weight remained stable.

Thus, weight loss by an older person of initially low body weight is associated with a particularly bad outcome. This may occur because such weight loss is more likely to be unintentional than weight loss by overweight, older people (see later discussion) and because sarcopenia is more likely to result when already lean older people lose weight. This additive adverse effect is of concern, because the tendency for older people to lose weight is variable, with lean individuals probably most at risk [22].

An unresolved issue is whether only unintentional weight loss has harmful effects in older people. This is important when it comes to advising older, overweight people about whether they should attempt to lose weight. Obesity is common in older people. According to recent large surveys, approximately 71% of Americans 60 years or older and 60% of those 65 years or older were overweight (BMI $\geq$ 25 kg/m^2), whereas approximately 32% of those 60 years or older and 20% of those 65 years or older were obese (BMI $\geq$ 30 kg/m^2) [23,24]. The prevalence of obesity in older people is increasing rapidly, in parallel with the dramatic increase in rates in younger adults. The prevalence of obesity (BMI $\geq$ 30 kg/m^2) among people in the United States older than 60 years increased from 20% to 32% between 1988–1994 and 1999–2000 [25] and from 11.4% to 15.5% between 1991 and 2000 among those older than 70 years [26]. As in younger adults, obesity in older adults is associated with absolute and relative increases in mortality and morbidity, although the relative increase in the risk for death associated with being obese is not as great in older adults. There is evidence that weight loss by overweight older people is associated with improved quality of life; in the Nurses Health Study, weight loss in initially overweight women was associated with improved physical function and vitality as well as decreased bodily pain [27]. The effects of deliberate weight loss by overweight older adults on mortality have not been established. Therefore, the potential benefits of weight loss must be balanced against the association—repeatedly detected in large population studies—between all-cause weight loss and increased mortality in older people, even those who are initially overweight.

Studies demonstrating an association between weight loss and increased mortality in older people largely have examined all-cause weight loss, whether intentional or unintentional. There is little doubt that unintentional weight loss is not good for the elderly. Although some study results have been interpreted to show increased mortality after even intentional weight loss in older people [10], it is difficult to determine what proportion of weight loss labeled intentional was instead unintentional. On balance, it seems that intentional weight loss by initially overweight older people has no significant effect [28,29] or even beneficial effects on mortality. In the US National Health Interview Survey, for example, which followed 20,847 adults with a mean age of 54 years for 9 years, all-cause weight loss was associated with a significant increase in mortality, as in other studies [30]. Reported attempted weight loss, however, even if unsuccessful, was associated with a 24% reduction in mortality, as was successful, intentional weight loss. There was no interaction between weight loss intention and age in the effect on mortality, consistent with a prolongation of life by intended weight loss in older as well as young adults. Therefore, the available evidence seems to provide no evidence of harm and suggests that it is safe to recommend weight loss to overweight older people with obesity-related morbidities, particularly reduced mobility and function.

There are many reasons why unintentional weight loss in older people has adverse effects, particularly when it leads to protein-energy malnutrition (PEM). Undernutrition per se has numerous adverse effects (see later discussion). Weight loss also can be a marker and consequence of illness, such as a malignancy, which is independently responsible for the poor outcome. Such illnesses may be multiple, interactive, and difficult to detect. Inflammatory conditions are important causes, acting by way of cachectic effects of increased cytokines (see later discussion).

Prevalence of undernutrition in older people

PEM is common in the elderly. Studies in developed countries found that up to 15% of community-dwelling and home-bound elderly, between 23% and 62% of hospitalized patients, and up to 85% of nursing homes residents suffer from the condition [3].

Adverse effects of undernutrition in older people

PEM is associated with impaired muscle function, decreased bone mass, immune dysfunction, anemia, reduced cognitive function, poor wound healing, delayed recovery from surgery, and, ultimately, increased mortality. Epidemiologic studies demonstrated that PEM was a strong independent predictor of mortality in elderly people, regardless of whether they lived in the community [31] or in a nursing home [32], were patients in a hospital [33], or had been discharged from the hospital in the last 1 to 2 years [34]. The increased mortality in elderly people who have PEM is increased further in the presence of other medical diseases, such as renal failure, cardiac failure, and cerebrovascular disease. For example, in one study, the 9-month mortality among patients older than 70 years, who did not have cancer and who were admitted to a medical ward in Sweden, was 44% in malnourished patients who did not have cardiac failure, but 80% in malnourished patients who had cardiac failure [33].

Causes of undernutrition in older people

An overview of appetite regulation

Central factors

The central feeding system is dependent on the stimulatory effect of neurotransmitters, including the opioids, noradrenaline, neuropeptide Y (NPY), the orexins, galanin, and ghrelin, and the inhibitory effect of corticotrophin-releasing factor, serotonin, cholecystokinin (CCK), and possibly, insulin.

Peripheral factors

The short-term peripheral satiety system largely is driven by gastrointestinal mechanisms. In the longer term, factors such as leptin and cytokines (see later discussion) become more important. Gastrointestinal sensory and motor functions are important in the regulation of satiation. Sensory signals induced by distension by food contribute to initial sensations of fullness during a meal. These sensations are mediated by way of vagal mechanisms from mechanoreceptors situated within the stomach wall. In young adult humans, gastric distension, using a barostat, reduces food intake by up to 30%. Distension of the distal stomach (antrum) is related to increased sensations of fullness and is likely to be more important than distension of the proximal stomach (fundus). After eating, the stomach relaxes by a process of receptive relaxation, resulting in decreased intragastric pressure and increased gastric volume. This relaxation is particularly marked in the proximal stomach and results in a proximal fundic reservoir where food is retained. Not long before it is emptied into the small intestine, food is propelled distally from the fundus into the antrum. The extent of antral filling and distension relates more closely to feelings of fullness and satiety than does proximal gastric distension.

Studies in animals and humans demonstrated a relationship between postprandial satiety and the rate of gastric emptying. Slowing of gastric emptying may reduce appetite and food intake by increasing and prolonging antral distension and by prolonging the effect of small intestinal satiety signals. People who have gastroparesis often exhibit symptoms of early satiety, loss of appetite, nausea, and vomiting; studies in animals and humans showed that there is a relationship between postprandial satiation and the rate of gastric emptying.

Once food enters the small intestine, mechano- and chemoreceptors relay signals to the hypothalamus, resulting in the cessation of food intake. These signals are mediated by the release of gastrointestinal peptide hormones, including CCK, peptide YY (PYY), and glucagon-like peptide (GLP)-1. Several gastrointestinal and pancreatic hormones, including CCK, GLP-1, and amylin, have feedback effects on the stomach to slow gastric emptying—an effect associated with increased fullness and reduced food intake—by increasing and prolonging gastric distension and prolonging the effect of small intestinal satiety signals. Feedback signals from peripheral fat cells, by way of leptin and possibly tumor necrosis factor α (TNF-α), as well as absorption of nutrients from the gut also contribute to satiation.

The causes of undernutrition in older people often are multiple and interacting. There is an age-related impairment in homeostatic responses, which together with a physiologic reduction in appetite and food intake ("the anorexia of aging"), seems to increase susceptibility and predisposes to the development of undernutrition when pathologic factors (see later discussion) are superimposed.

Age-related impairment of homeostasis

Healthy aging is associated with a physiologic decline in energy (food) intake and a reduction in function of homeostatic mechanisms that work in younger people to restore food intake in response to anorectic insults. As an illustration of the latter, Roberts and colleagues [35] underfed young and old men by 3.17 MJ/d (?750 kcal/d) for 21 days, during which time the young and old men lost weight. After the underfeeding period the men were allowed to eat ad libitum. The young men ate more than at baseline (before underfeeding) and quickly returned to normal weight, whereas the old men did not compensate, returned only to their baseline intake, and did not regain the weight that they had lost. The combination of age-related physiologic anorexia and impaired homeostasis means that older people do not respond as well as do young adults to acute undernutrition. Consequently, after an anorectic insult (eg, major surgery), older people are likely to take longer than young adults to regain the weight lost, remain undernourished longer, and are more susceptible to subsequent superimposed illnesses, such as infections.

The physiologic anorexia of aging

The anorexia of aging has many interacting causes, and these have not been defined fully. Several probable and possible causes are described below and summarized in Box 1.

Declining senses of taste and smell

Taste and smell are important in making eating pleasurable. The sense of taste probably deteriorates with age, although not all studies confirm this. There is stronger evidence that the sense of smell deteriorates, particularly after age 50 years. In one study, more than 60% of subjects aged 65 to 80 years and more than 80% of subjects aged 80 years or older had major reductions in their sense of smell compared with less than 10% of those younger than 50 years [36]. The decline in sense of smell decreases food intake in the elderly and may influence the type of food eaten; several studies showed a strong correlation between impaired sense of smell and reduced interest in

---

Box 1. Possible factors contributing to the physiologic anorexia of aging

Diminished sense of smell and taste
Reduced sensory-specific satiety
Increased cytokine activity
Alterations in gastrointestinal function
    Delayed gastric emptying
    Altered gastric food distribution
Hormonal
Increase appetite/food intake
Opioids: decreased activity; not proven in humans
Testosterone: decreased activity with age
Ghrelin: possible decreased activity with aging (unproven)
NPY: possible decreased activity with aging (little evidence)

Decrease appetite/food intake
Cocaine-amphetamine-regulated transcript: possible increased
    central levels (rodent)
CCK: increased circulating levels, increased cerebrospinal fluid
    levels, increased sensitivity to satiating effects
Leptin: situation complex: circulating levels increased in men but
    possible leptin resistance
PYY: possible increased activity (little evidence)

and intake of food. Consistent with this is the observation that aging is associated with a less varied, more monotonous diet.

Reduced sensory-specific satiety

Sensory-specific satiety is the normal decline in pleasantness of the taste of a particular food after it has been consumed. Sensory-specific satiety leads to a decrease in the consumption of a previously eaten food and a tendency to shift consumption to other food choices during a meal. This acts to promote the intake of a more varied, nutritionally balanced diet. Older people have a reduced capacity to develop sensory-specific satiety [37], perhaps because of reduced senses of smell and taste. In turn, reduced sensory-specific satiety may favor the consumption of a less varied diet and the development of micronutrient deficiencies.

The aging gut

Aging is associated with cell loss in the myenteric plexus of the human esophagus and a decline in conduction velocity within visceral neurones. The consequent reduction in sensory perception may contribute to reduced food intake by inhibiting the positive stimuli for feeding. The elderly frequently complain of increased fullness and early satiation during a meal. This also may be related to changes in gastrointestinal sensory function; aging is associated with reduced sensitivity to gastrointestinal tract distension. If anything, reduced sensitivity to the satiating effects of distension might be expected to increase, not decrease, food intake in older people. Nevertheless, proximal gastric distension has similar effects on food intake in healthy older and young adults, and the role, if any, of impairment of gastric sensory function in causing the anorexia of aging is unknown.

Aging probably is associated with impaired receptive relaxation of the gastric fundus. As a result, for any given gastric volume there is more rapid antral filling and distension and earlier satiety. This impaired gastric accommodation response in the elderly may be due to altered fundic nitric oxide (NO) concentrations. Peripheral NO causes receptive and adaptive relaxation of the stomach, leading to dilation of the fundus and, ultimately, slower gastric emptying. Therefore, the increase in NO with aging may contribute to the slower gastric emptying observed in the elderly. Most, but not all, studies indicated that gastric emptying slows slightly, but significantly, with increasing age. Clarkston and colleagues [2] found that healthy older subjects were less hungry and more satiated after a meal than were young subjects, and postprandial hunger was inversely related to the rate of gastric emptying. The effects of aging on the gastric emptying rate may require ingestion of a large energy content, because small meals have not been shown to cause different emptying rates in old compared with young individuals. In part, delayed gastric emptying in older people may result from enhanced release of small intestinal hormones, such as CCK (see later discussion).

In contrast, it seems that age has little, if any, effect on small intestinal or colonic motor function, and oro-cecal and whole gut transit time are not affected in the healthy elderly. Healthy older people do have slower phase III migration velocities and more frequent "propagated contractions" in the small intestine, but no differences in the duration of postprandial motility or amplitude or frequency of fasting or postprandial pressure waves.

Age-related changes in hormones and neurotransmitters: a selective review

Central

Opioids. Endogenous opioids play a role in mediating the short-term sensory reward response to food. Exogenous administration of opioid agonists increased food intake in animals and opioid antagonists decreased food intake in animals and adult humans [38]. There is evidence that aging is associated with a reduced opioid feeding drive (for review see Ref. [3]). Elderly patients who have idiopathic, senile anorexia have lower plasma and cerebrospinal fluid (CSF) β-endorphin concentrations than do normal weight, aged-matched controls [39]. Intraperitoneal (IP) morphine injection increases food intake in young but not old mice, whereas IP naloxone decreases food intake in young but not older rats. Healthy older men were less sensitive to the inhibitory effects of subcutaneous naloxone on fluid intake than were young men [40]. In one small study of feeding in humans, the suppression of food intake by naloxone was nonsignificantly greater in the older adults than in young adults: 16% versus 8% [38].

Neuropeptide Y. NPY is synthesized in the peripheral nervous system and brain and strongly stimulates food intake. There is preliminary evidence from animal studies that aging may be associated with reduced NPY activity, perhaps more in males than in females. Old rats have lower levels of arcuate nucleus prepro NPY mRNA than do young rats and hypothalamic NPY levels decrease with aging in male, but not female, rats. Studies in humans, however, suggest, if anything, increased NPY activity with increasing age. CSF NPY levels increase with healthy aging in woman, and plasma and CSF levels are increased in elderly people who have idiopathic anorexia [39]. In rats, the feeding response to hypothalamic NPY injections diminishes with aging, whereas the stimulation of feeding by intracerebroventricular NPY administration in mice does not diminish with age. The effects of NPY administration in humans have not been reported. Therefore, there is no convincing evidence for involvement of NPY in the human anorexia of aging.

Galanin. Galanin is a peptide hormone located in the brain and periphery, which stimulates food intake. Declining galanin levels are unlikely to contribute to the anorexia of aging [41], but reduced sensitivity to galanin might. The effect of aging on the stimulation of feeding by galanin has not been reported in humans, but older women (although not men) display a reduced growth hormone secretory response to galanin compared with young adults [42].

Orexins (hypocretins). Orexin A and B (hypocretin-1 and -2) are neuropeptides that are synthesized in the hypothalamus and involved with feeding and sleep. Orexin deficiency causes narcolepsy in animals and humans and hypophagia and weight loss in animals [43], whereas orexin increases food intake (for review see Ref. [44]). Most evidence does not support declining orexin activity as a cause of the anorexia of aging. Plasma orexin concentrations apparently increase, not decrease, with age in healthy humans [43], although the effect of age on brain and receptor levels and the sensitivity to orexin is not known.

Cocaine-amphetamine–regulated transcript. Cocaine-amphetamine–regulated transcript (CART) is a peptide that is distributed widely through the brain, including the hypothalamus. In animals, central CART administration reduces feeding and blocks NPY-induced feeding. Sohn and colleagues [45] reported that arcuate nucleus CART mRNA levels were higher and NPY mRNA levels were lower in healthy old rates compared with young male rats, whereas testosterone treatment of castrate, older rats significantly decreased CART mRNA levels and increased NPY mRNA levels. This suggests that in males there is aging-related increased central activity of CART and reduced activity of NPY, both mediated by the normal age-related decline in testosterone. This is an intriguing possibility, but the effects of aging on CART in female animals have not been reported, nor have those in humans.

Peripheral hormones, including gut peptides
Cholecystokinin. CCK is present in the hypothalamus, cortex, and midbrain and is released from the lumen of the intestine in response to nutrients, particularly fat and protein, in the gut. Exogenous CCK administration decreases food intake in animals and humans. This is probably a physiologic effect, because the suppression of food intake occurs with the administration of doses producing plasma CCK concentrations within the physiologic range, and administration of CCK antagonists increases food intake in animals and young, adult humans [46]. CCK also slows gastric emptying.

The satiating effects of CCK seem to increase with age. In most studies, plasma CCK concentrations were higher in healthy older adults than in young adults [47]. Elderly people who had idiopathic anorexia had significantly higher plasma levels and nonsignificantly higher CSF levels of CCK than did healthy, age-matched controls [39]. Intraperitoneal CCK suppresses food intake more in old than young rats and mice. Intravenous

CCK-8 administration acutely suppressed food intake twice as much in older healthy human adults compared with young healthy human adults (31% versus 15%, $P = .02$) [47]. The combination of increased circulating CCK concentrations and enhanced sensitivity to CCK suggests that CCK may be a cause of the anorexia of aging and raises the possibility of using CCK antagonists to increase energy intake in undernourished older people.

Glucagon-like peptide-1. GLP-1 is released by the lining of the intestine in response to nutrient ingestion, particularly carbohydrates. It stimulates insulin secretion and, together with gastric inhibitory peptide, is one of the incretin hormones. It also slows gastric emptying. Administration of GLP-1 to humans increased feelings of fullness and reduced food intake [48]. Studies have not found a consistent effect of aging on plasma GLP-1 concentrations [49], and the effects of aging on the satiating effects of GLP-1 are unknown.

Peptide YY. PYY is a peptide hormone present in the brain and released from the bowel in response to fat and carbohydrate in the small intestine. Administration of PYY to rodents reduced food intake and body weight [50]. Intravenous infusion of PYY to normal weight and obese humans younger than 50 years of age, in doses that produce postprandial blood levels, reduced short-term food intake by approximately 30% [51]. This suppression may be mediated by the associated suppression of ghrelin levels, whereas leptin, insulin, and GLP-1 are unaltered. Therefore, increased PYY activity could contribute to the anorexia of aging; however, although fasting and postprandial plasma PYY levels were higher in older people in one study [52], no effect of age was found in another study [49]. Furthermore, the suppression of food intake by PYY that was reported previously [50,51] has been difficult to reproduce and, therefore, confirm in subsequent studies [53]. Sensitivity to the appetite-stimulating effects of PYY may decline with age; although the effects of aging on the sensitivity to PYY in humans have not been reported, senescent rats have a reduced feeding response to NPY administration [54].

Leptin. Leptin is produced predominantly in adipose tissue and circulates in amounts directly related to the size of fat stores. It suppresses appetite and food intake. Congenital leptin deficiency in humans is a rare cause of morbid obesity associated with hyperphagia, and leptin treatment produces substantial weight loss in these people. Most obese people, however, have elevated circulating leptin concentrations consistent with their increased fat mass. Leptin resistance probably is a feature of most human obesity, and leptin administration to obese people has resulted in only minor weight loss.

Animal studies have not shown an age-related increase in circulating leptin concentrations. Plasma leptin concentrations in humans often increase with aging, to a large extent because of the increased fat mass that also accompanies aging; however, most, but not all [55], studies showed that adjustment for fat mass removes this effect [56]. In men, however, some studies showed an increase in circulating leptin levels, even allowing for fat mass. This probably is due to age-related decreases in circulating testosterone concentrations; because plasma leptin levels are inversely related to plasma testosterone, testosterone therapy reduces, and inhibition of testosterone production increases, circulating leptin levels [57].

Little is known about the effects of aging on sensitivity to the effects of leptin. Fasting usually suppresses plasma leptin concentrations dramatically, thus stimulating hunger. Reduced suppression of leptin levels by fasting has been reported in aging rats. Conversely, food intake, fat mass, and insulin action are suppressed less by leptin administration in older rats than in young rats. This suggests that aging may be accompanied by leptin resistance, which would tend to increase food intake.

Ghrelin. Ghrelin stimulates feeding and growth hormone release. It is present in the hypothalamus, but the gastric mucosa is the main site of production. Circulating ghrelin concentrations increase with fasting and with diet-induced weight loss in obese subjects and are elevated in underweight, undernourished young and older subjects. In contrast, circulating concentrations decrease after the ingestion of food, particularly fat and carbohydrate, and are reduced in obese people. These changes are consistent with compensatory responses to, rather than causes of, these altered nutritional states. Therefore, it seems unlikely that reduced ghrelin activity contributes significantly to the anorexia and weight loss in markedly undernourished older subjects. Nevertheless, the effects of aging and undernutrition on the sensitivity to ghrelin have not been reported, and ghrelin resistance may occur in these states. In support of this, older subjects are less sensitive to the growth hormone-releasing effects of intravenous ghrelin than are young adults [58].

The effect of healthy aging on circulating ghrelin concentrations has not been clarified, but probably is minimal. Although one study of adults up to 64 years of age found an increase in plasma ghrelin concentrations with increasing age, there was no relationship with age per se when a multivariate analysis was performed [59]. Another study found no difference in fasting and postprandial serum ghrelin concentrations between healthy older adults (mean age 78 years) and young adults [55]. Two small studies reported that circulating ghrelin concentrations were 20% [60] and 35% [61] lower in healthy older adults (69–87 and 67–91 years, respectively) than in young adults; the latter figure was statistically significant. These observed changes may have been due to increasing body fat, which is associated with reduced circulating ghrelin levels, because the older subjects had higher BMIs than did the young subjects in both studies. Studies involving body composition analysis are needed to assess the effects of aging per se on ghrelin.

Insulin. Human aging tends to be associated with increased fasting and postprandial circulating insulin concentrations [62]. Insulin had satiating effects, at least in animal studies, and particularly when administered centrally [63]. Therefore, increased insulin activity could be a cause of reduced food intake in older people; however, this may be unlikely. The evidence for a satiating role of insulin in humans is limited. Short-term, peripheral, euglycemic insulin infusions did not affect appetite or food intake in humans [64]. Moreover, age-associated increases in insulin concentrations are due mainly to insulin resistance resulting from increased adiposity, and only to a small extent to aging itself.

Testosterone and other androgens. Circulating androgen concentrations decline with aging. This may contribute to the development of sarcopenia and the decrease in functional status that occurs with aging. Although androgen replacement therapy generally is advocated for men who have marked androgen deficiency, there is no consensus about its use in elderly men with less severe aging-related declines in androgen concentrations or in elderly women.

Studies of androgen replacement have been performed in healthy, older men who had androgen deficiency; although benefits were seen in muscle mass and, in some cases, strength, there is no good evidence that this leads to improvements in functional status (for review see Refs. [65,66]). Two small studies reported functional benefits when testosterone was administered in supraphysiologic doses to older, frail men. Amory and colleagues [67] gave older men—with a mean total testosterone within the normal range—testosterone, 600 mg, intramuscularly (IM) weekly for 4 weeks, before elective knee replacement surgery; they found significant increases in their ability to stand postoperatively and trends to improvements in walking and stair climbing compared with placebo-treated men. Bakhshi and colleagues [68] gave testosterone, 100 mg IM, or placebo weekly to older men with low-normal testosterone levels in a rehabilitation program; they found significant increases in grip strength and the function independence measure after testosterone but not placebo.

In women, serum concentrations of testosterone and the adrenal androgens gradually and progressively decline from the decade preceding the menopause. Even if testosterone therapy does not increase food intake in older, undernourished people, it may provide functional benefits by treating the associated sarcopenia; studies to examine this are underway.

Cytokines

Age-associated increases in the production or effect of satiating cytokines may contribute to the anorexia of aging [69]. Cytokines are secreted in response to significant stress, often due to malignancy or infection. Circulating concentrations of the cytokines interleukin (IL)-1, IL-6, and TNF-α are increased in cachectic patients who have cancer or AIDS. They decrease food intake and reduce body weight by way of several central and peripheral pathways. Blockade of these cytokines (eg, TNF in mice with TNF-producing sarcomas) significantly attenuates weight loss in high-stress conditions that are associated with cachexia.

Aging itself may be a form of stress. It is associated with stress-like changes in circulating hormonal patterns: increased cortisol and catecholamines and decreased sex hormones and growth hormone. In turn, increased cortisol and catecholamine levels stimulate the release of IL-6 and TNF-α [69], whereas sex hormones inhibit IL-6. IL-1 and IL-6 levels are elevated in older people who have cachexia, whereas plasma IL-6 concentrations apparently increase as a function of normal aging and correlate inversely with levels of functional ability in elderly people [70]. Thus, increased cytokine levels, which result from the "stress" of aging per se or the amplified stressful effects of other pathologies, may provide an explanation for some of the decline in appetite and body weight that occurs in many older people.

Pathologic anorexia and undernutrition in older people

PEM is particularly likely to develop in the presence of other "pathologic" factors, many of which become more common with increased age (Box 2). Most are responsive to treatment, at least in part, so recognition is important. Older people are more likely than young adults to live alone, and social isolation and loneliness have been associated with decreased appetite and energy intake in the elderly [71]. Elderly people tend to consume substantially more food (sometimes up to 50% more) during a meal when eating in the company of friends than when eating alone. The simple measure of having older people eat in company rather than alone may be effective in increasing their energy intake.

Depression is a common problem in older people, present in 2% to 10% of community-dwelling older people and a much greater proportion of those in institutions [72]. Depression is more likely to manifest as reduced appetite and weight loss in the elderly than in younger adults and is an important cause of weight loss and undernutrition in this group, accounting for up to 30% to 36% of the total in medical outpatients and nursing home residents. [73,74]. Undernutrition per se, particularly if it produces folate deficiency, may worsen depression [75]. Treatment of depression is effective in producing weight gain and improving other nutritional indices [76].

Many older people no longer have their own teeth. Poor dentition and ill-fitting dentures may limit the type and quantity of food eaten. Complaints of problems with chewing, biting, and swallowing are common among nursing home residents, and those with dentures are more likely than those with their own teeth to have poor protein intake [77]. The elderly often take multiple medications, which increases the risk for drug interactions that can cause anorexia.

Box 2. Pathologic causes of undernutrition in older people

Social factors
Poverty
Inability to shop, prepare, and cook meals or to feed oneself
Living alone/social isolation/lack of social support network
Failure to cater to ethnic and other food preferences in
    institutionalized individuals

Psychologic factors
Depression
Dementia/Alzheimer's disease
Alcoholism
Bereavement

Medical factors
Cardiac failure
Chronic obstructive pulmonary disease
Infection
Cancer
Alcoholism
Poor dentition
Dysphagia
Rheumatoid arthritis
Malabsorption syndromes
Gastrointestinal symptoms
    Dyspepsia
    Helicobacter pylori infection/atrophic gastritis
    Vomiting/diarrhea/constipation
    Parkinson's disease
Hypermetabolism (eg, hyperthyroidism)
Medications - multiple

Diagnosis of undernutrition in older people

Multiple methods have been used to diagnose undernutrition in older people (for review see Ref. [20]), and there is no gold standard. Probably the most important thing is to be aware of the possible diagnosis. It is important to weigh older people at regular intervals, particularly those in nursing homes or other institutions, because weight loss, particularly unintentional loss of greater than 5%, is a key indicator. BMI less than 22 kg/m^2 suggests undernutrition, which is particularly likely if the BMI is less than 18.5 kg/m^2, even at weight stability.

Various diagnostic instruments have been developed that rely on differing combinations of anthropometric measures; questions regarding weight loss, food intake, and medications; and measurement of blood parameters; among those associated with a risk for undernutrition and poor outcome are reduced serum albumin, hematocrit, lymphocyte count, and serum folate [78]. Among the most widely used outpatient screening tools for undernutrition risk are the Mini Nutritional Assessment [79], the Functional Assessment of Anorexia Cachexia Therapy [80], and the Seniors in the Community Risk Evaluation for Eating and Nutrition tool [81]. Even the most simple of these tools can provide useful information; for example, the Simplified Nutritional Appetite Questionnaire, which consists of four questions on appetite, timing of eating, frequency of meals, and taste, has a high sensitivity and specificity (both > 75%) in predicting future 5% weight loss in older people [82].

Management

Underlying causes, particularly depression and problems with dentition, should be identified and corrected where possible (see Box 2). Adequate intake of vitamins and minerals should be ensured by supplements including vitamin D and calcium unless contraindicated. Target weight gains should be set, and the intake of nutritional food should be increased if possible by offering more food, improving the social setting of food intake (eg, eating in company, not alone), and encouraging the older person to eat. If target weight gains are not achieved or the deficiency is severe, protein and energy nutritional supplements should be added, preferably providing at least 400 kcal/d. In undernourished older people they have been shown—by meta-analysis of controlled trials—to produce weight gain, to be free of side effects, and to reduce mortality by up to 34% among patients in short-term hospital care (odds ratio, 0.66; 95% CI, 0.49–0.90) [83,84]. The effects of supplements on function are less clear, although they may improve cognitive function [85]. These supplements are best ingested between meals because this reduces the compensatory suppression of food at usual meal times [74,86]. Various forms of tube feeding may be required for severe undernutrition, particular when swallowing is impaired or not possible.

There may be a limited role for orexigenic drugs to promote weight gain in undernourished older patients, but study results are sparse [87]. Megestrol acetate is a progestational agent that increases appetite and has been shown to produce weight gain in cancer-related anorexia, HIV/AIDS, and other conditions that are characterized by increased cytokine activity, although weight is gained disproportionately as fat [87]. When megestrol, 800 mg/d, was administered for 12 weeks to undernourished nursing home residents in a placebo-controlled trial, there was no significant weight gain during that time; however, there was a significant increase in weight in the 12 weeks after ceasing it [88]. Although usually well tolerated, megestrol can produce fluid retention, flushing, adrenal insufficiency, and an increased rate of deep vein thromboses. Testosterone levels are reduced in men, and testosterone probably should be coadministered with megestrol in men. Dronabinol is a cannabis derivative, which can stimulate appetite, improve mood, and aid pain relief. Its effects in undernourished older people are not well characterized, and its use is associated with delirium and occasional nausea. The 6-week administration of dronabinol, 2.5 mg twice daily, to older patients who had Alzheimer's disease was associated with a 0.5- to 1-kg greater weight gain than was placebo in one study [89]. It is hoped that the identification of specific causes of the anorexia of aging will enable the development of targeted treatments. Examples might include CCK antagonists or oral analogs of ghrelin.

References

[1] Wurtman JJ, Lieberman H, Tsay R, et al. Calorie and nutrient intakes of elderly and young subjects measured under identical conditions. J Gerontol 1988;43(6):B174–80.

[2] Clarkston WK, Pantano MM, Morley JE, et al. Evidence for the anorexia of aging: gastrointestinal transit and hunger in healthy elderly vs. young adults. Am J Physiol 1997;272(1 Pt 2): R243–8.

[3] Morley JE. Anorexia of aging: physiologic and pathologic. Am J Clin Nutr 1997;66(4): 760–73.

[4] Briefel RR, McDowell MA, Alaimo K, et al. Total energy intake of the US population: the Third National Health and Nutrition Examination Survey, 1988–1991. Am J Clin Nutr 1995; 62(Suppl 5):1072S–80S.

[5] Koehler KM. The New Mexico Aging Process Study. Nutr Rev 1994;52(8 Pt 2):S34.

[6] Sjogren A, Osterberg T, Steen B. Intake of energy, nutrients and food items in a ten-year cohort comparison and in a six-year longitudinal perspective: a population study of 70- and 76-year-old Swedish people. Age Ageing 1994;23(2):108–12.

[7] Villareal DT, Apovian CM, Kushner RF, et al. Obesity in older adults: technical review and position statement of the American Society for Nutrition and NAASO, The Obesity Society. Am J Clin Nutr 2005;82(5):923–34.

[8] Wallace JI, Schwartz RS, LaCroix AZ, et al. Involuntary weight loss in older outpatients: incidence and clinical significance. J Am Geriatr Soc 1995;43(4):329–37.

[9] Schoenborn CA, Adams PF, Barnes PM. Body weight status of adults: United States, 1997–98. Adv Data 2002;(330):1–15.

[10] Newman AB, Yanez D, Harris T, et al. Weight change in old age and its association with mortality. J Am Geriatr Soc 2001;49(10):1309–18.

[11] Prentice AM, Jebb SA. Beyond body mass index. Obes Rev 2001;2(3):141–7.

[12] Beaufrere B, Morio B. Fat and protein redistribution with aging: metabolic considerations. Eur J Clin Nutr 2000;54(Suppl. 3):S48–53.

[13] Cree MG, Newcomer BR, Katsanos CS, et al. Intramuscular and liver triglycerides are increased in the elderly. J Clin Endocrinol Metab 2004;89(8):3864–71.

[14] Melton LJ 3rd, Khosla S, Riggs BL. Epidemiology of sarcopenia. Mayo Clin Proc 2000; 75(Suppl):S10–2 [discussion: S12–3].

[15] Janssen I, Baumgartner RN, Ross R, et al. Skeletal muscle cutpoints associated with elevated physical disability risk in older men and women. Am J Epidemiol 2004;159(4): 413–21.

[16] Manson JE, Willett WC, Stampfer MJ, et al. Body weight and mortality among women. N Engl J Med 1995;333(11):677–85.

[17] Calle EE, Thun MJ, Petrelli JM, et al. Body-mass index and mortality in a prospective cohort of U.S. adults. N Engl J Med 1999;341(15):1097–105.

[18] Somes GW, Kritchevsky SB, Shorr RI, et al. Body mass index, weight change, and death in older adults: the systolic hypertension in the elderly program. Am J Epidemiol 2002;156(2): 132–8.
[19] Heiat A, Vaccarino V, Krumholz HM. An evidence-based assessment of federal guidelines for overweight and obesity as they apply to elderly persons. Arch Intern Med 2001;161(9): 1194–203.
[20] Omran ML, Morley JE. Assessment of protein energy malnutrition in older persons, part II: laboratory evaluation. Nutrition 2000;16(2):131–40.
[21] Potter JF, Schafer DF, Bohi RL. In-hospital mortality as a function of body mass index: an age-dependent variable. J Gerontol 1988;43(3):M59–63.
[22] Rumpel C, Harris TB, Madans J. Modification of the relationship between the Quetelet index and mortality by weight-loss history among older women. Ann Epidemiol 1993;3(4):343–50.
[23] Li F, Fisher KJ, Harmer P. Prevalence of overweight and obesity in older U.S. adults: estimates from the 2003 Behavioral Risk Factor Surveillance System survey. J Am Geriatr Soc 2005;53(4):737–9.
[24] Ogden CL, Carroll MD, Curtin LR, et al. Prevalence of overweight and obesity in the United States, 1999-2004. JAMA 2006;295(13):1549–55.
[25] Flegal KM, Carroll MD, Ogden CL, et al. Prevalence and trends in obesity among US adults, 1999-2000. JAMA 2002;288(14):1723–7.
[26] Mokdad AH, Bowman BA, Ford ES, et al. The continuing epidemics of obesity and diabetes in the United States. JAMA 2001;286(10):1195–200.
[27] Fine JT, Colditz GA, Coakley EH, et al. A prospective study of weight change and health-related quality of life in women. JAMA 1999;282(22):2136–42.
[28] Yaari S, Goldbourt U. Voluntary and involuntary weight loss: associations with long term mortality in 9,228 middle-aged and elderly men. Am J Epidemiol 1998;148(6):546–55.
[29] Wannamethee SG, Shaper AG, Lennon L. Reasons for intentional weight loss, unintentional weight loss, and mortality in older men. Arch Intern Med 2005;165(9):1035–40.
[30] Gregg EW, Gerzoff RB, Thompson TJ, et al. Intentional weight loss and death in overweight and obese U.S. adults 35 years of age and older. Ann Intern Med 2003;138(5):383–9.
[31] Campbell AJ, Spears GF, Brown JS, et al. Anthropometric measurements as predictors of mortality in a community population aged 70 years and over. Age Ageing 1990;19(2):131–5.
[32] Morley JE, Silver AJ. Nutritional issues in nursing home care. Ann Intern Med 1995;123(11): 850–9.
[33] Cederholm T, Jagren C, Hellstrom K. Outcome of protein-energy malnutrition in elderly medical patients. Am J Med 1995;98(1):67–74.
[34] Sullivan DH, Walls RC, Lipschitz DA. Protein-energy undernutrition and the risk of mortality within 1 y of hospital discharge in a select population of geriatric rehabilitation patients. Am J Clin Nutr 1991;53(3):599–605.
[35] Roberts SB, Fuss P, Heyman MB, et al. Control of food intake in older men. JAMA 1994; 272(20):1601–6.
[36] Doty RL, Shaman P, Applebaum SL, et al. Smell identification ability: changes with age. Science 1984;226(4681):1441–3.
[37] Rolls BJ, McDermott TM. Effects of age on sensory-specific satiety. Am J Clin Nutr 1991; 54(6):988–96.
[38] MacIntosh CG, Sheehan J, Davani N, et al. Effects of aging on the opioid modulation of feeding in humans. J Am Geriatr Soc 2001;49(11):1518–24.
[39] Martinez M, Hernanz A, Gomez-Cerezo J, et al. Alterations in plasma and cerebrospinal fluid levels of neuropeptides in idiopathic senile anorexia. Regul Pept 1993;49(2):109–17.
[40] Silver AJ, Morley JE. Role of the opioid system in the hypodipsia associated with aging. J Am Geriatr Soc 1992;40(6):556–60.
[41] Baranowska B, Radzikowska M, Wasilewska-Dziubinska E, et al. Relationship among leptin, neuropeptide Y, and galanin in young women and in postmenopausal women. Menopause 2000;7(3):149–55.

[42] Giustina A, Licini M, Bussi AR, et al. Effects of sex and age on the growth hormone response to galanin in healthy human subjects. J Clin Endocrinol Metab 1993;76(5):1369–72.

[43] Matsumura T, Nakayama M, Nomura A, et al. Age-related changes in plasma orexin-A concentrations. Exp Gerontol 2002;37(8–9):1127–30.

[44] Kirchgessner AL. Orexins in the brain-gut axis. Endocr Rev 2002;23(1):1–15.

[45] Sohn EH, Wolden-Hanson T, Matsumoto AM. Testosterone (T)-induced changes in arcuate nucleus cocaine-amphetamine-regulated transcript and NPY mRNA are attenuated in old compared to young male brown Norway rats: contribution of T to age-related changes in cocaine-amphetamine-regulated transcript and NPY gene expression. Endocrinology 2002; 143(3):954–63.

[46] Beglinger C, Degen L, Matzinger D, et al. Loxiglumide, a CCK-A receptor antagonist, stimulates calorie intake and hunger feelings in humans. Am J Physiol Regul Integr Comp Physiol 2001;280(4):R1149–54.

[47] MacIntosh CG, Morley JE, Wishart J, et al. Effect of exogenous cholecystokinin (CCK)-8 on food intake and plasma CCK, leptin, and insulin concentrations in older and young adults: evidence for increased CCK activity as a cause of the anorexia of aging. J Clin Endocrinol Metab 2001;86(12):5830–7.

[48] Flint A, Raben A, Astrup A, et al. Glucagon-like peptide 1 promotes satiety and suppresses energy intake in humans. J Clin Invest 1998;101(3):515–20.

[49] MacIntosh CG, Andrews JM, Jones KL, et al. Effects of age on concentrations of plasma cholecystokinin, glucagon-like peptide 1, and peptide YY and their relation to appetite and pyloric motility. Am J Clin Nutr 1999;69(5):999–1006.

[50] Batterham RL, Cowley MA, Small CJ, et al. Gut hormone PYY(3-36) physiologically inhibits food intake. Nature 2002;418(6898):650–4.

[51] Batterham RL, Cohen MA, Ellis SM, et al. Inhibition of food intake in obese subjects by peptide YY3-36. N Engl J Med 2003;349(10):941–8.

[52] Johns CE, Newton JL, Westley BR, et al. Human pancreatic polypeptide has a marked diurnal rhythm that is affected by ageing and is associated with the gastric TFF2 circadian rhythm. Peptides 2006;27(6):1341–8.

[53] Boggiano MM, Chandler PC, Oswald KD, et al. PYY3-36 as an anti-obesity drug target. Obes Rev 2005;6(4):307–22.

[54] Blanton CA, Horwitz BA, Blevins JE, et al. Reduced feeding response to neuropeptide Y in senescent Fischer 344 rats. Am J Physiol Regul Integr Comp Physiol 2001;280(4):R1052–60.

[55] Di Francesco V, Zamboni M, Zoico E, et al. Unbalanced serum leptin and ghrelin dynamics prolong postprandial satiety and inhibit hunger in healthy elderly: another reason for the "anorexia of aging". Am J Clin Nutr 2006;83(5):1149–52.

[56] Baumgartner RN, Waters DL, Morley JE, et al. Age-related changes in sex hormones affect the sex difference in serum leptin independently of changes in body fat. Metabolism 1999; 48(3):378–84.

[57] Hislop MS, Ratanjee BD, Soule SG, et al. Effects of anabolic-androgenic steroid use or gonadal testosterone suppression on serum leptin concentration in men. Eur J Endocrinol 1999; 141(1):40–6.

[58] Broglio F, Benso A, Castiglioni C, et al. The endocrine response to ghrelin as a function of gender in humans in young and elderly subjects. J Clin Endocrinol Metab 2003;88(4): 1537–42.

[59] Purnell JQ, Weigle DS, Breen P, et al. Ghrelin levels correlate with insulin levels, insulin resistance, and high-density lipoprotein cholesterol, but not with gender, menopausal status, or cortisol levels in humans. J Clin Endocrinol Metab 2003;88(12):5747–52.

[60] Sturm K, MacIntosh CG, Parker BA, et al. Appetite, food intake, and plasma concentrations of cholecystokinin, ghrelin, and other gastrointestinal hormones in undernourished older women and well-nourished young and older women. J Clin Endocrinol Metab 2003; 88(8):3747–55.

[61] Rigamonti AE, Pincelli AI, Corra B, et al. Plasma ghrelin concentrations in elderly subjects: comparison with anorexic and obese patients. J Endocrinol 2002;175(1):R1–5.

[62] Fraze E, Chiou YA, Chen YD, et al. Age-related changes in postprandial plasma glucose, insulin, and free fatty acid concentrations in nondiabetic individuals. J Am Geriatr Soc 1987;35(3):224–8.

[63] Wynne K, Stanley S, McGowan B, et al. Appetite control. J Endocrinol 2005;184(2): 291–318.

[64] Chapman IM, Goble EA, Wittert GA, et al. Effect of intravenous glucose and euglycemic insulin infusions on short-term appetite and food intake. Am J Physiol 1998;274(3 Pt 2): R596–603.

[65] Morley JE. Androgens and aging. Maturitas 2001;38(1):61–71 [discussion: 71–3].

[66] Nair KS, Rizza RA, O'Brien P, et al. DHEA in elderly women and DHEA or testosterone in elderly men. N Engl J Med 2006;355(16):1647–59.

[67] Amory JK, Chansky HA, Chansky KL, et al. Preoperative supraphysiological testosterone in older men undergoing knee replacement surgery. J Am Geriatr Soc 2002;50(10):1698–701.

[68] Bakhshi V, Elliott M, Gentili A, et al. Testosterone improves rehabilitation outcomes in ill older men. J Am Geriatr Soc 2000;48(5):550–3.

[69] Yeh SS, Schuster MW. Geriatric cachexia: the role of cytokines. Am J Clin Nutr 1999;70(2): 183–97.

[70] Roubenoff R, Harris TB, Abad LW, et al. Monocyte cytokine production in an elderly population: effect of age and inflammation. J Gerontol A Biol Sci Med Sci 1998;53(1):M20–6.

[71] Walker D, Beauchene RE. The relationship of loneliness, social isolation, and physical health to dietary adequacy of independently living elderly. J Am Diet Assoc 1991;91(3): 300–4.

[72] Evers MM, Marin DB. Mood disorders. Effective management of major depressive disorder in the geriatric patient. Geriatrics 2002;57(10):36–40 [quiz: 41].

[73] Morley JE, Kraenzle D. Causes of weight loss in a community nursing home. J Am Geriatr Soc 1994;42(6):583–5.

[74] Wilson MM, Vaswani S, Liu D, et al. Prevalence and causes of undernutrition in medical outpatients. Am J Med 1998;104(1):56–63.

[75] Morris MS, Fava M, Jacques PF, et al. Depression and folate status in the US population. Psychother Psychosom 2003;72(2):80–7.

[76] Thomas P, Hazif-Thomas C, Clement JP. Influence of antidepressant therapies on weight and appetite in the elderly. J Nutr Health Aging 2003;7(3):166–70.

[77] Sahyoun NR, Otradovec CL, Hartz SC, et al. Dietary intakes and biochemical indicators of nutritional status in an elderly, institutionalized population. Am J Clin Nutr 1988;47(3): 524–33.

[78] Fuhrman MP, Charney P, Mueller CM. Hepatic proteins and nutrition assessment. J Am Diet Assoc 2004;104(8):1258–64.

[79] Guigoz Y, Lauque S, Vellas BJ. Identifying the elderly at risk for malnutrition. The Mini Nutritional Assessment. Clin Geriatr Med 2002;18(4):737–57.

[80] Ribaudo JM, Cella D, Hahn EA, et al. Re-validation and shortening of the Functional Assessment of Anorexia/Cachexia Therapy (FAACT) questionnaire. Qual Life Res 2000;9(10): 1137–46.

[81] Keller HH, McKenzie JD, Goy RE. Construct validation and test-retest reliability of the seniors in the community: risk evaluation for eating and nutrition questionnaire. J Gerontol A Biol Sci Med Sci 2001;56(9):M552–8.

[82] Wilson MM, Thomas DR, Rubenstein LZ, et al. Appetite assessment: simple appetite questionnaire predicts weight loss in community-dwelling adults and nursing home residents. Am J Clin Nutr 2005;82(5):1074–81.

[83] Milne AC, Avenell A, Potter J. Meta-analysis: protein and energy supplementation in older people. Ann Intern Med 2006;144(1):37–48.

[84] Milne AC, Potter J, Avenell A. Protein and energy supplementation in elderly people at risk from malnutrition. Cochrane Database Syst Rev 2005;(2):CD003288.

[85] Manders M, de Groot LC, van Staveren WA, et al. Effectiveness of nutritional supplements on cognitive functioning in elderly persons: a systematic review. J Gerontol A Biol Sci Med Sci 2004;59(10):1041–9.

[86] Wilson MM, Purushothaman R, Morley JE. Effect of liquid dietary supplements on energy intake in the elderly. Am J Clin Nutr 2002;75(5):944–7.

[87] Morley JE. Orexigenic and anabolic agents. Clin Geriatr Med 2002;18(4):853–66.

[88] Yeh SS, Wu SY, Lee TP, et al. Improvement in quality-of-life measures and stimulation of weight gain after treatment with megestrol acetate oral suspension in geriatric cachexia: results of a double-blind, placebo-controlled study. J Am Geriatr Soc 2000;48(5):485–92.

[89] Volicer L, Stelly M, Morris J, et al. Effects of dronabinol on anorexia and disturbed behavior in patients with Alzheimer's disease. Int J Geriatr Psychiatry 1997;12(9):913–9.

ELSEVIER
SAUNDERS

CLINICS IN
GERIATRIC
MEDICINE

Clin Geriatr Med 23 (2007) 757–767

The Aging Gut: Physiology

John E. Morley, MB, BCh[a,b,*]

[a]Division of Geriatric Medicine, Saint Louis University Medical Center,
Saint Louis University School of Medicine, 1402 South Grand Boulevard,
M238, St. Louis, MO 63104, USA
[b]Geriatric Research, Education and Clinical Center, St. Louis VA Medical Center,
Jefferson Barracks Division, GRECC, #1 Jefferson Barracks Drive,
11G/JB, St. Louis MO 63125, USA

Aging of the gastrointestinal tract is less obvious than seen in other organs, such as the brain. Most of the changes that occur are of small magnitude and are rarely noticed unless an excessive stress is placed on the gut. The major exception to this seems to be the physiologic anorexia of aging that plays a major role in weight loss with aging and makes older persons highly vulnerable to developing cachexia [1]. It often is difficult to distinguish true physiologic changes that occur with aging and subclinical disease processes as is illustrated in discussing the changes in swallowing and the increased propensity to develop aspiration pneumonia as we age. Another example of this physiology–disease interface is postprandial hypotension.

The physiologic anorexia of aging

The concept of a physiologic anorexia of aging was first enunciated clearly in 1988, although it had been recognized since the time of the ancient Romans [2]. This anorexia is more marked in men than in women. This physiologic anorexia involves multiple small changes, such as those in taste and smell; altered fundal compliance; altered secretion of gastrointestinal hormones; alterations in autonomic nervous system feedback to the central nervous system; alterations in the fat hormone leptin and in steroid hormones; and changes in the central nervous system in response to food intake [3]. The complexities of these changes are summarized briefly in the next few paragraphs.

* Division of Geriatric Medicine, Saint Louis University Medical Center, Saint Louis University School of Medicine, 1402 South Grand Boulevard, M238, St. Louis, MO 63104.
    E-mail address: morley@slu.edu

0749-0690/07/$ - see front matter © 2007 Elsevier Inc. All rights reserved.
doi:10.1016/j.cger.2007.06.002

Much of the human experience of taste actually is due to the sensations produced by food in the mouth stimulating the retronasal olfactory receptors. With aging there is a marked deterioration of olfactory function beginning in the fifth decade [4]. By the age of 80 years, most individuals have less smell identification ability than 5- to 9-year-olds. Whether these changes are truly physiologic or due to environmental insults, repeated viral infections, or neurodegenerative pathology is uncertain. Sinus disease and Alzheimer's disease are associated with marked decreases in olfactory ability. Direct taste testing has shown a decline in the four primary tastes (salt, bitter, sweet, and sour) with aging [5]. Also, older persons lose the increased sensitivity of the tongue tip that is seen in younger persons [6]. Cigarette smoking, medications, xerostomia, and local inflammatory conditions can interfere with taste acuity. Diabetics often lose the taste for glucose. Severe zinc deficiency also can lead to loss of taste acuity. The exact role of chemosensory dysfunction in producing the physiologic anorexia of aging is unknown, but it seems to be minor [7].

A major component of satiation is related to food stretching the antrum of the stomach [8]. With aging there is a decline in the adaptive compliance of the fundus of the stomach, possibly due to a decrease in nitric oxide production in response to food [9,10]. This leads to a more rapid escape of food from the fundus into the antrum. Thus, antral stretch occurs earlier, resulting in early satiation [11,12].

Fat in the duodenum leads to the release of cholecystokinin (CCK) [13]. CCK acts as a satiety hormone [14]. With aging in humans there is an increased release of CCK, basally and in response to fat [15,16]. In addition, CCK is a more potent inhibitor of feeding in older persons and animals [17,18].

Leptin, a hormone produced from adipocytes, produces satiation in animals; its levels increase with aging in men because of the decline in testosterone [19–21]. It has been postulated that this effect of testosterone on leptin is the reason for the increased anorexia that occurs in aging men compared with women [22].

Many of the orexigenic neuropeptides seem to produce their effects within the central nervous system by stimulating nitric oxide synthase [23–27]. The decline in nitric oxide production with aging also may play a role in the anorexia of aging [10].

It is now well recognized that this physiologic anorexia of aging places older persons at major risk for having severe decreases in food intake when they are stressed [28–30]. In addition, mild chronic cytokine excess, such as occurs in frailty, can lead to a further decrease in food intake [31–36].

Postprandial hypotension

Substantial decreases in blood pressure following a meal were demonstrated to occur in elderly persons who did not have evidence of autonomic neuropathy [37]. This decrease in blood pressure occurs more often in the morning and is more sensitive to carbohydrate, but it also occurs with other macronutrients [38–40]. Rate of nutrient entry into the duodenum may be more important than the actual nutrient [41]. The major cause seems to be due to the release of a gastrointestinal peptide [42], most likely calcitonin gene-related peptide [43]. A low dose of a nitric oxide synthase inhibitor reverses postprandial hypotension in older persons [44]. Young persons who have diabetes mellitus also develop postprandial hypotension [45]. Acarbose, an alpha-1-glucosidose inhibitor, attenuates postprandial hypotension [46].

Pharyngoesophageal function

Dysphagia and the associated aspiration pneumonia occur with increasing frequency as we age. Physiologically in older persons, there is a prolongation of the oropharyngeal phase and a delay in the opening of the upper esophageal sphincter. The fluid volume necessary to induce pharyngeal swallows is greater in older persons, and older persons require a greater volume of fluid to stimulate the pharyngogluttal closure reflex [47]. In older persons, the bolus head often descends further below the tongue base before the swallowing reflex is initiated [48,49]; however, this is not associated with aspiration. In older persons, hypopharyngeal pressure wave is increased in amplitude and duration [50]. This is associated with decreased hypopharyngeal acceleration and an increase in transsphincteric pressure [51].

Aspiration pneumonia occurs when the older person has a combination of abnormalities in the swallowing reflex and a lack of protective reflexes, such as the cough reflex. These abnormalities do not seem to be present in highly functional older persons [52]. Elderly persons with small basal ganglia infarcts have abnormalities in their swallowing reflexes [53]. The pharyngeal and tracheal epithelium is heavily innervated by substance P–containing nerves. Substance P depletion results in a decrease in the cough response and the swallowing reflex. It seems that deterioration of substance P–induced reflexes plays an important role in "silent" aspiration in older persons [54]. Angiotensin-converting enzyme (ACE) inhibitors block the breakdown of substance P [55]. ACE inhibitors increase the cough reflex and enhance the swallowing reflex [56,57]. The ACE DD allele is associated with an increased risk for aspiration pneumonia [25]. Poor oral hygiene further increases the risk for aspiration pneumonia because of an increase in pathogenic bacteria in the oropharynx [58].

Soergel and colleagues [59] found that esophageal abnormalities were so common in older persons that they suggested the use of the term "presbyesophagus"; however, these abnormalities are much less common in the truly healthy elderly. In the healthy elderly, there are small increases in esophageal amplitude in the distal esophagus and a higher pressure needed to

MORLEY

produce secondary peristalsis [60]. No systematic changes in lower esophageal pressure have been reported in healthy elderly [61]. Older persons may
have longer duration of acid reflux than younger persons [62].

Gastrointestinal motility

Gastric emptying is unchanged when the meal consists of less than 500
kcal, but is slowed when a greater amount of calories are given [63]. The
small intestine transit rate is not altered with aging [64]. Similarly, migratory
motor complexes are not different between young and older persons [65].

The increase in intestinal transit time that occurs with aging seems to be
predominantly due to an increase in colon transit time [66]. In rats, the
increase in colon transit time is associated with an increased diameter of
the colon and a decreased in vitro response to electrical and cholinergic
stimulation [67]. These changes most probably are related to the loss of
enteric neurons, especially cholinergic ones, with aging [68]. In older persons
with slow transit constipation or dysmotility, there is an increase in
amphophilic/polyglucoson smooth muscle inclusion bodies [69,70].

There is a marked increase in fecal incontinence, from 3.7% to 27%, with
aging [71]. Frail older persons in long-term care settings can have a prevalence of fecal incontinence as high as 50%; however, most of these changes
seem to be due to disease and cognitive impairment. Physiologically, older
persons have lower mean basal and squeeze anal pressures [72]. These
changes are particularly present in older women, possibly related to the
trauma of childbirth. Older women also require less rectal pressure to
produce relaxation of the anal sphincter.

Gastric acid and mucosa

Gastric acid and pepsinogen secretion increase with aging in persons who
do not have disease [73,74]. Atrophic gastritis occurs commonly with aging
with a prevalence of approximately 20%. *Helicobacter pylori* infection is
associated with a decrease in gastric acid secretion.

Aging is associated with an increase in gastric mucosa proliferation;
however, the gastric mucosa seems to be more susceptible to injury. Prostaglandin (PG) levels, such as PGE_2 and PGF2 alpha, are lower in biopsy
specimens from the stomach and the duodenum [75].

Intestinal absorption

Despite the numerous factors that can alter intestinal absorption,
minimal meaningful changes in absorption have been demonstrated in older
humans. These changes are summarized in Box 1; however, there can be
major effects of disease (eg, chronic gastritis and bacterial overgrowth)
and medications on micronutrient absorption. Loss of intrinsic factor leads
to vitamin B_{12} deficiency (pernicious anemia). When older persons are losing

---

Box 1. Changes in intestinal absorption with aging

Reduced
  Carbohydrate
  Protein
  Triglycerides
  Folate
  Vitamin B_{12}
  Vitamin D
  Calcium

No change
  Thiamine
  Riboflavin
  Niacin
  Vitamin K
  Zinc
  Magnesium
  Iron

Increased
  Cholesterol
  Vitamin A
  Vitamin C

---

weight, pancreatic insufficiency and celiac disease may be causing malabsorption.

Intestinal microflora

There is increasing awareness that the commensal intestinal antibiotics play an important role in maintaining the intestinal defensive barrier. Translocation of pathogenic bacteria from the gut into the circulation or lymphatics can lead to release of endotoxins, such as lipopolysaccharides. These activate macrophages to produce excess cytokines, such as tumor necrosis factor α and interleukin (IL)-6 [76]. This leads to sarcopenia, anorexia, and anemia. IL-6 also releases hepciclin from the liver, which inhibits the ferroportens, thus decreasing absorption of iron from the intestine.

There are apparent physiologic changes in gut bacteria in older persons. Overall, there is a decrease in the total number of bifidobacteria, accompanied by an increase in species diversity [77,78]. Fungi and enterobacteria tend to increase. These changes result in an increased propensity of older persons to develop *Clostridium difficile* diarrhea [79].

Gastrointestinal peptides

Aging alters the circulating levels of several gastrointestinal hormones (Table 1). These hormonal changes can result in changes in gastrointestinal related function, such as the anorexia of aging and postprandial hypotension. The levels of the incretins, inhibitory peptide and glucagons-like peptide I, are unaltered with healthy aging but decrease when the older person develops diabetes. This results in a decrease in insulin secretion and a worsening of the diabetes [80]. Insulin levels are increased in an attempt to overcome the insulin resistance that occurs with aging. Amylin levels increase above those of middle-aged persons and approximate those of young persons [81]. This may play a role in the anorexia of aging [82].

Several gut peptides enhance memory and improve the ability to recall old memories. These include CCK, amylin, and ghrelin [83–85]. This is in keeping with the finding that if an animal learns a task and then eats, it improves the animal's ability to remember the task [86,87].

Pancreas, liver, and gallbladder

The volume of pancreatic secretion and a decline in enzyme (lipase, trypsin, and phospholipase) output occur with aging [88–90]. These changes

Table 1
The effects of aging on gastrointestinal hormones

Hormone	Function	Aging effect
Gastrin	Gastric acid secretion	Increased
Ghrelin	Increased food intake and growth hormone	No change
Cholecystokinin	Satiation Gallbladder secretion Pancreatic enzyme secretion	Increased
Secretion	Pancreatic enzyme secretion Bicarbonate secretion	Unknown
Gastric inhibitory peptide	Insulin secretion Slows gastric emptying	No change
Glucagon-like peptide	Insulin secretion Slows gastric emptying	No change
Pancreatic polypeptide	Inhibits pancreatic secretion	Increased
Somatostatin	Inhibits gut secretion, intestinal motility, and peptide hormone secretion	Increased
Motilin	Gastric emptying Migratory motor complexes	Increased
Insulin	Glucose regulation	Increased
Amylin	Inhibits insulin Satiation	Increased above middle age levels
Calcitonin gene-related peptide	Postprandial hypotension	No change or increased

have no clear effect on fat or protein absorption. Fibrotic changes in the pancreas occur commonly in older persons and are associated with ductal papillary hyperplasia [91]. On ultrasound, this is associated with increased echogeneity of the pancreas and increased pancreatic duct diameter (up to 3 mm) [92].

Liver volume decreases by a third with aging [93–95]. Small changes in serum alanine aminotransferase (ALT) occur with aging. In women, levels continue to increase with age, whereas in men levels only increase up to 50 years of age [96]. In frail older persons, ALT levels show a bell-shaped curve with lower levels in the old-old [97]. Although most liver function shows no change with aging, there is a general decline in the P450 enzyme system in animals [98]. This leads to delayed metabolism of many of the medications given to older persons. There is a marked increase in interindividual variability in enzyme activity with aging, and some of the microsomal enzymes, such as CYP3A, are more affected than others [93]. Also, there is a greater decline in the activity of rapid metabolism than for poor metabolizers with aging [99]. The minimal effects of aging on liver physiology can be discerned by the fact that livers from donors older than 80 years of age can be transplanted satisfactorily [100].

The biliary duct is dilated with aging as a result of increased connective tissue [101]. The upper limit for a normal bile duct in older persons should be 8.5 mm. Lithogenicity of bile salts increases with aging, leading to an increased propensity to develop gallstones.

References

[1] Morley JE, Thomas DR, Wilson MM. Cachexia: pathophysiology and clinical relevance. Am J Clin Nutr 2006;83:735–43.
[2] Morley JE, Silver AJ. Anorexia in the elderly. Neurobiol Aging 1988;9:9–16.
[3] Morley JE. Anorexia of aging: physiologic and pathologic. Am J Clin Nutr 1997;66:760–73.
[4] Boyce JM, Shone GR. Effects of ageing on smell and taste. Postgrad Med J 2006;82:239–41.
[5] Weiffenbach JM, Cowart BJ, Baum BJ. Taste intensity perception in aging. J Gerontol 1986;41:460–8.
[6] Matsuda T, Doty RL. Regional taste sensitivity to NaCl: relationship to subject age, tongue locus and area of stimulation. Chem Senses 1995;20:283–90.
[7] Schiffman SS. Taste and smell losses with age. Bol Asoc Med P R 1991;83:411–4.
[8] Jones KL, Doran SM, Hveem K, et al. Relation between postprandial satiation and antral area in normal subject. Am J Clin Nutr 1997;66:127–32.
[9] Morley JE, Kumar VB, Mattammal MB, et al. Inhibition of feeding by a nitric oxide synthase inhibitor: effects of aging. Eur J Pharmacol 1996;31:15–59.
[10] Sun WM, Doran S, Lingenfelser T, et al. Effects of glyceryl trinitrate on the pyloric motor response to intraduodenal triglyceride infusion in humans. Eur J Clin Invest 1996;26:657–64.
[11] Sun WM, Doran S, Jones KL, et al. Effects of nitroglycerin on liquid gastric emptying and antropyloroduodenal motility. Am J Physiol 1998;275(5 Pt I):G1173–8.
[12] Rolland Y, Kim MJ, Gammack JK, et al. Office management of weight loss in older persons. Am J Med 2006;119:1019–26.
[13] Morley JE. Minireview. The ascent of cholecystokinin (CCK)—from gut to brain. Life Sci 1982;30:479–93.

[14] Silver AJ, Flood JF, Song AM, et al. Evidence for a physiological role for CCK in the regulation of food intake in mice. Am J Physiol 1989;256(3 Pt 2):R646–52.

[15] McIntosh CG, Horowitz M, Verhagen MA, et al. Effect of small intestinal nutrient infusion on appetite, gastrointestinal hormone release, and gastric myoelectrical activity in young and older men. Am J Gastroenterol 2001;96:997–1007.

[16] MacIntosh CG, Andrews JM, Jones KL, et al. Effects of age on concentrations of plasma cholecystokinin, glucagon-like peptide 1, and peptide YY and their relation to appetite and pyloric motility. Am J Clin Nutr 1999;69:999–1006.

[17] McIntosh CG, Morley JE, Wishart J, et al. Effect of exogenous cholecystokinin (CCK)-8 on food intake and plasma CCK, leptin, and insulin concentrations in older and young adults: evidence for increased CCK activity as a cause of the anorexia of aging. J Clin Endocrinol Metab 2001;86:5830–7.

[18] Silver AJ, Flood JF, Morley JE. Effect of gastrointestinal peptides on ingestion in old and young mice. Peptide 1988;9:221–5.

[19] Morley JE, Perry HM 3rd, Baumgartner RP, et al. Leptin, adipose tissue and aging—is there a role for testosterone? J Gerontol A Biol Sci Med Sci 1999;54:B99–107.

[20] Perry HM 3rd, Morley JE, Horowitz M, et al. Body composition and age in African-American and Caucasian women: relationship to plasma leptin levels. Metabolism 1997;46:1399–405.

[21] Sih R, Morley JE, Kaiser FE, et al. Testosterone replacement in older hypogonadal men: a 12-month randomized controlled trial. J Clin Endocrinol Metab 1997;82:1661–7.

[22] Wilson MM, Morley JE. Aging and energy balance (review). J Appl Physiol 2003;95:1728–36.

[23] Morley JE, Flood JF. Evidence that nitric oxide modulates food intake in mice. Life Sci 1991;49:707–11.

[24] Farr SA, Banks WA, Kumar VB, et al. Orexin-A-induced feeding is dependent on nitric oxide. Peptides 2005;26:759–65.

[25] Morimoto S, Okaishi K, Onishi M, et al. Deletion allele of the angiotensin-converting enzyme gene as a risk factor for pneumonia in elderly patients. Am J Med 2002;112:89–94.

[26] Gaskin FS, Farr SA, Banks WA, et al. Ghrelin-induced feeding is dependent on nitric oxide. Peptides 2003;24:913–8.

[27] Morley JE, Alshaher MM, Farr SA, et al. Leptin and neuropeptide Y (NPY) modulate nitric oxide synthase: further evidence for a role of nitric oxide in feeding. Peptides 1999;20:595–600.

[28] Morley JE. Is weight loss harmful to older men? Aging Male 2006;9:135–7.

[29] Thomas DR, Zdrowski CD, Wilson MM, et al. Malnutrition in subacute care. Am J Clin Nutr 2002;75:308–13.

[30] Chapman IM, MacIntosh CG, Morley JE, et al. The anorexia of aging. Biogerontology 2002;3:67–71.

[31] Morley JE, Perry HM 3rd, Miller Dk. Editorial: something about frailty. J Gerontol A Biol Sci Med Sci 2002;57:M698–704.

[32] Morley JE. Anorexia, sarcopenia and aging. Nutrition 2001;17:660–3.

[33] Morley JE, Baumgartner RN. Cytokine-related aging process. J Gerontol A Biol Sci Med Sci 2004;59:M924–9.

[34] Morley JE, Kim MJ, Haren MT, et al. Frailty and the aging male. Aging Male 2005;8:135–40.

[35] Morley JE, Haren MT, Rolland Y, et al. Frailty. Med Clin North Am 2006;90:837–47.

[36] Roubenoff R. Catabolism of aging: is it an inflammatory process? Curr Opin Clin Nutr Metab Care 2003;6:295–9.

[37] Morley JE. Postprandial hypotension—the ultimate Big Mac attack [editorial]. J Gerontol A Biol Sci Med Sci 2001;56:M741–3.

[38] Jansen RW, Kelly-Gagnon MM, Lipsitz LA. Intraindividual reproducibility of postprandial and orthostatic blood pressure changes in older nursing-home patients: relationship with chronic use of cardiovascular medications. J Am Geriatr Soc 1996;44:383–9.

[39] Jones KL, Tonkin A, Horowitz M, et al. Rate of gastric emptying is a determinant of postprandial hypotension in non-insulin-dependent diabetes mellitus. Clin Sci 1998;94: 65–70.

[40] Gentilcore D, Jones KL, O'Donovan DG, et al. Postprandial hypotension—novel insights into pathophysiology and therapeutic implications. Curr Vasc Pharmacol 2006;4:161–71.

[41] Jones KL, O'Donovan D, Russo A, et al. Effects of drink volume and glucose load on gastric emptying and postprandial blood pressure in healthy older subjects. Am J Physiol Gastrointest Liver Physiol 2005;289:G240–8.

[42] Jansen RW, Lipsitz LA. Postprandial hypotension: epidemiology, pathophysiology, and clinical management. Ann Intern Med 1995;122:286–95.

[43] Edwards BJ, Perry HM 3rd, Kaiser FE, et al. Relationship of age and calcitonin gene-related peptide to postprandial hypotension. Mech Ageing Dev 1996;87:61–73.

[44] Gentilcore D, Visvanathan R, Russo A, et al. Role of nitric oxide mechanisms in gastric emptying of, and the blood pressure and glycemic responses to, oral glucose in healthy older subjects. Am J Physiol Gastrointest Liver Physiol 2005;288:G1227–32.

[45] Kim MJ, Rolland Y, Cepeda O, et al. Diabetes mellitus in older men. Aging Male 2006;9: 139–47.

[46] Gentilcore D, Bryant B, Wishart JM, et al. Acarbose attenuates the hypotensive response to sucrose and slows gastric emptying in the elderly. Am J Med 2005;118:1289.

[47] Shaker R, Ren J, Bardan E, et al. Pharyngoglottal closure reflex: characterization in healthy young, elderly and dysphagic patients with predeglutitive aspiration. Gerontology 2003;49: 12–20.

[48] Stephen JR, Taves DH, Smith RC, et al. Bolus location at the initiation of the pharyngeal stage of swallowing in healthy older adults. Dysphagia 2005;20:266–72.

[49] Ren J, Shaker R, Zamir Z, et al. Effect of age and bolus variables on the coordination of the glottis and upper esophageal sphincter during swallowing. Am J Gastroenterol 1993;88: 665–9.

[50] Bardan E, Kern M, Arndorfer RC, et al. Effect of aging on bolus kinematics during the pharyngeal phase of swallowing. Am J Physiol Gastrointest Liver Physiol 2006;290: G458–65.

[51] Cook IJ, Weltman MD, Wallace K, et al. Influence of aging on oral-pharyngeal bolus transit and clearance during swallowing: scintigraphic study. Am J Physiol 1994;266(6 Pt 1): G972–7.

[52] Katsumata U, Sekizawa K, Ebihara T. Aging effects on the cough reflex. Chest 1995;107: 290–1.

[53] Ebihara S, Saito H, Kanda A, et al. Impaired efficacy of cough in patients with Parkinson disease. Chest 2003;124:1009–15.

[54] Ebihara T, Takahashi H, Ebihara S, et al. Capsaicin troche for swallowing dysfunction in older people. J Am Geriatr Soc 2005;53:824–8.

[55] Skidgel RA, Erdos EG. Cleavage of peptide bonds by angiotensin I converting enzymes. Agents Actions Suppl 1987;22:289–307.

[56] Okaishi K, Morimoto S, Fukuo K, et al. Reduction of risk of pneumonia associated with use of angiotensin I converting enzyme inhibitors in elderly inpatients. Am J Hypertens 1999;12(8 Pt 1):778–83.

[57] Nakayama K, Sekizawa K, Sasaki H. ACE inhibitor and swallowing reflex. Chest 1998;113: 1425–7.

[58] Yoneyama T, Yoshida M, Ohrui T, et al. Oral care reduces pneumonia in older patients in nursing homes. J Am Geriatr Soc 2002;50:430–3.

[59] Soergel KH, Zboralske FF, Amberg JE. Presbyesophagus: esophageal motility in nonagenarians. Clin Invest 1964;43:1472–9.

[60] Orr WL, Chen LL. Aging and neural control of the GI tract: IV clinical and physiological aspects of gastrointestinal motility and aging. J Physiol 2002;540:673–9.

[61] Shaw DW, Cook IJ, Gabb M. Influence of normal aging on oral pharyngeal and upper esophageal sphincter function during swallowing. Am J Physiol 1995;268:G238–96.

[62] Smout AJ, Breedig KM, van der Zouw L, et al. Physiological gastroesophageal reflux and esophageal motor activity studied with a new system for 24 hour recording and automated analysis. Dig Dis Sci 1981;34:372–8.

[63] Clarkston WK, Pantano MM, Morley JE, et al. Evidence for the anorexia of aging: gastrointestinal transit and hunger in healthy elderly vs. young adults. Am J Physiol 1997;272(1 Pt 2):R243–8.

[64] Madsen JL, Graff J. Effects of ageing on gastrointestinal motor function. Age and Ageing 2004;33:154–9.

[65] Husebye E, Engedal K. The patterns of motility are maintained in the human small intestine throughout the process of aging. Scand J Gastroenterol 1992;27:347–406.

[66] Vagra F. Transit time changes with age in the gastrointestinal tract of the rat. Digestion 1976;14:319–24.

[67] McDougal JN, Miller MS, Banks TF, et al. Age related changes in colonic function in rats. Am J Physiol 1984;274:9542–6.

[68] Wade PR, Cowen T. Neurodegeneration: a key factor in the ageing gut. Neurogastroenterol Motil 2004;16(Suppl 1):19–23.

[69] Knowles CH, Nickols CD, Scott SM, et al. Smooth muscle inclusion bodies in slow transit constipation. J Pathol 2001;193:390–7.

[70] Knowles CH, Nickols CD, Feakins R, et al. A systematic analysis of polyglucosan bodies in the human gastrointestinal tract in health and disease. Acta Neuropathol (Berl) 2003;105:410–3.

[71] Tariq SH, Morley JE, Prather CM. Fecal incontinence in the elderly patient. Am J Med 2003;115:217–27.

[72] Fox JC, Fletcher JG, Zinsmeister AR, et al. Effect of aging on anorectal and pelvic floor functions in females. Dis Colon Rectum 2006;49:1726–35.

[73] Goldschmiedt M, Barnet CC, Schwarz BE, et al. Effect of age on gastric acid secretion and serum gastrin concentrations in healthy men and women. Gastroenterology 1992;102:2181–2.

[74] Kekki M, Samloff IM, Sipponen P, et al. Increase of serum pepsinogen I with age in females with normal gastric mucosa but not in males, possibly due to increase in acid-pepsin secreting area. Scan J Gastroenterol Suppl 1991;186:62–4.

[75] Goto H, Sugiyama S, Ohara A, et al. Age-associated decreases in prostaglandin contents in human gastric mucosa. Biochem Biophys Res Commun 1992;186:1443–8.

[76] Pirlich M, Norman K, Lochs H, et al. Role of intestinal function in cachexia. Curr Opin Clin Nutr Metab Care 2006;9:603–6.

[77] Hopkins MJ, Sharp R, MacFarlane GT. Age and disease related changes in intestinal bacterial populations assessed by cell culture, 16S rRNA abundance, and community cellular fatty acid profiles. Gut 2001;48:198–205.

[78] Hopkins MJ, MacFarlane GT. Evaluation of 16s rRNA and cellular fatty acid profiles as markers of human intestinal bacterial growth in the chemostat. J Appl Microbiol 2000;89:668–77.

[79] Gorbach SL, Nahas L, Lerner PI, et al. Studies of intestinal microflora. I. Effects of diet, age, and periodic sampling on numbers of fecal microorganisms in man. Gastroenterology 1967;53:845–55.

[80] Morley JE. An overview of diabetes mellitus in older persons. Clin Geriatr Med 1999;15:211–24.

[81] Edwards BJ, Perry HM, Kaiser FE, et al. Age-related changes in amylin secretion. Mech Ageing Dev 1996;86:39–51.

[82] Edwards BJ, Morley JE. Amylin. Life Sci 1992;51:1899–912.

[83] Morley JE, Flood JF, Farr SA, et al. Effects of amylin on appetite regulation and memory. Can J Physiol Pharmacol 1995;73:1042–6.

[84] Diano S, Farr SA, Benoit SC, et al. Ghrelin controls hippocampal spine synapse density and memory performance. Nat Neurosci 2006;9:381–8.

[85] Flood JF, Morley JE. Cholecystokinin receptors mediate enhanced memory retention produced by feeding and gastrointestinal peptides. Peptides 1989;10:809–13.

[86] Flood JF, Morley JE. Effects of bombesin and gastrin-releasing peptide on memory processing. Brain Res 1988;460:314–22.

[87] Morley JE. Food for thought. Am J Clin Nutr 2001;74:567–8.

[88] Laugier R, Bernard JP, Berthezene P, et al. Changes in pancreatic exocrine secretion with age: pancreatic exocrine secretion does decrease in the elderly. Digestion 1991;50:202–11.

[89] Matsumoto S, Harada H, Tanaka J, et al. Aging and exocrine pancreatic function. Nippon Ronen Igakkai Zasshi 1989;26:146–52.

[90] Ishibashi T, Matsumoto S, Harada H, et al. Aging and exocrine pancreatic function evaluated by the recently standardized secretin test. Nippon Ronen Igakkai Zasshi 1991; 28:599–605.

[91] Detlefsen S, Sipos B, Feyerabend B, et al. Pancreatic fibrosis associated with age and ductal papillary hyperplasia. Virchows Arch 2005;447:800–5.

[92] Glaser J, Stienecker K. Pancreas and aging: a study using ultrasonography. Gerontology 2000;46:93–6.

[93] Schmucker DL. Liver function and phase I drug metabolism in the elderly: a paradox. Drugs Aging 2001;18:837–51.

[94] Wakabayashi H, Nishiyama Y, Ushiyama T, et al. Evaluation of the effect of age on functioning hepatocyte mass and liver blood flow using liver scintigraphy in preoperative estimations for surgical patients: comparison with CT volumetry. J Surg Res 2002;106: 246–53.

[95] Regev A, Schiff ER. Liver disease in the elderly. Gastroenterol Clin North Am 2001;30: 547–63.

[96] Leclercq I, Horsmans Y, De Bruyere M, et al. Influence of body mass index, sex and age on serum alanine aminotransferase (ALT) level in healthy blood donors. Acta Gastroenterol Belg 1999;62:16–20.

[97] Elinav E, Ben-Dov IZ, Ackerman E, et al. Correlation between serum alanine aminotransferase activity and age: an inverted U curve pattern. Am J Gastroenterol 2005;100:2201–4.

[98] Woodhouse K. Drugs and the liver. Part III: ageing of the liver and the metabolism of drugs. Biopharm Drug Dispos 1992;13:311–20.

[99] Ishizawa Y, Yasui-Furukori N, Takahata T, et al. The effect of aging on the relationship between the cytochrome P450 2C19 genotype and omeprazole pharmacokinetics. Clin Pharmacokinet 2005;44:1179–89.

[100] Zapletal CH, Faust D, Sullstein C, et al. Does the liver ever age? Results of liver transplantation with donors above 80 years of age. Transplant Proc 2005;37:1182–5.

[101] Bachar GN, Cohen M, Belenky A, et al. Effect of aging on the adult extrahepatic bile duct: a sonographic study. J Ultrasound Med 2003;22:879–82.

CLINICS IN
GERIATRIC
MEDICINE

ELSEVIER
SAUNDERS

Clin Geriatr Med 23 (2007) 769–784

Gastrointestinal Bleeding in Older Adults

Syed H. Tariq, MD, FACP[a],*, George Mekhjian, MD[b]

[a]Division of Geriatric Medicine, Department of internal medicine,
St. Louis University School of Medicine, Room M-238, 1402 South Grand,
St. Louis, MO 63104, USA
[b]Internal Medicine, St. Anthony's Hospital, 3550 College, Suite B, Alton, IL 62002, USA

Gastrointestinal bleeding could results from multiple lesions in the gastrointestinal tract. Bleeding could vary greatly in volume, such as massive or insignificant, and may be clinically apparent or hidden. Bleeding could manifest either from upper gastrointestinal tract or lower gastrointestinal alone or a combination of both. Bleeding could be apparent or occult. With occult bleeding, the patient is unaware of the bleeding and finding the cause could be challenging. Bleeding distal to the ligament of Treitz is termed lower gastrointestinal bleeding (LGIB).

Incidence and mortality

Gastrointestinal bleeding is a common geriatric problem [1,2]. In the United States, approximately 350,000 patients are hospitalized for upper gastrointestinal bleeding (UGIB) each year [3] and 355 to 45% are 60 years of age or older [4]. The annual incidence of UGIB ranges between 50 to 150 per 100,000 population per year [5], with women aged 60 years and older accounting for 60% [6]. The mortality of UGIB has remained approximately 6% to 10% for the past 6 decades [5,7–9]. No difference in morbidity and mortality has been reported between young and old adults [10,11].

The exact incidence of LGIB is not known, but the annual incidence of hospitalization is approximately 20 to 27 episodes per 100,000 persons per year [12,13]. A 200-fold increase of LGIB is seen with advancing age from the third to ninth decades [12]. Little information exists on racial difference in LGIB. Most patients who have LGIB have favorable outcomes despite advance age and other comorbid conditions [14,15].

* Corresponding author.
  E-mail address: tariqsh@slu.edu (S.H. Tariq).

0749-0690/07/$ - see front matter © 2007 Elsevier Inc. All rights reserved.
doi:10.1016/j.cger.2007.07.002   geriatric.theclinics.com

The mortality for LGIB is 4% to 10% or greater [16,17] and is more common when associated with severe bleeding and in those undergoing emergent surgery [13,18,19]. Hospitalized patients admitted for other causes who experience bleeding have significantly higher mortality than those admitted with LGIB (23% versus 2.4%). One study reported death in 19% of the population studied. The independent predictors of all cause mortality were increasing age, duration of hospital stay, and number of comorbid conditions [20]. Box 1 summarizes the factors predictive of mortality in older adults.

Economic impact

The economic burden of LGIB is not known but is presumably significant higher given the prevalence of this disorder in older adults. Thomas and colleagues [21,22] estimated that diverticular hemorrhage alone cost $1.3 billion in 2001. The average case cost for a patient who has LGIB in Canada was $4832 (SD = 7187) [23]. The estimated direct and indirect cost of peptic ulcer disease exceeds $9 billion a year [24].

Causes of gastrointestinal bleeding

In elderly individuals, esophagitis and gastritis in combination with peptic ulcer disease account for 70% to 91% of hospital admissions for UGIB. A greater percentage of Mallory-Weiss tears, gastrointestinal varices, and gastropathy are seen in the younger population.

Tables 1 and 2 [15,25–55] summarize the causes of UGIB and LGIB. The prevalence of UGIB varies by cause, with gastric ulcer accounting for 5% to 43%; duodenal ulcer, 6% to 42%; gastritis, 6% to 42%; esophagitis, 2% to 15%; esophageal varices, 1% to 20%, Mallory-Weiss tear, 1% to 16%; and other combinations of lesions, between 2% and 17%. The common causes of LGIB also vary, with diverticular bleeding accounting for 17% to 56%; angiodysplasia, 3% to 30%; hemorrhoids, 3% to 28%; and polyps, 2% to 30%.

Box 1. Clinical factors that predict mortality in older adults

Hemodynamic instability
Bleeding manifested as hematemesis or hematochezia
Failure of blood to clear with gastric lavage
Age older than 60 years
Coagulopathy
Presence of underlying serious medical condition
Hospitalization

Table 1
Causes of upper gastrointestinal bleeding by location

Author	GU	DU	E	G	D	EV	AVM	MW	GCA	ND	OTH
Palmer [47]	16	28	7	12	—	19	—	5	—	7	6
Crook, et al [46]	9	42	—	11	—	—	—	1	2	12	5
Allen, et al [45]	27	25	—	25	1	6	1	1	—	10	3
Sagawa, et al [44]	18	11	2	42	1	5	1	15	4	—	—
Cotton, et al [43]	27	21	7	9	1	3	1	1	2	14	—
Katon and Smith [42]	15	23	13	9	—	16	—	8	15	4	—
Paull, et al [41]	20	32[e]	—	20	5	6	—	6	4	—	17
Katz, et al [40][d,e,f]	5	23	0	22	0	17	—	—	—	22	11
	7	8	4	37	9	7	—	—	—	18	10
Lee and Dagradi [39]	43[d,e,f]	—	—	19	—	—	—	—	—	—	—
Katz, et al [38]	3	21[f]	—	36	—	16	—	—	—	14	13
Dagradi, et al [8]	31[d,e,f]	—	—	34	—	16	—	6	2	11	—
Antler, et al [1][g]	29	21	14	17	0	12	—	2	2	—	—
Peterson, et al [37]	18	22	—	6	—	20	—	16	2	12	—
Silverstein, et al [36]	22	23	13	30	9	15	0.5	8	4	—	7
Brolin and Stremple [35]	10	23	—	34	—	12	—	—	—	15	6
Bansal, et al [34]	25	25	—	22	—	1	—	—	9	3	14
Borch, et al [33]	—	—	—	11	—	—	—	—	—	—	—
Tabiban and Sutton [32][a]	24	19	15	5	—	25	—	6	0.4	5	2
	22	33	9	3	—	20	1	8	3	1	3
Vreeburg, et al [10]	12	20	7	5	—	9	1	5	3	22	7
Segal, et al [11][b]	35	38	11	7	—	11	—	3	1	—	—
Zimmerman, et al [21][c]	21	36	11	7	—	6	—	—	—	—	—
Wilcox and Clark [12]	26	24	4	7	—	9	—	6	—	4	10
Tariq, et al [19,26]	14	6	10	24	13	7	9	3	—	—	16

Abbreviations: AVM, angiodysplasia; D, duodenitis; DU, duodenal ulcer; E, esophagitis; EV, esophageal varices; G, Gastritis; GCA, gastric cancer; GU, gastric ulcer; MW, Mallory-Weiss tear; ND, no abnormality detected; OTH, others.
[a] First row includes patients in the county hospital and the second row includes patients in community hospital.
[b] Only patients ≥ 60 years reported.
[c] Both patient groups added (60–69 years and ≥80 years).
[d] Peptic ulcer.
[e] Pyloroduodenal ulcer.
[f] Chronic peptic ulcer.
[g] Only patients aged ≥55 years are included.

In up to 40% of patients who have LGIB, more than one potential bleeding source will be noted [56] and the stigmata of recent bleeding in LGIB are infrequently identified [57,58]. Therefore, no definitive source will be found in a large percentage of patients [59,60].

Clinical presentation

Determining accurate clinical presentation in older people may occasionally be difficult because of poor vision or cognition. Hematemesis, melena,

Table 2
Comparison of lower gastrointestinal bleeding by location

Author	D	CCA	AVM	H	IBD	P	C	CU	ND	O
Boley et al [15][a]	34	8	—	7	1	11	3	—	12	17
Boley et al [15][b]	43	5	20	—	1	4	2	—	11	14
Caos et al [56]	23	3	20	—	—	14	1	—	23	9
Leitman and Paul [18]	26	7	24	2	4	2	6	—	—	9
Jensen and Machicado [27]	17	11	30	—	—	2	9	—	6	14
Makela et al [38]	19	10	6	28	8	11	4	—	27	13
Richter et al [16]	47	10	12	3	3	—	3	—	14	2
Peura et al [29]	30	8	10	—	8	9	6	—	—	28
Longstreth [20]	42	9	3	5	2	4	14	—	12	10
Wilcox and Clark [12]	56	7	5	3	2	2	2	10	4	5
Tariq et al [25,26][c]	29	4	6	25	—	30	4	2	—	—

Abbreviations: AVM, angiodysplasia; C, colitis; CCA, colon carcinoma; CU, colonic ulcers; D, diverticulosis; H, hemorrhoids; IBD, inflammatory bowel disease, ND, no diagnosis; O, others; P, polyp.
[a] Minor bleeding.
[b] Major bleeding.
[c] Percentages of all patients.

and hematochezia are the most common manifestations of gastrointestinal bleeding [61,62]. Hematemesis is defined as vomiting of blood and is caused by UGIB from the esophagus, stomach, or proximal small bowel. Blood may be bright red or may be old and have a similar appearance to coffee grounds. Melena is defined as passage of black, tarry, and foul-smelling stools. The black, tarry character of melena is caused by the degradation of blood in the more proximal colon. Hematochezia refers to bright red blood from the rectum that may or may not be mixed with the stool. Occult gastrointestinal bleeding denotes bleeding that is not apparent to the patient because of its small amount. However, patient and physician reports of stool color are often inaccurate and inconsistent [63]. In addition to causing bright red bleeding, significantly proximal lesions can be found on colonoscopy [64]. The manifestation of gastrointestinal bleeding varies with underlying medical problems; for example, a patient who has underlying ischemic heart disease may present with chest pain after brisk bleeding. Severe gastrointestinal bleeding may exacerbate coexisting heart failure, hypertension, renal disease, diabetes, and pulmonary disease. Some patients who experience chronic blood loss may present with signs of anemia (weakness, pallor, dizziness, fatigue) or cirrhosis and portal hypotension. Gastrointestinal bleeding can also cause hepatic encephalopathy in patients who have existing liver disease or who develop hepatorenal syndrome.

Clinical course

The hospital course of gastrointestinal bleeding is similar in young and older adults with respect to endoscopic therapy for bleeding and rebleeding, need for admission to intensive care, blood transfusion requirements, need for surgery, and length of hospital stay [1,10]. The length of hospital stay shortened from 1970 to 1980 and into the 1990s. In 1992 and 1994, the mean hospital stay for UGIB in older adults (age >60 years) was 6 days compared with 5.6 days in those younger than 60 years. Table 2 describes factors that predict ulcer rebleeding and mortality in older adults. The need for surgery is higher for adherent clots, nonbleeding vessels, and arterial bleeding compared with clean base and flat spot. Mortality rates are also higher for arterial bleeding than for clean base bleeding [6,65,66].

Evaluation and management of gastrointestinal bleeding

Initial evaluation and clinical outcomes

The first step in the management is to assess the severity of bleeding. Orthostatic changes usually suggest 10% to 20% loss in circulatory volume; although supine hypotension suggests greater than 20% volume loss. Hypotension with a systolic blood pressure less than 100 mm Hg or baseline tachycardia suggests significant hemodynamic compromise that requires urgent volume resuscitation. Bleeding could also be classified in three categories depending on percent of blood loss. In massive gastrointestinal bleeding, the loss of blood is approximately 20% to 25%, moderate is 10% to 20%, and minor is less than 10% blood loss. All patients require a complete history and physical examination, including platelet counts, prothrombin time, partial thromboplastin time, liver function tests, renal functions, and complete blood counts. Determination of blood group typing and crossing 2 to 4 units of blood should be performed urgently.

Strate and Syngal [67] identified seven independent predictors of severity in acute LGIB. These factors include hypotension, tachycardia, syncope, nontender abdominal examination, bleeding within 4 hours of presentation, aspirin use, and more than two morbid diseases. These predictors can help classify patient into three risk groups. Patients who have more than three risk factors have an 84% risk for severe bleeding, those who had one to three risk factors had a 43% risk, and those who had no risk factors had a 9% risk [68]. Velayos and colleagues [69] prospectively studied patients admitted with LGIB and identified three predictors of severity and adverse outcome (initial hematocrit less than 35%, abnormal vital signs, and gross blood on rectal examination). These predictive tools will help guide the initial triage of patients who have LGIB and provide a more standardized and cost-effective approach to this disorder.

Excluding upper gastrointestinal bleeding

Excluding UGIB is important because 2% to 15% of patients who have presumed LGIB have UGIB. Nasogastric lavage is a quick and safe procedure, but to avoid unnecessary patient discomfort, it should be reserved for patients who have evidence of brisk bleeding in whom an upper endoscopy is not anticipated. Nasogastric lavage containing gross blood, 25% blood-tinged fluid, or strongly guaiac-positive dark fluid was found to have 80% sensitivity for detecting bleeding above the ligament of Treitz, and positive and negative predictive values of 93% and 99%, respectively [70]. The presence of bile increases the sensitivity of nasogastric lavage [27], although the correlation between the presence of a bilious aspirate verses the presence of bile acids has been questioned [71]. The blood urea nitrogen to creatinine ratio is a noninvasive test also used to help distinguish upper versus colonic sources of bleeding. In one study, a ratio of 33 or higher had a sensitivity of 96% for UGIB, although overlap was observed with LGIB, especially in patients who had UGIB without hematemesis [72]. Esophagogastroduodenoscopy (EGD) remains the gold standard for excluding an upper gastrointestinal source in patients presenting with severe bleeding, especially those who have hemodynamic instability.

Restoration of intravascular volume is established by inserting two large-bore intravenous peripheral lines with an 18-gauge catheter or a central venous line. Fluids used for resuscitation include normal saline, lactated Ringer's solution, or 5% hetastarch and blood transfusion as soon as it is available to improve the oxygen-carrying capacity. Patients who are in shock may require volume administration using infusion devices or vasopressors if clinically indicated.

Correction of coagulopathy is absolutely necessary. Parental vitamin K may be used to prolong prothrombin time. Platelets may be transfused if clinically indicated. The airway may need to be protected in patients who have decreased in mental status (shock, encephalopathy), massive hematemesis, or active variceal hemorrhage.

History

A detailed history could point toward a possible diagnosis. Pain in the epigastric region relieved with food or antacid suggests peptic ulcer disease. Weight loss and anorexia may suggest gastrointestinal malignancy, but in the geriatric population the most common cause of weight loss is depression. Dysphagia can be caused by stricture or cancer of the esophagus. Patients who have inflammatory bowel disease or infectious colitis usually present with bloody diarrhea, fever, and abdominal pain. Occult blood or hematochezia could be the first sign of colon cancer or polyps. Painless lower gastrointestinal bleeding can also be seen in diverticulosis, angiodysplasia, or ulcerated cancerous lesion. Blood on the surface of stool or on toilet paper suggests internal hemorrhoids. Determining patient cognitive ability with the Mini-mental status examination [73] or Saint Louis University Mental Status examination [74] is equally important. If a patient is demented, then obtaining the history from the caregiver accompanying the patient or the nursing home staff is advisable.

Drug history is important, especially the use of aspirin, nonsteroidal anti-inflammatory drugs (NSAIDs), and anticoagulation drugs. The medical history may also help to elucidate a specific bleeding source. Key points include antecedent constipation or diarrhea (hemorrhoids, colitis), the presence of diverticulosis (diverticular bleeding), receipt of radiation therapy (radiation enteritis), recent polypectomy (postpolypectomy bleeding), and vascular disease/hypotension (ischemic colitis).

Physical examination

A detailed physical examination starting with inspection of the nose and throat is important to exclude bleeding in this area. Physicians should look for signs of chronic liver failure (eg, spider angiomas, hepatosplenomegaly, ascites, jaundice) and arteriovenous malformation, especially of the mucous membranes, which may be associated with hereditary hemorrhagic telangiectasia (Rendu-Osler-Weber syndrome), in which multiple angiomas of the gastrointestinal tract are associated with recurrent bleeding. Cutaneous nail bed and gastrointestinal telangiectasia may be associated with connective tissue disease or scleroderma. A digital rectal examination is important to feel for masses and fissures and to obtain a sample of stool, to be tested chemically. Physicians must also comment on the color of stools.

Presence of selected physical findings, including respiratory failure (57%), jaundice (42%), mental confusion (31.2%), shock (30%), congestive heart failure (28%), and postural blood pressure change (14%), are related to increased mortality in patients who have gastrointestinal bleeding. Similarly, the presence of certain diseases process, including renal 29.4%, liver 24.6%, neoplasm 24.3%, central nervous system 23.5%, and lung 22.6%, are responsible for increased mortality; [6]. The presence of abdominal tenderness on examination may indicate an ischemic colitis or inflammatory bowel disease, in contrast with bleeding diverticula or angiodysplasia [75]. Rectal examination helps identify anorectal lesions and confirm stool color. However, positive findings on rectal examination do not preclude a concomitant abnormal finding on colonoscopy [76]. Despite presenting features and findings on physical examination, most patients who have LGIB require a full examination of the colon.

EGD can be performed at the bedside or in the gastrointestinal suites and is the preferred method of investigation and therapy for UGIB. It has the highest diagnostic accuracy and therapeutic capacity, and low morbidity. It can be performed early in the clinical course, after the patient is hemodynamically stabilized. Box 2 summarizes the endoscopic risks factors for bleeding. Barium radiographs have no role in acute UGIB. Endoscopy has a sensitivity of 92% for identifying the site of UGIB, compared with 54% for barium radiography, and a specificity approaching 100%. Retained blood and clots in the stomach may limit the sensitivity of endoscopy. In this situation, vigorous gastric lavage using a large-bore orogastric tube is

---

Box 2. Endoscopic risk factors for rebleeding

Clean base (5%)
Flat spot (10%)
Adherent clot (22%)
Nonbleeding vessel (43%)
Arterial bleeding (55%)

---

critical before the procedure. Endoscopy has the added advantage of guiding biopsies to test for *Helicobacter pylori* infection and to diagnose malignancy. Barium radiography is contraindicated in acute UGIB because it interferes with subsequent endoscopy, angiography, or surgery.

In patients who have nonvariceal UGIB who have persistent or recurrent bleeding determined through nasogastric lavage or endoscopy, endoscopic therapy reduces both morbidity and mortality. The major methods may be divided into thermal coagulation, injection therapy, and mechanical compression. The most common thermal methods use electrical current (multipolar or bipolar electrode) or direct application of a heated device (heater probe) to seal the vessel with thermal energy. Using these methods, hemostasis can be achieved in 90% of patients who have active bleeding, and rebleeding rates are significantly reduced by more than 50%.

The least expensive method of endoscopic therapy for UGIB is to inject the bleeding site with saline or diluted epinephrine. This approach yields initial results that are generally similar to those of thermal therapy but may not be as effective for long-term hemostasis. Thermal therapy and injection can be combined to control bleeding and treat the lesion definitively. Mechanical methods to treat bleeding include hemostatic clips and the use of rubber band ligation. Both methods seem to have an efficacy similar to thermal therapy. In the few patients who have recurrent bleeding after initial endoscopic therapy, a second attempt has a significant success rate and can reduce the need for surgery.

Medical therapy

The most common causes of peptic ulcer disease are *H pylori* infection and NSAID use. NSAIDs should be discontinued and *H pylori* infection should be treated in all patients who have bleeding ulcers. Data are now compelling that profound acid suppression reduces rebleeding in patients who have high-risk endoscopic stigmata for rebleeding. Studies using high doses of intravenous and oral omeprazole have shown a significant improvement in outcome (eg, rebleeding, hospital stay, transfusion requirement) compared with histamine$_2$ (H$_2$) receptor antagonists. This effect is likely caused by improved coagulation and platelet aggregation through increased intragastric pH. Vigorous acid suppression should be provided to all patients who have acute UGIB.

Nonulcer acute upper gastrointestinal bleeding

Variceal bleeding is the most common cause of nonulcer UGIB. The approach to variceal bleeding is a combination of pharmacologic (octreotide, somatostatin), endoscopic (band ligation, sclerotherapy), and mechanical (balloon tamponade) approaches.

Most nonpeptic ulcer, nonvariceal causes of UGIB can be treated using the same endoscopic modalities described earlier with similar success. The most common causes is a tear at the gastroesophageal junction, called a Mallory-Weiss tear. Mallory-Weiss bleeding usually stops spontaneously, but persistent bleeding should be treated in a manner similar to bleeding from peptic ulcers. Dieulafoy's lesion, which is an aberrant submucosal artery that erodes into the lumen of the stomach, is a rare cause of recurrent vigorous UGIB. Tumors also are rare (<1%) causes of acute UGIB. Vascular lesions may rarely present as acute bleeding, but more commonly cause chronic, low-grade blood loss. Diffuse bleeding from gastric erosions, which can occur in critically ill patients, does not respond to endoscopic therapy but can usually be prevented with prophylactic treatment.

Colonoscopy is performed if lower gastrointestinal bleeding is suspected as a cause of bleeding. Recent studies have shown that colonoscopy, particularly when performed early (within 12–24 hours of admission), is safe and effective [27,57,77,78]. Colonoscopy is undoubtedly the best test for confirming the source of LGIB. The diagnostic yield of colonoscopy ranges from 45% to 95% [57,58].

Early performance of colonoscopy has been shown to reduce length of hospital stay independent of other factors, such as severity of bleeding and comorbid illness, and therefore should decrease treatment costs. Emergency colonoscopy is considered within 12 to 24 hours of admission [57,77,79]. Evidence suggests, although not overwhelmingly, that earlier performance leads to more diagnostic and therapeutic opportunities [79] and reduces length of stay [16,79]. However, urgent colonoscopy is difficult to orchestrate and logistical factors, such as time of admission, seem to play a significant role in determining whether patients will undergo endoscopic or radiographic intervention [67]. Colonoscopy is best performed in patients whose condition has clinically stabilized and who can tolerate adequate bowel purge. For good results, patients should be able to drink adequate bowel preparation. Many patients find polyethylene glycol (PEG)-based preparations difficult to take because of the large volume of fluid they are required to consume. In a randomized prospective trail comparing sodium phosphate and PEG, Thomson and colleagues [65] randomized 116 predominantly elderly patients to receive either sodium phosphate (n = 61) or PEG (n = 55) bowel preparations before colonoscopy. The sodium phosphate preparation was found to be slightly more tolerable than PEG. No significant side effects were experienced among all patients. However, 91% of patients who had previously taken PEG found sodium phosphate easier to take. The colonoscopists found no difference in the overall quality of the bowel preparation. Sodium phosphate was a safe and effective bowel preparation for colonoscopy in this carefully selected group of patients, and was preferred by patients who had previously taken PEG. In another clinical trial involving 124 consecutive patients aged 75 years or older scheduled for colonoscopy, Lashner and colleagues [66] randomized 63 patients to take GoLYTELY (17 inpatient, 33 outpatient, and 13 cancelled colonoscopies) and 61 to take the enema preparation (17 inpatient, 30 outpatient, and 14 cancelled colonoscopies). Although both preparations were adequate, the enema preparation was superior in outpatients, whereas GoLYTELY was superior in inpatients. Both outpatients and inpatients tolerated the enema preparation better. Contrary to previous reports of a significant advantage with GoLYTELY, patients aged 75 years or older did not experience this advantage and seemed to tolerate enemas better than GoLYTELY with little difference in adequacy of the preparation.

However, complication rates for colonoscopy in LGIB are low, and bowel preparation itself seems to be safe. A review of 13 studies found an overall complication rate of 1.3% [61]. The most commonly reported complications are fluid overload and bowel perforation.

Radionuclide scintigraphy

When colonoscopy is negative and LGIB is suspected, a radionuclide scintigraphy is considered. Two methods are used, one that uses technetium-99m (Tc-99m) sulfur colloid and the other using Tc-99m–labeled red blood cells (tagged red blood cell scan). Radiolabeled red blood cells have a longer half-life, and therefore repeat scans can be performed for recurrent bleeding after a single injection. In addition, red cell scans may localize bleeding anywhere outside the splenic area. Sulfur collide is simple to prepare and is rapidly cleared from the circulation, although bleeding detection rates are not different.

Bleeding rates as low as 0.05 to 0.1 mL/min can be detected [62]. When the test is positive, it is accurate in approximately 80% of cases. Approximately 20% of the localization is false-positive, which precludes the use of this test alone for surgical resection of the bowel. Radionuclide scintigraphy is used for two purposes: to localize the bleeding site before surgical resection and as a screening test before angiography.

Arteriography allows localization and potential therapy for gastrointestinal bleeding when the bleeding rate exceeds 0.5 mL/min [81]. It can determine the cause of bleeding, such as diverticula or angiodysplasia. Complications occur in 0% to 10% of patients undergoing angiography, although adverse events are inconsistently reported in the literature. The most common complications seem to be hematoma or bleeding at the catheter site [82,83], and other adverse events include arterial dissection, catheter site infection, loss of pedal pulses, and contrast reaction [80,84]. Myocardial and intestinal ischemia, renal failure, and cardiac arrhythmias have been reported with the use of vasopressin infusion [18,80,84]. Localized bowel ischemia and infarction are concerns with therapeutic embolization [18,84]. Technologic advances in coaxial catheter techniques, embolization materials, and nonionic contrast agents promise to reduce complication rates in diagnostic and therapeutic angiography.

Barium enema cannot detect superficial lesions or confirm a definitive bleeding source and may miss important pathology [79,85]. In one study, 46% of patients undergoing barium enema were found to have significant lesions at colonoscopy, including 20 malignancies. Furthermore, barium contrast may complicate subsequent colonoscopy or angiography.

Small bowel evaluation is indicated when upper and lower endoscopies fail to identify a source of bleeding. Capsule endoscopy is the newest technology for evaluating the gastrointestinal tract and has a clear role in identifying small intestinal or obscure gastrointestinal bleeding. The diagnostic yield in patients who have overt bleeding and negative upper and lower endoscopies ranges from 40% to 90% [86,87]. Capsule endoscopy has proven superior to other modalities used for detecting obscure gastrointestinal bleeding. The diagnostic yield of capsule endoscopy ranges from 55% to 70% versus 25% to 30% for push endoscopy [88,89]. Costamagna and colleagues [90] found that a source of obscure bleeding was found in 31% of patients who underwent capsule endoscopy, and in only 5% of those who underwent barium small bowel radiographs. Colonic sources of bleeding are difficult to evaluate through capsule endoscopy because of retained stool, limited battery life, and poor field of vision because of the colon's large diameter. Technologic advancements in capsule endoscopy are likely to improve diagnostic accuracy and may facilitate procedural interventions.

Small-bowel enteroscopes are used when radiologic evaluation suggests a jejunal bleeding source or for recurrent (obscure) gastrointestinal bleeding when conventional endoscopy is unrevealing.

Surgery is considered when blood transfusion requirement exceeds 4 to 6 units over 24-hours or 10 units overall, and when more than two to three recurrent bleeding episodes occur from the same course. Performing EGD before emergent total colectomy is prudent. The extent of comorbid conditions and the degree of bleeding must be factored in when considering surgery. Some procedure are discussed briefly, but details are provided by gastroenterology textbooks or journals.

Transjugular intrahepatic portosystemic shunts (TIPS) have been used in the treatment of complications of portal hypertension. TIPS is used to control acute variceal bleeding and prevent variceal rebleeding when pharmacologic and endoscopic therapy have failed. TIPS is also helpful in patients who have refractory ascites with adequate hepatic reserve and renal function who do not experience response to a large-volume paracentesis. Other indications for TIPS are Budd-Chiari syndrome uncontrolled with medical therapy, severe portal hypertensive gastropathy, refractory hepatic hydrothorax, and hepatorenal syndrome. The major limiting factors for TIPS success are shunt dysfunction and hepatic encephalopathy. Shunt stenosis is the most important cause of recurrent complications of portal hypertension; therefore, a surveillance program to monitor shunt patency is mandatory.

Shunt surgery (portacaval or distal splenorenal shunt) should be considered in patients who have good hepatic reserve if they fail to experience response to endoscopic or pharmacologic therapy, have difficulty returning for follow-up visits, have increased risk for death from recurrent bleeding, or live away from medical care. The morbidity and mortality are high with this procedure, as is the risk for postoperative encephalopathy.

Balloon tamponade has an important role in the therapy of variceal hemorrhage. It is used temporarily to stabilize patients when more definite therapy is available. The most commonly used balloon tamponades are the Sengstaken-Blakemore tube and the Minnesota tubes, which have a gastric and esophageal balloon.

Stress ulcer is encountered in patients who are in the intensive care unit and on ventilation for more than 48 hours with coagulopathy, sepsis, burns, and cerebrovascular events. Prophylactic therapy should be administered in patients who are at increased risk. H_2 receptor antagonist, sucralfate, and proton pump inhibitors can be used.

Diverticulosis is usually seen on endoscopy, but bleeding develops in approximately 5% of patients who have diverticula. Bleeding usually stops in these patients 80% of the time but may reoccur. Persistent bleeding may require intra-arterial vasopressin at angiography or even surgical resection.

Aortoenteric fistula is an uncommon but lethal cause of gastrointestinal bleeding. Patients who have aortoenteric fistula usually have a history of aortic graft surgery and present with bleeding after surgery. The fistula site is usually aortoduodenal but can be anywhere in the small and large intestine. The classic presentation is precursor bleed hours to weeks before massive gastrointestinal bleeding. Recognizing this condition is essential, because undiagnosed cases could be fatal. Endoscopy with examination of the fourth portion of the duodenum is essential and should be performed immediately. Angiography or CT scanning may show leak at the graft site. A negative study does not exclude an aortoenteric fistula; if suspicion is high, a surgical consultation is absolutely necessary.

Radiation proctitis/colitis results years after exposure to radiation therapy. Intermittent hematochezia results from aberrant superficial mucosal vasculature in the distal colon. Treatment is usually supportive and laser photocoagulation of the mucosal telangiectasias.

Hemorrhoids are the most common cause of outpatient causes of hematochezia. Treatment is usually avoiding constipation through a fiber-rich

diet and supportive care. Surgical and endoscopic banding of the hemorrhoids is also available.

Summary

Gastrointestinal bleeding is a common geriatric problem. The incidence
of gastrointestinal bleeding is approximately 35% to 45% in people aged
60 years and older. The incidence of LGIB is unknown. The causes of gastrointestinal bleeding in elderly individuals vary in different studies, and its
diagnosis and management is similar to young adults in several ways.

References

[1] Antler AS, Pitchumoni CS, Thomas E, et al. Gastrointestinal bleeding in the elderly, morbidity, mortality and causes. Am J Surg 1981;142:271–3.
[2] Allen R, Dykes P. A study of the factors influencing mortality rates from gastrointestinal
hemorrhage. Q J Med 1976;45:533–50.
[3] Papp JP. Management of upper gastrointestinal bleeding. Clin Geriatr Med 1991;7:255–64.
[4] Reinus JF, Brandt LJ. Upper and lower gastrointestinal bleeding in the elderly. Gastroenterol Clin North Am 1990;19:293–318.
[5] Gilbert DA. Epidemiology of upper gastrointestinal bleeding. Gastrointest Endosc 1990;36:
S8–13.
[6] Silverstein FE, Gilbert DA, Tedesco FJ. The national ASGE Survey of upper gastrointestinal bleeding: II. Clinical prognostic factors. Gastrointest Endosc 1981;27:80–93.
[7] Warren JR, Marshall JB. Unidentified curved bacilli on gastric epithelium in active chronic
gastritis. Lancet 1983;1:1273–5.
[8] Dagradi AE, Ruiz RA, Weingarten ZG. Influence of emergency endoscopy on the management and outcomes of patients with upper gastrointestinal hemorrhage. Am J Gastroenterol
1979;72:403–15.
[9] Velanovich V. The spectrum of helicobacter pylori in upper gastrointestinal diseases. Am
Surg 1996;62:60–3.
[10] Vreeburg EM, Snel P, De Bruijne JD, et al. Acute upper gastrointestinal bleeding in the Am-
sterdam area: incidence, diagnosis, and clinical outcome. Am J Gastroenterol 1997;92(2):
236–42.
[11] Segal WN, Cello JP. Hemorrhage in the upper gastrointestinal tract in the older patient. Am
J Gastroenterol 1997;92(1):42–6.
[12] Wilcox CM, Clark WS. Causes of upper and lower gastrointestinal bleeding. The Grady hospital experience. South Med J 1999;92(1):44–50.
[13] Browder W, Cerise EJ, Litwin MS. Impact of emergency angiography in massive lower gastrointestinal hemorrhage. Ann Surg 1986;204:530–6.
[14] Bokhari M, Vernava AM, Ure T, et al. Diverticular hemorrhage in the elderly—is it well
tolerated? Dis Colon Rectum 1996;39:191–5.
[15] Boley SJ, DiBiase A, Brandt LJ, et al. Lower intestinal bleeding in the elderly. Am J Surg
1979;137:57–64.
[16] Richter JM, Christensen MR, Kaplan LM, et al. Effectiveness of current technology in the
diagnosis and management of lower gastrointestinal hemorrhage. Gastrointest Endosc 1995;
41:93–8.
[17] Schiller KF, Truelove SC, Williams DG. Hematemesis and melena, with special reference to
factors influencing the outcome. BMJ 1970;2:7–14.
[18] Leitman IM, Paul DE. Shires111 GT. Evaluation and management of massive lower gastrointestinal hemorrhage. Am Surg 1989;209(2):175–80.

[19] Levy R, Barto W, Gani J. Retrospective study of the utility of nuclear scintigraphic-labelled red cell scanning for lower gastrointestinal bleeding. ANZ J Surg 2003;73:205–9.

[20] Longstreth GF. Epidemiology and out come of patients hospitalized with acute lower gastrointestinal hemorrhage: a population based study. Am J Gastroenterol 1997;92(3):419–24.

[21] Thomas S, Wong R, Das A. Economic burden of acute diverticular hemorrhage in the U.S.: a nationwide estimate [abstract W1290]. Presented at the 105th Annual Meeting of the American Gastroenterological Association. New Orleans, May 15–20, 2004.

[22] Zimmerman J, Shohat V, Tsvang E, et al. Esophagitis is a major cause of upper gastrointestinal hemorrhage in the elderly. Scand J Gastroenterol 1997;32:906–9.

[23] Comay D, Marshall JK. Resource utilization for acute lower gastrointestinal hemorrhage: the Ontario GI Bleed study. Can J Gastroenterol 2002;16:677–82.

[24] Del Valle J. Acid peptic disorders. In: Yamada T, Alpers DH, editors. Textbook of gastroenterology. Philadelphia: Lippincott Williams & Wilkins; 2003. p. 1322–76.

[25] Tariq SH, Zia N, Khan Y, et al. Causes of gastrointestinal bleeding in older persons. J Invest Med 1999;47:254A.

[26] Tariq SH, Zia N, Omran ML, et al. Gastritis is the most common cause of gastrointestinal bleeding in older persons. J Am Geriatr Soc 2000;48:S53.

[27] Jensen DM, Machicado GA. Diagnosis and treatment of severe hematochezia. The role of urgent colonoscopy after purge. Gastroenterology 1988;95:1569–74.

[28] Makela JT, Kiviniemi H, Laitinen S, et al. Diagnosis and treatment of acute lower gastrointestinal bleeding. Scand J Gastroenterol 1993;28:1062–6.

[29] Peura DA, Lanza FL, Gostout CJ, et al. The American College of Gastroenterology Bleeding Registry: preliminary findings. Am J Gastroenterology 1997;6:924–8.

[30] Zimmerman J, Shohat V, Tsvang E, et al. Esophagitis is a major cause of upper gastrointestinal hemorrhage in the elderly. Scand J Gastroenterol 1997;32:906–9.

[31] Segal WN, Cello JP. Hemorrhage in the upper gastrointestinal tract in the older patient. Am J Gastroenterol 1997;92(1):42–6.

[32] Tabibian N, Sutton FM. Gastritis: a common source of acute bleeding in the upper gastrointestinal tract? South Med J 1990;83(4):769–70.

[33] Borch K, Jansson L, Sjodahal R, et al. Haemorrhagic gastritis. Incidence, etiological factors, and prognosis. Acta Chir Scand 1988;154(3):211–4.

[34] Bansal SK, Gautam PC, Sahi SP, et al. Upper gastrointestinal haemorrhage in the elderly: a record of 92 patients in a joint geriatric/surgical unit. Age Ageing 1987;16:279–84.

[35] Brolin RE, Stremple JF. Emergency operation for upper gastrointestinal hemorrhage. Am Surg 1982;7:302–8.

[36] Silverstein FE, Gilbert DA, Tedesco FJ, et al. The national ASGE survey on upper gastrointestinal bleeding. I. Study design and baseline data. Gastrointest Endosc 1981;27(2):73–9.

[37] Peterson WL, Barnett CC, Smith HJ, et al. Routine early endoscopy in upper gastrointestinal-tract bleeding a randomized control trial. N Engl J Med 1981;304(16):925–9.

[38] Katz D, Pitchumoni CS, Thomas E, et al. The endoscopic diagnosis of upper gastrointestinal hemorrhage changing concepts of etiology and management. Am J Dig Dis 1976;21:2182–9.

[39] Lee ER, Dagradi AE. Hemorrhagic erosive gastritis: a clinical study. Am J Gastroenterol 1975;63(3):202–8.

[40] Katz D, Pitchumoni CS, Thomas E, et al. Endoscopy in the upper gastrointestinal bleeding then and now changing concepts of bleeding sources. Gastrointest Endosc 1975;21(3):109–11.

[41] Paull A, Van Deth AG, Grant K. Combined endoscopy in upper gastrointestinal haemorrhage. Aust N Z J Med 1974;4:12–5.

[42] Katon RM, Smith FW. Panendoscopy in the early diagnosis of acute upper gastrointestinal bleeding. Gastroenterology 1973;65(5):728–34.

[43] Cotton PB, Rosenberg MT, Axon AT, et al. Early endoscopy of oesophagus, stomach, and duodenal bulb in patients with haematemesis and melaena. Br Med J 1973;2(5865):505–9.

[44] Sagawa C, Werner MH, Hayes DF, et al. Early endoscopy a guide to therapy for acute hemorrhage in the upper gastrointestinal tract. Arch Surg 1973;107:133–7.

[45] Allen HM, Block MA, Schuman BM. Gastroduodenal endoscopy management of acute upper gastrointestinal hemorrhage. Arch Surg 1973;106:450–5.

[46] Crook JN, Gray LW, Nance FC, et al. Upper gastrointestinal bleeding. Ann Surg 1972; 175(5):771–9.

[47] Palmer ED. The vigorous diagnostic approach to upper gastrointestinal tract hemorrhage. A 23-year prospective study of 1400 patients. JAMA 1969;207(8):1477–80.

[48] Fleiss JL. Statistical methods for rates and proportions. New York: John Wiley and sons; 1973. p. 146–7.

[49] Dooley CP, Cohn H, Fitzgibbons PL, et al. Prevalence of Helicobacter pylori infection and histologic gastritis in asymptomatic persons. N Engl J Med 1989;321(23):1562–6.

[50] Al-Assi MT, Genta RM, Karttunen TJ, et al. Ulcer site and complications in relation to Helicobacter Pylori infection and NSAID use. Endoscopy 1996;28:229–33.

[51] Kalogeropoulos NK, Whitehead R. Campylobacter-like organisms and candida in peptic ulcer and similar lesions of the upper gastrointestinal tract: a study of 247 cases. J Clin Pathol 1988;41:1093–8.

[52] Niemela S, Karttunen T, Lehtola J. Campylobacter like organism in patients with gastric ulcer. Scand J Gastroenterol 1987;22:487–90.

[53] Graham DY, Hepps KS, Ramirez FC, et al. Treatment of helicobacter pylori reduces the rate of rebleeding in peptic ulcer disease. Scand J Gastroenterol 1993;28:939–42.

[54] Bramley PM, Masson JW, McKnight G. The role of an open access-bleeding unit in the management of colonic hemorrhage: a 2-year prospective study. Scand J Gastroenterol 1996;31: 764–9.

[55] Yovarski RT, Wong RKH, Madonovitch C. Analysis of 3,294 cases of upper gastrointestinal bleeding in military medical facilities. Am J Gastroenterol 1995;90(4):568–73.

[56] Caos A, Benner KG, Manier J, et al. Colonoscopy after Golytely preparation in acute rectal bleeding. J Clin Gastroenterol 1986;8(1):46–9.

[57] Jensen DM, Machicado GA, Jutabha R, et al. Urgent colonoscopy for the diagnosis and treatment of severe diverticular hemorrhage. N Engl J Med 2000;342:78–82.

[58] Bloomfeld RS, Rockey DC, Shetzline MA. Endoscopic therapy of acute diverticular hemorrhage. Am J Gastroenterol 2001;96:2367–72.

[59] Al Qahtani AR, Satin R, Stern J, et al. Investigative modalities for massive lower gastrointestinal bleeding. World J Surg 2002;26:620–5.

[60] Zuckerman GR, Prakash C. Acute lower intestinal bleeding. Part II: etiology, therapy, and outcomes. Gastrointest Endosc 1999;49:228–38.

[61] Zuckerman GR, Prakash C. Acute lower intestinal bleeding: part I: clinical presentation and diagnosis. Gastrointest Endosc 1998;48:606–17.

[62] Alavi A, Dann RW, Baum S, et al. Scintigraphic detection of acute gastrointestinal bleeding. Radiology 1977;124:753–6.

[63] Zuckerman GR, Trellis DR, Sherman TM, et al. An objective measure of stool color for differentiating upper from lower gastrointestinal bleeding. Dig Dis Sci 1995;40: 1614–21.

[64] Fine KD, Nelson AC, Ellington RT, et al. Comparison of the color of fecal blood with the anatomical location of gastrointestinal bleeding lesions: potential misdiagnosis using only flexible sigmoidoscopy for bright red blood per rectum. Am J Gastroenterol 1999;94:3202–10.

[65] Thomson A, Naidoo P, Crotty B. Bowel preparation for colonoscopy: a randomized prospective trail comparing sodium phosphate and polyethylene glycol in a predominantly elderly population. J Gastroenterol Hepatol 1996;11(2):103–7.

[66] Lashner BA, Winans CS, Blackstone MO. Randomized clinical trial of two colonoscopy preparation methods for elderly patients. J Clin Gastroenterol 1990;12(4):405–8.

[67] Strate LL, Syngal S. Predictors of utilization of early colonoscopy vs. radiography for severe lower intestinal bleeding. Gastrointest Endosc 2005;61:46–52.

[68] Strate L, Saltzman J, Ookubo R, et al. Validation of a clinical prediction rule for severe acute lower intestinal bleeding. Am J Gastroenterol 2005;100:1821–7.

[69] Velayos FS, Williamson A, Sousa KH, et al. Early predictors of severe lower gastrointestinal bleeding and adverse outcomes: a prospective study. Clin Gastroenterol Hepatol 2004;2: 485–90.

[70] Luk GD, Bynum TE, Hendrix TR. Gastric aspiration in localization of gastrointestinal hemorrhage. JAMA 1979;241:576–8.

[71] Cuellar RE, Gavaler JS, Alexander JA, et al. Gastrointestinal tract hemorrhage. The value of a nasogastric aspirate. Arch Intern Med 1990;150:1381–4.

[72] Chalasani N, Clark WS, Wilcox CM. Blood urea nitrogen to creatinine concentration in gastrointestinal bleeding: a reappraisal. Am J Gastroenterol 1997;92:1796–9.

[73] Folstein MF, Folstein SE, McHugh PR. "Mini-mental state." A practical method for grading the cognitive state of patients for the clinician. J Psychiatr Res 1975;12:189–98.

[74] Tariq SH, Tumosa N, Chibnall JT, et al. The Saint Louis University mental status examination and the mini-mental status examination for detecting dementia and mild neurocognitive disorder—a pilot study. Am J Geriatr Psychiatry 2006;14(11):900–10.

[75] Strate LL, Orav EJ, Syngal S. Early predictors of severity in acute lower intestinal tract bleeding. Arch Intern Med 2003;163:838–43.

[76] Graham DJ, Pritchard TJ, Bloom AD. Colonoscopy for intermittent rectal bleeding: impact on patient management. J Surg Res 1993;54:136–9.

[77] Chaudhry V, Hyser MJ, Gracias VH, et al. Colonoscopy: the initial test for acute lower gastrointestinal bleeding. Am Surg 1998;64:723–8.

[78] Strate LL, Syngal S. Timing of colonoscopy: impact on length of hospital stay in patients with acute lower intestinal bleeding. Am J Gastroenterol 2003;98:317–22.

[79] Colacchio TA, Forde KA, Patsos TJ, et al. Impact of modern diagnostic methods on the management of active rectal bleeding. Ten-year experience. Am J Surg 1982;143:607–10.

[80] Jensen DM, Machicado GA. Colonoscopy for diagnosis and treatment of severe lower gastrointestinal bleeding. Routine outcomes and cost analysis. Gastrointest Endosc Clin N Am 1997;7:477–98.

[81] Steer ML, Silen W. Diagnostic procedures in gastrointestinal hemorrhage. N Engl J Med 1983;309:646–50.

[82] Pennoyer WP, Vignati PV, Cohen JL. Mesenteric angiography for lower gastrointestinal hemorrhage: are there predictors for a positive study? Dis Colon Rectum 1997;40:1014–8.

[83] Cohn SM, Moller BA, Zieg PM, et al. Angiography for preoperative evaluation in patients with lower gastrointestinal bleeding: are the benefits worth the risks? Arch Surg 1998;133: 50–5.

[84] Vernava AM, Moore BA, Longo WE, et al. Lower gastrointestinal bleeding. Dis Colon Rectum 1997;40:846–58.

[85] Tedesco FJ, Waye JD, Raskin JB, et al. Colonoscopic evaluation of rectal bleeding: a study of 304 patients. Ann Intern Med 1978;89:907–9.

[86] Pennazio M, Santucci R, Rondonotti E, et al. Outcome of patients with obscure gastrointestinal bleeding after capsule endoscopy: report of 100 consecutive cases. Gastroenterology 2004;126:643–53.

[87] Rastogi A, Schoen RE, Slivka A. Diagnostic yield and clinical outcomes of capsule endoscopy. Gastrointest Endosc 2004;60:959–64.

[88] Adler DG, Knipschield M, Gostout C. A prospective comparison of capsule endoscopy and push enteroscopy in patients with GI bleeding of obscure origin. Gastrointest Endosc 2004; 59:492–8.

[89] Ell C, Remke S, May A, et al. The first prospective controlled trial comparing wireless capsule endoscopy with push enteroscopy in chronic gastrointestinal bleeding. Endoscopy 2002; 34:685–9.

[90] Costamagna G, Shah SK, Riccioni ME, et al. A prospective trial comparing small bowel radiographs and video capsule endoscopy for suspected small bowel disease. Gastroenterology 2002;123:999–1005.

ELSEVIER
SAUNDERS

CLINICS IN
GERIATRIC
MEDICINE

Clin Geriatr Med 23 (2007) 785–808

Gastric Emptying, Diabetes, and Aging

Paul Kuo, MBBS,
Christopher K. Rayner, MBBS, PhD, FRACP,
Michael Horowitz, MBBS, PhD, FRACP*

*Discipline of Medicine, Royal Adelaide Hospital, North Terrace, Adelaide,
South Australia 5000, Australia*

In addition to temporarily storing ingesta, the stomach, together with the small intestine, represents an important regulatory "checkpoint" in nutrient processing, and the two together form one of the major neuroendocrine units in the body. Current information about how these functions are affected by healthy aging is limited, although it is well recognized that factors associated with older age, including comorbid medical conditions and medications, can influence upper gut motor and sensory function.

Gastric emptying is a major determinant of postprandial glycemia [1], and slowing of gastric emptying by either pharmacologic or nonpharmacologic means, has the capacity to reduce postprandial glycaemic excursions in both healthy subjects [2] and patients with diabetes [3,4]. Manipulation of gastric emptying, therefore, represents a therapeutic strategy in the management of diabetes. Cross-sectional studies have established that gastric emptying is delayed in some 50% of adults with long-standing type 1 or type 2 diabetes [5]; however, there is a lack of information about elderly people with diabetes. Gastric emptying appears to be slightly slower in older people (those in their 60s and 70s) than young people, while information in the very old (those age 80 or above) is scarce. This article focuses on the interactions between gastric emptying and diabetes, how each is influenced by the process of aging, and the implications for patient management.

Normal regulation of gastric emptying

The proximal stomach accommodates ingesta, which are ground into 1-mm to 2-mm sized particles in the distal stomach before emptying into

---

* Corresponding author.
E-mail address: michael.horowitz@adelaide.edu.au (M. Horowitz).

0749-0690/07/$ - see front matter © 2007 Elsevier Inc. All rights reserved.
doi:10.1016/j.cger.2007.06.009

the small intestine [6]. Gastric emptying is determined by the integration of motor activities in the proximal and distal stomach, as well as the pylorus and the proximal small intestine [6]. Tonic and phasic contractions located to the pylorus act to retard gastric emptying [5,6].

During fasting, patterns of gastric and small intestinal motility are cyclical, termed the migrating motor complex (MMC). Depolarization of specialized pacemaker cells, the interstitial cells of Cajal, which are situated mainly along the greater curvature of the stomach, set an underlying electrical rhythm that determines the maximum frequency of contractions [5]. Each cycle contains three phases: I—motor quiescence (lasting approximately 40 minutes), II—irregular contractions (lasting approximately 50 minutes), and III—regular, high amplitude contractions occurring at a maximal rate of 3 per minute in the stomach and 10 to 12 per minute in the small intestine (lasting approximately 5–10 minutes) [7]. The MMC functions as an "intestinal housekeeper" that "sweeps" intraluminal contents aborally from the distal stomach to the terminal ileum [8].

Ingestion of food disrupts the MMC and produces a postprandial pattern that aids the trituration and propulsion of chyme [9]. Postprandially, the rate of gastric emptying is tightly regulated, as a result of neural and hormonal feedback triggered by the interaction of nutrients with the small intestine [5]. This feedback is caloric load-dependent, relates to the length of small intestine exposed to nutrient, and regulates the overall rate of emptying to about 2 kcal/min to 3 kcal/min [6]. The presence of nutrients in the small intestine is associated with relaxation of the gastric fundus, suppression of antral contractions, and stimulation of tonic and phasic pyloric contractions [6]. The main hormones involved include cholecystokinin (CCK), glucagon-like peptide-1 (GLP-1), peptide YY (PYY), and amylin [9–11]. The neural feedback involves both intrinsic (the enteric nervous system) and extrinsic (the autonomic and central nervous systems) components. Nitric oxide, an important inhibitory neurotransmitter in the gut, plays a role in the neural feedback pathway (Fig. 1) [12,13].

Gastric emptying is also influenced by the physical and chemical composition of a meal [9], with solids emptying in a linear fashion after an initial lag phase, high nutrient liquids emptying in a linear fashion, and nonnutrient liquids emptying in a monoexponential pattern [9,14]. Liquids empty more rapidly than solids, reflecting the need for the latter to be ground into small particles before emptying [7].

Effect of diabetes on gastric emptying

Delayed gastric emptying occurs in about 30% to 50% of outpatients with long-standing type 1 and type 2 diabetes [5,15], and can be associated with upper gut symptoms, as well as have implications for glycemic control, nutrition, drug absorption, quality of life, and health resource consumption [5,7,16,17]. In most cases, the magnitude of the delay in gastric emptying is

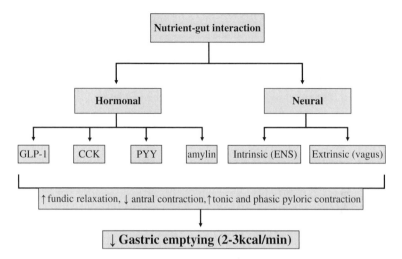

Fig. 1. Normal regulation of gastric emptying. Nutrient-gut interactions in the small intestine set off both hormonal and neural feedback responses which slow subsequent gastric emptying by a variety of mechanisms, so that the overall rate of gastric emptying approximates 2 kcal/min to 3 kcal/min. Amylin is indirectly involved, as it is cosecreted with insulin by the pancreas, while the other hormones are secreted by the small intestine in response to nutrient exposure. Hormones shown are Glucagon-like peptide-1 (GLP-1), cholecystokinin (CCK), peptide YY (PYY); enteric nervous system is ENS.

modest and there is a poor correlation between symptoms, such as nausea and vomiting, with the rate of gastric emptying [6]. Limited data suggest that moderately delayed gastric emptying is associated with a good long-term prognosis [18]. Abnormally rapid gastric emptying occurs in a minority of patients, most of whom have "early" type 2 diabetes [19,20]. Gastroparesis is usually arbitrary, defined by a rate of emptying more than two standard deviations from the healthy mean [6,21]. More recently, the nonspecific term "diabetic gastropathy" has been used to denote abnormal motor or sensory function of the upper gut in patients with diabetes [22].

The motor dysfunctions responsible for disordered gastric emptying in diabetes are heterogeneous and include impaired meal-induced relaxation of the gastric fundus [23], increased pyloric motor activity [24], fewer antral contractions [25], and impaired antroduodenal coordination [26]. Disturbances of the gastric electrical rhythm, measured by electrogastrography, also occur frequently [27].

There is no direct measure of gastrointestinal autonomic function, and cardiovascular autonomic tests are generally used as a surrogate marker, but the validity of such an approach is controversial. Diabetic gastroparesis is often attributed to irreversible autonomic neuropathy, but the association is weak and inconsistent [28,29]. Numerous histologic abnormalities have been documented in the gastrointestinal tract of animals with diabetes [30–34], but relatively few have been documented in human beings. There is, however, evidence of a loss of interstitial cells of Cajal in patients with medically-refractory gastroparesis [35], and gastric myopathy in a small group of type 1 diabetes patients [36].

Acute changes in the blood glucose concentration have reversible effects on the motility of the entire gastrointestinal tract [15]. Even modest elevation in blood glucose to 8 mmol/L slows gastric emptying in both healthy subjects and patients with type 1 diabetes, when compared with a blood glucose of 4 mmol/L [37,38], while substantial increases in blood glucose to 16 mmol/L to 20 mmol/L slow gastric emptying of both solids and liquids markedly [39,40]. Furthermore, insulin-induced hypoglycemia (blood glucose approximately 2.6 mmol/L) accelerates gastric emptying in type 1 diabetes patients [41], even in those with delayed gastric emptying during euglycemia.

The mechanisms mediating the effects of glycemia on gastrointestinal function are incompletely understood. In animal models, acute hyperglycemia causes reversible inhibition of vagal efferent activity [42], and glucose responsive neurons have been identified in both the central [43] and enteric [44] nervous systems. In healthy human beings, cardiovascular autonomic function is impaired during hyperglycemia [45], but whether this equates to a similar impairment in gastrointestinal autonomic function is not known. A significant role for insulin appears unlikely given that euglycemic hyperinsulinemia has no effect on gastric emptying [46], and that hyperglycemia delays gastric emptying in type 1 (insulin deficient) diabetes patients.

Effect of gastric emptying on diabetes

Strict glycemic control reduces the risk of long-term micro- and macrovascular complications of type 1 and type 2 diabetes [47–49]. Postprandial, as opposed to fasting, glycemia, is now recognized to be a major determinant of overall glycemic control, as indicated by glycated hemoglobin (HbA1c) [50]. This is hardly surprising given that human beings spend most of their lives in the postprandial or postabsorptive state [51]. Postprandial glycemia appears to be an independent determinant of cardiovascular disease and mortality, even in people without diabetes [52,53]. Improved overall glycemic control can be achieved by lowering postprandial glucose levels, even at the expense of higher fasting levels [54]. The traditional emphasis on primarily controlling fasting glycemia is therefore inappropriate, and postprandial glycemia should be a major focus of diabetes management (Fig. 2).

The rate of gastric emptying accounts for at least one third of the variation in the postprandial glycemic response [1,55]. Delayed gastric emptying is now recognized as a risk factor for hypoglycemia in insulin-treated patients—probably because the delay in nutrient delivery leads to a mismatch with the actions of exogenous insulin [56]. On the other hand, in patients with type 2 diabetes who are not treated with insulin, slowing gastric emptying by adding guar gum [1], increasing dietary fiber (especially the

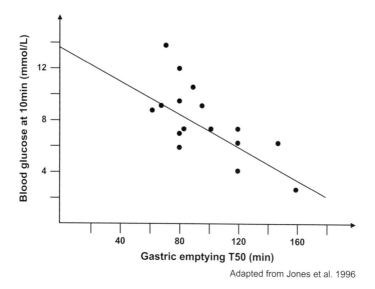

Adapted from Jones et al. 1996

Fig. 2. Relationship between gastric emptying and postprandial glycemia in type 2 diabetes mellitus.

soluble type) [57], or consuming an oil "preload" before a carbohydrate-containing meal [58], is associated with an improvement in the postprandial glycemic profile. Pharmacologic agents, such as GLP-1 and its analogs (eg, exenatide) [59–61], the amylin analog pramlintide [62], the oral proteinase potato II inhibitor [63], cholecystokinin-8 [64], and even morphine [65], have all been shown to slow gastric emptying and attenuate the postprandial rise in blood glucose in type 2 diabetes.

Gastric emptying and aging

Gastrointestinal function, in general, and especially that of the stomach and the small intestine, is relatively preserved during healthy aging [66–68]. Studies on the effect of aging on gastric emptying have yielded conflicting information, with reports that emptying is slowed [69–73], accelerated [67], or unchanged [68]. A variety of techniques have been used to measure gastric emptying, some less than ideal [69,74], and published studies have involved very different subject populations [74,75], or included those with significant medical comorbidities [72]. Despite these limitations, the overall weight of evidence supports the notion that healthy aging is associated with a modest slowing of gastric emptying, although the rate generally remains within the normal range of the young (Fig. 3) [70,71,75,76]. Nonetheless, slowing of gastric emptying can potentially influence postprandial glycemia; reduced transpyloric flow in the healthy elderly is associated with an attenuation of the initial rise in postprandial blood glucose concentrations, when compared with the young [77].

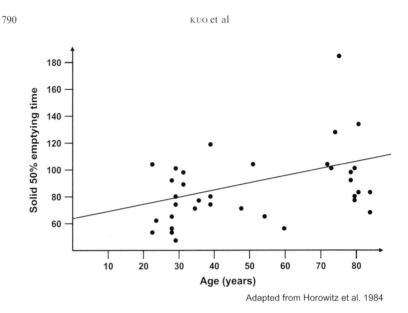

Adapted from Horowitz et al. 1984

Fig. 3. Relationship between the solid 50% emptying time and age in 35 subjects, where r = 0.42, and P<.01.

The mechanisms underlying the slowing of gastric emptying with aging are uncertain. Autonomic nerve dysfunction is more prevalent in the older population, but its correlation with delayed gastric emptying is poor [71]. Postprandial antral contraction frequency, measured by scintigraphy, is preserved in older age [68]. The healthy elderly have greater stimulation of phasic pyloric contractions during intraduodenal lipid infusion when compared with the young, and these contractions act as a brake to gastric emptying [78,79]. There are conflicting data as to whether the gastric electrical rhythm is affected by age [80–83]. Plasma concentrations of CCK are higher both before and after meals in older people, potentially contributing to the age-related slowing in gastric emptying [79], while GLP-1 and PYY levels are similar [79]. Older subjects also appear to have greater slowing of gastric emptying in response to a lipid-containing liquid meal when compared with younger subjects [73].

Other changes in gastroduodenal function related to aging

Healthy older subjects, compared with the young, report less hunger before and after a meal [71,84,85]. The higher fasting CCK levels potentially contribute to reduced preprandial hunger [85,86], while slower gastric emptying [69–71], delayed proximal gastric accommodation [87], and increased postprandial antral volume [71,84], may be relevant postprandially. Conversely, the healthy elderly experience less fullness, discomfort, and bloating, but greater hunger, in response to proximal gastric distension, when compared with the young [87].

As indicated above, healthy aging is associated with changes in gastrointestinal hormone release. In addition to higher fasting plasma CCK levels [79,85,86] and a greater postprandial increase [79], when compared with young subjects the elderly are more sensitive to the suppressive effects of CCK on energy intake [85]. GLP-1, PYY, and amylin concentrations are similar in young and old subjects [79,81,88], and while fasting ghrelin levels appear lower (by 20%–35%) in the elderly than in the young [86,89], this may in part relate to a higher body mass index of the elderly in some studies [89–91]. Conversely, others have reported a rise in ghrelin levels with increasing age, although the correlation was weak (r = 0.27) [91].

Changes in gastric secretory and mucosal function have also been described in older aged subjects, including reduced mucosal prostaglandin concentrations [92], diminished bicarbonate [93] and pepsin [94] secretion, and probably decreased protective quality of the gastric mucus, caused by a significantly increased parietal-to-mucus cell ratio [95] and reduced gastric mucosal surface hydrophobicity [96]. In animal models, both basal gastric blood flow and the capacity for mucosal repair in response to injury are impaired in older age [97,98]. The effect of aging on gastric acid secretion is controversial, with findings of increased [99], decreased [100–103], or unchanged [94,104–106] secretion, although earlier studies often did not take into account the presence of chronic atrophic gastritis, and preceded the discovery of Helicobacter pylori, both of which are more prevalent with age. Overall, the more recent, better-designed studies indicate no change in gastric acid secretion with healthy aging. Serum gastrin levels also appear unchanged [105]. In the small intestine, transit does not appear to be affected by age [68], while mucosal integrity and permeability, as assessed by the lactulose-mannitol absorption test, appears preserved (Box 1) [107].

In human beings, age-related neuronal loss has been described in the myenteric plexus of the gastrointestinal tract, involving the esophagus [108], small intestine [109], and colon [110], although not in the stomach [111]; in animal models, all regions of the gastrointestinal tract, including the stomach, are affected [111]. In rats, the rate of neuronal loss is linear in the small and large intestines, but later and more abrupt in the stomach [112]. Data relating to the effect of aging on the extrinsic neural supply to the gastrointestinal tract are conflicting in animals, while no significant change has been detected in human beings [111,113]. Information on the effect of aging on gastrointestinal smooth muscle is scarce, and no human data are available. One report indicated decreased relaxation of the rat gastric fundus in response to vasoactive intestinal peptide, and an increased response to exogenous nitric oxide [114].

Diabetes and aging

Normal aging is associated with decreased glucose tolerance [115–117], because of a combination of increased peripheral insulin resistance,

---

Box 1. Changes in gastroduodenal function in the elderly

Motor
- Moderate slowing of gastric emptying
- Delayed postprandial proximal gastric accommodation
- Increased postprandial antral volume

Sensory
- Reduced pre- and postprandial hunger
- Reduced fullness, distension, and bloating in response to proximal gastric distension

Hormonal
- Increased fasting and postprandial rise of plasma CCK
- Decreased plasma ghrelin level
- Increased suppression of food intake in response to exogenous CCK

Mucosal
- Decreased mucosal prostaglandin
- Decreased bicarbonate secretion
- Decreased pepsin secretion

---

decreased pancreatic beta-cell function [118,119] and, possibly, delayed postprandial suppression of hepatic glucose production [120]. In Western populations it has been estimated that at least 20% of people aged 65 years and over have diabetes [121], with the majority being type 2, characterized by peripheral insulin resistance and, to a much lesser extent, insulin deficiency. These people are frequently overweight or obese. The impact of diabetes in the older population is uncertain, because in this group there is little information about long-term outcome, although in octogenarians, in contrast to all other younger age groups, glycemic control does not worsen with a longer duration of diabetes [122], implying a different natural history.

Insulin is normally secreted in a pulsatile manner, consisting of rapid, low amplitude pulses occurring at 8 to15 minute intervals, which inhibit hepatic glucose production, and ultradian pulses of larger amplitude, occurring at 60 to 140 minute intervals, which stimulate peripheral glucose uptake [123]. The effect of aging on insulin secretion is controversial. The issue is complicated by differences in the methodology used, and uncontrolled variables, including body composition, insulin sensitivity, levels of physical fitness, androgen and growth hormone levels, and insulin/C-peptide clearance. Most studies have found the insulin response to intravenous glucose to be impaired in healthy older subjects [118,124–127], but changes in response to oral glucose are less well defined [120,127,128]. The normal pattern of insulin release appears to be disturbed in older age, leading to a reduction in the frequency and amplitude of both rapid and ultradian insulin pulses [116,129–131]. Potential mechanisms include impaired pancreatic conversion of proinsulin to insulin [127], and decreased beta-cell sensitivity to glucose-dependent insulinotropic polypeptide (GIP) [117,132–134]. Like GLP-1, GIP secretion is not diminished with aging [81] and may in fact be increased [133,134]. Similar disturbances of insulin secretion have been described in both elderly [131] and nonelderly [123,135] type 2 diabetes patients, but compared with the healthy elderly, older type 2 patients have a greater impairment in basal and pulsatile insulin secretion during hyperglycemia induced by a glucose clamp, as well as reduced insulin burst mass, and increased irregularity of insulin release [131].

The etiology of insulin resistance in age-associated glucose intolerance is poorly defined. Insulin resistance seems likely to relate to altered body composition rather than to age per se [136–141]. Increased visceral fat, which is associated with increased insulin resistance [142–145], increases with age [144,145], and in aged mice its surgical removal results in the restoration of insulin sensitivity [146]. Caloric restriction probably prevents the development of type 2 diabetes in mice [147] by reducing visceral fat formation [146]. Other mechanisms proposed to explain age-related insulin resistance and glucose intolerance include an impairment in noninsulin-mediated glucose uptake [148], age-related decline in cellular mitochondrial

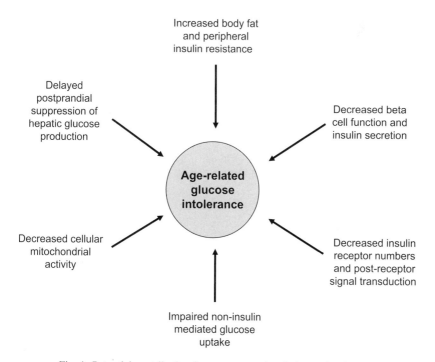

Fig. 4. Potential contributing factors to age-related glucose intolerance.

function [149], reduced insulin receptor numbers [150], and impaired postreceptor signal transduction (Fig. 4) [150].

One study suggested seasonal variations in insulin sensitivity among the elderly, independent of changes in body weight, with higher insulin resistance in summer as compared with winter, although the follow-up period was only 12 months [151]. This is in contrast to a previous study in healthy young men, where no seasonal variation in insulin sensitivity was detected [152]. Furthermore, low—rather than high—levels of vitamin D have been associated with insulin resistance [153].

In recent years, a distinct subtype of type 2 diabetes has been recognized, characterized by normal body weight and affecting both younger and older individuals [154–156]. This group has been termed the "lean type 2" or "type $1^1/_2$" [157], because of the presence of features of both type 1 and type 2 diabetes, but the prevalence of this form of diabetes has not been adequately defined. Compared to patients with type 2 diabetes, type $1^1/_2$ patients typically have much milder degrees of peripheral insulin resistance, but are predominantly insulin deficient [158,159]. Furthermore, compared with their lean middle-aged counterparts, lean, elderly type 2 patients have even less insulin resistance, and normal—as opposed to increased—hepatic glucose production [154]. Little information exists regarding optimal management of these cases, but early insulin replacement has been advocated [154,159]. Data regarding the prevalence of ischemic heart disease, retinopathy, or nephropathy among lean type 2 patients are scarce. The prevalence of autonomic neuropathy in these patients appears similar to the obese [160], but the severity may not be as great [161].

Hyperglycemia is an important cause of impaired cognition in older adults, independent of vascular pathology, affecting processing speed and verbal memory [162]. It is associated with an increased risk of developing dementia [163,164], especially when combined with other risk factors, including the apolipoprotein E4 gene [164]. Good glycemic control, instituted before the age of 70, has been advocated to help prevent this cognitive decline [165,166]. Even among young healthy subjects, abnormal glucose regulation is associated with impaired ability to perform cognitive tasks [167]. In older type 2 diabetes patients there is an improvement in cognitive function as their glycemic control improves [168,169], although no such benefit was observed in the absence of pre-existing cognitive deficit [170]. Improved postprandial glycemia, independent of fasting glucose and HbA1c levels, has also been shown to improve cognitive function in older type 2 patients [171]. Diabetes is associated with brain atrophy, independent of vascular pathology, as measured by magnetic resonance imaging [172,173].

Decreased skeletal muscle strength has also been described in older people with type 2 diabetes [174], predisposing them to falls and injuries. It is associated particularly with a long duration of diabetes (greater or equal to 6 years) and poor glycemic control (HbA1c greater than 8%) [174].

Management of delayed gastric emptying and diabetes in the elderly

Available evidence supports both a mild delay in gastric emptying and impaired glucose tolerance associated with healthy aging. However, the significance of this evidence and optimal management remain controversial. Most drugs are absorbed in the small intestine with minimal absorption in the stomach [175]. Therefore, delayed gastric emptying can potentially impact on the absorption of oral drugs [5,175,176]. In healthy subjects, slowing in gastric emptying induced by hyperglycemia resulted in a 50% reduction in the rate of oral glipizide absorption [177], while intramuscular injections of opioid drugs caused a delay in gastric emptying and slowed the absorption of oral paracetamol [178]. Steady-state concentrations for the majority of drugs are, however, unlikely to be affected [5]. The slowing of gastric emptying associated with aging may therefore affect drug absorption, although there was no difference in paracetamol absorption in healthy older subjects compared with the younger subjects [179–181]. Given that age-related slowing of gastric emptying is modest, it may only affect drugs with a very narrow therapeutic index, or when very rapid onset of effect is desired. However, it is important to realize that gastric emptying in older people is affected not only by changes of aging per se, but also by multiple other factors associated with older age, including comorbid medical conditions and medications, which can have a much greater impact (Box 2).

Gastrointestinal complaints are common among the elderly [182], and factors including increased use of medications, such as aspirin and nonsteroidal anti-inflammatory drugs [183], and increased prevalence of Helicobacter pylori infection [184] can all contribute. It is not known whether slowed gastric emptying associated with healthy aging is a significant contributor to upper gut symptoms, and the role of prokinetic agents in this situation is uncertain.

The management of diabetes in the older population has predominantly been based on extrapolation from younger patients, with few studies specifically targeting the elderly. Managing diabetes in older individuals poses extra challenges because of altered pharmacokinetics, polypharmacy with increased potential for drug interactions, reduced physiologic reserve, and declining physical and cognitive function in managing their own care. Liver function is relatively preserved, but renal function declines significantly with age, making calculation of glomerular filtration rate and appropriate drug dosage adjustment mandatory [185].

In older adults with impaired glucose tolerance, both lifestyle changes (diet and exercise) and pharmacologic interventions (metformin and acarbose) have been shown to decrease the risk of progression to type 2 diabetes [186–188]. An intensive lifestyle modification program, aiming for at least 7% weight loss and 150 minutes of exercise per week, was particularly effective in those 60 or above, achieving over 70% reduction in the progression to type 2 diabetes during an average follow-up of

---

Box 2. Factors potentially causing delayed gastric emptying

Acute
Drugs (anticholinergics, opiates, calcium-channel blockers,
  levodopa, alcohol, octreotide, nicotine, cannabis)
Viral infection (gastroenteritis, Herpes zoster)
Postoperative state
Critical illness
Electrolyte or metabolic disturbances (hyperglycemia,
  hypokalemia, hypomagnesemia)

Chronic
Diabetes mellitus
Idiopathic (including functional dyspepsia)
Gastroesophageal reflux disease
Achalasia
Surgery (vagotomy, heart or lung transplantation)
Connective tissue diseases (systemic sclerosis, polymyositis/
  dermatomyositis, amyloidosis, systemic lupus erythematosis)
Metabolic and endocrine causes (chronic liver or renal failure,
  hyper- or hypothyroidism, Addison's disease, porphyria)
Chronic idiopathic intestinal pseudo-obstruction
Malignancy
Neuromuscular diseases (head trauma, stroke, brain tumor,
  brainstem or spinal cord lesions, Parkinson's disease,
  myotonic and muscular dystrophies, autonomic degeneration)
Infection (HIV, Chaga's disease)
Irradiation
Anorexia nervosa

2.8 years, compared with 11% reduction with metformin [187]. In a population study, a high dietary intake of whole grains, cereal fiber, and magnesium was also associated with a reduced risk of developing type 2 diabetes in older women [188]. In older men with glucose intolerance, endurance exercise training for 12 weeks improved skeletal muscle glucose transporter-4 protein expression and decreased the intramuscular triglyceride concentration [189].

Screening for diabetes in older people is controversial, particularly regarding the timing of testing, the method and reference ranges used, and whether screening should be undertaken at all. The American Diabetes Association currently recommends testing all people over 45 years old at 3-year intervals [121]. Lifestyle modification is the initial management of choice for type 2 diabetes in the elderly, involving dietary changes [190] and realistic exercise programs [191]. In those who are obese, a low energy diet (800 kcal/d) for 20 to 24 days leads to significant weight loss and improvement in glycemic profile, regardless of the duration of diabetes [192]. However, pharmacotherapy is still needed in a majority of patients to optimize glycemia [49]. In addition to improving glycemic control, lifestyle modification has the benefit of improving other cardiovascular risk factors and reducing fracture risk; diabetes in older women is independently associated with an increased risk of both falls [193] and fractures [194], despite having normal or increased bone mass.

Older people are particularly susceptible to severe hypoglycemia because of reduced hypoglycemic awareness. Compared with the young, older healthy men are more prone to develop cognitive impairment during hypoglycemia [195]. Indeed, the threshold for cognitive impairment may be higher than for symptoms [195], and cognitive recovery is slower after the blood glucose returns to the euglycemic range [195]. Potential secondary complications include motor vehicle accidents, falls and fractures, myocardial infarction, and stroke [196]. Avoidance of hypoglycemia is therefore a priority in the elderly.

Strategies to improve postprandial glycemia by modulating gastric emptying aim to optimize the coordination between nutrient delivery and insulin availability. The specific strategies, therefore, are likely to differ depending on the requirement for exogenous insulin. For type 2 diabetes patients managed by oral medication or diet alone, it may be advantageous to slow gastric emptying to match endogenous insulin output, which is frequently deficient in the early postprandial phase, but subsequently relatively normal. Conversely, for those receiving exogenous insulin, gastric emptying may need to be either slowed or accelerated to match the peak activity of insulin.

Analogs of GLP-1, such as exenatide, appear promising in the treatment of type 2 diabetes in the elderly [197–199]. Given acutely, analogs of GLP-1 slow gastric emptying [3,200], suppress glucagon secretion [201], improve insulin secretion in response to hyperglycemia [198], and increase both insulin-mediated [202] and noninsulin-mediated [199] peripheral glucose uptake. In addition, their benefits appear to be maintained after prolonged therapy (up to 3 months) [131,197]. Furthermore, long-term therapy is associated with HbA1c levels comparable to those in patients using oral hypoglycemic agents, but with a much lower incidence of hypoglycemic events due to the glucose-dependent nature of GLP-1, and probably a narrower range of glycemic excursions [197]. In lean elderly type 2 diabetes patients, where the blood glucose was acutely elevated to 15 mmol/L, the administration of exogenous GLP-1 did not cause hypoglycemia [203], providing evidence for the safety of such treatment in those with relatively intact insulin sensitivity. It is not clear whether individuals with delayed gastric emptying before therapy will derive as much benefit from GLP-1 and its analogs as those whose emptying is in the normal range, given that the predominant mechanism of action of GLP-1 is by slowing of gastric emptying [204,205]. Furthermore, there are insufficient data as to whether the side effect profile of GLP-1 and its analogs will be affected by differences in age, upper gastrointestinal symptoms, or the rate of gastric emptying before therapy.

Management of diabetic gastroparesis is traditionally centered around the use of prokinetic agents, such as metoclopramide, domperidone, erythromycin, and cisapride, which have all been shown to improve symptoms and quality of life [5–7,206]. In recent years, numerous new agents have appeared, including 5-HT$_4$ agonists tegaserod and mosapride [207,208], ghrelin [209], the dopamine (D$_2$) antagonist levosulpiride [210,211], as well as intrapyloric botulinum toxin injection [212] and gastric electrical stimulation [213–216], with the latter showing promise in medically refractory cases. The newer treatments are currently not recommended as first-line. Because of the potential for cardiac arrhythmias [217], cisapride is now only available through special access schemes in certain countries. Concerns over antimicrobial resistance associated with long term erythromycin use [218], and central nervous system side effects of metoclopramide [217], especially in the older population, probably makes domperidone the agent of first choice.

Summary

Gastric emptying in healthy aging appears modestly slowed, although in general, remains within the normal range for the young population. Its effect on drug absorption appears to be minor, and data relating delayed emptying to gastrointestinal symptoms in this population are lacking. However, delayed gastric emptying in the older population is more likely to be clinically relevant when related to comorbid medical conditions and medications, rather than healthy aging (see Box 2).

The incidence of diabetes, especially type 2 diabetes, increases with age and is likely to be caused by a combination of factors, including decreased insulin secretion, altered body composition with increased insulin resistance, and changes in the pattern of food intake, rate of metabolism, hepatic glucose production, and insulin clearance.

The addition of the factor of age to the already complex interactions between gastric emptying and glycemic control, makes management of both diabetes and abnormal gastric emptying in the elderly all the more challenging. Data on gastric emptying and diabetes in older age groups are lacking, especially in the very elderly (80 years and older). More research is indicated, particularly in very old, type 2 diabetes patients.

References

[1] Russo A, Stevens JE, Wilson T, et al. Guar attenuates fall in postprandial blood pressure and slows gastric emptying of oral glucose in type 2 diabetes. Dig Dis Sci 2003;48(7):1221–9.

[2] Gentilcore D, Hausken T, Horowitz M, et al. Measurements of gastric emptying of low- and high-nutrient liquids using 3D ultrasonography and scintigraphy in healthy subjects. Neurogastroenterol Motil 2006;18(12):1062–8.

[3] Dupre J, Behme MT, McDonald TJ. Exendin-4 normalized postcibal glycemic excursions in type 1 diabetes. J Clin Endocrinol Metab 2004;89(7):3469–73.

[4] Kolterman OG, Gottlieb A, Moyses C, et al. Reduction of postprandial hyperglycemia in subjects with IDDM by intravenous infusion of AC137, a human amylin analogue. Diabetes Care 1995;18(8):1179–82.

[5] Horowitz M, O'Donovan D, Jones KL, et al. Gastric emptying in diabetes: clinical significance and treatment. Diabet Med 2002;19(3):177–94.

[6] Rayner CK, Horowitz M. New management approaches for gastroparesis. Nat Clin Pract Gastroenterol Hepatol 2005;2(10):454–62 [quiz: 493].

[7] Horowitz M, Su YC, Rayner CK, et al. Gastroparesis: prevalence, clinical significance and treatment. Can J Gastroenterol 2001;15(12):805–13.

[8] Husebye E. The patterns of small bowel motility: physiology and implications in organic disease and functional disorders. Neurogastroenterol Motil 1999;11(3): 141–61.

[9] Gentilcore D, O'Donovan D, Jones KL, et al. Nutrition therapy for diabetic gastroparesis. Curr Diab Rep 2003;3(5):418–26.

[10] Little TJ, Horowitz M, Feinle-Bisset C. Role of cholecystokinin in appetite control and body weight regulation. Obes Rev 2005;6(4):297–306.

[11] Schmitz O, Brock B, Rungby J. Amylin agonists: a novel approach in the treatment of diabetes. Diabetes 2004;53(Suppl 3):S233–8.

[12] Desai KM, Sessa WC, Vane JR. Involvement of nitric oxide in the reflex relaxation of the stomach to accommodate food or fluid. Nature 1991;351(6326):477–9.

[13] Tack J, Demedts I, Meulemans A, et al. Role of nitric oxide in the gastric accommodation reflex and in meal induced satiety in humans. Gut 2002;51(2):219–24.

[14] Collins PJ, Horowitz M, Cook DJ, et al. Gastric emptying in normal subjects—a reproducible technique using a single scintillation camera and computer system. Gut 1983;24(12): 1117–25.

[15] Rayner CK, Samsom M, Jones KL, et al. Relationships of upper gastrointestinal motor and sensory function with glycemic control. Diabetes Care 2001;24(2):371–81.

[16] Bell RA, Jones-Vessey K, Summerson JH. Hospitalizations and outcomes for diabetic gastroparesis in North Carolina. South Med J 2002;95(11):1297–9.

[17] Gallar P, Oliet A, Vigil A, et al. Gastroparesis: an important cause of hospitalization in continuous ambulatory peritoneal dialysis patients and the role of erythromycin. Perit Dial Int 1993;13(Suppl 2):S183–6.

[18] Kong MF, Horowitz M, Jones KL, et al. Natural history of diabetic gastroparesis. Diabetes Care 1999;22(3):503–7.

[19] Phillips WT, Schwartz JG, McMahan CA. Rapid gastric emptying of an oral glucose solution in type 2 diabetic patients. J Nucl Med 1992;33(8):1496–500.

[20] Schwartz JG, Green GM, Guan D, et al. Rapid gastric emptying of a solid pancake meal in type II diabetic patients. Diabetes Care 1996;19(5):468–71.

[21] Jones MP, Maganti K. A systematic review of surgical therapy for gastroparesis. Am J Gastroenterol 2003;98(10):2122–9.

[22] Koch KL. Diabetic gastropathy: gastric neuromuscular dysfunction in diabetes mellitus: a review of symptoms, pathophysiology, and treatment. Dig Dis Sci 1999;44(6): 1061–75.

[23] Samsom M, Roelofs JM, Akkermans LM, et al. Proximal gastric motor activity in response to a liquid meal in type I diabetes mellitus with autonomic neuropathy. Dig Dis Sci 1998; 43(3):491–6.

[24] Mearin F, Camilleri M, Malagelada JR. Pyloric dysfunction in diabetics with recurrent nausea and vomiting. Gastroenterology 1986;90(6):1919–25.

[25] Thumshirn M, Bruninga K, Camilleri M. Simplifying the evaluation of postprandial antral motor function in patients with suspected gastroparesis. Am J Gastroenterol 1997;92(9): 1496–500.

[26] Fraser RJ, Horowitz M, Maddox AF, et al. Postprandial antropyloroduodenal motility and gastric emptying in gastroparesis—effects of cisapride. Gut 1994;35(2): 172–8.

[27] Mathur R, Pimentel M, Sam CL, et al. Postprandial improvement of gastric dysrhythmias in patients with type II diabetes: identification of responders and nonresponders. Dig Dis Sci 2001;46(4):705–12.

[28] Asakawa H, Onishi M, Hayashi I, et al. Comparison between coefficient of R-R interval variation and gastric emptying in type 2 diabetes mellitus patients. J Gastroenterol Hepatol 2005;20(9):1358–64.

[29] Jones KL, Russo A, Stevens JE, et al. Predictors of delayed gastric emptying in diabetes. Diabetes Care 2001;24(7):1264–9.

[30] Horvath VJ, Vittal H, Lorincz A, et al. Reduced stem cell factor links smooth myopathy and loss of interstitial cells of Cajal in murine diabetic gastroparesis. Gastroenterology 2006;130(3):759–70.

[31] Watkins CC, Sawa A, Jaffrey S, et al. Insulin restores neuronal nitric oxide synthase expression and function that is lost in diabetic gastropathy. J Clin Invest 2000;106(3): 373–84.

[32] Horvath VJ, Vittal H, Ordog T. Reduced insulin and IGF-I signaling, not hyperglycemia, underlies the diabetes-associated depletion of interstitial cells of Cajal in the murine stomach. Diabetes 2005;54(5):1528–33.

[33] Ordog T, Takayama I, Cheung WK, et al. Remodeling of networks of interstitial cells of Cajal in a murine model of diabetic gastroparesis. Diabetes 2000;49(10):1731–9.

[34] Anitha M, Gondha C, Sutliff R, et al. GDNF rescues hyperglycemia-induced diabetic enteric neuropathy through activation of the PI3K/Akt pathway. J Clin Invest 2006; 116(2):344–56.

[35] Forster J, Damjanov I, Lin Z, et al. Absence of the interstitial cells of Cajal in patients with gastroparesis and correlation with clinical findings. J Gastrointest Surg 2005;9(1): 102–8.

[36] Ejskjaer NT, Bradley JL, Buxton-Thomas MS, et al. Novel surgical treatment and gastric pathology in diabetic gastroparesis. Diabet Med 1999;16(6):488–95.

[37] Jones KL, Kong MF, Berry MK, et al. The effect of erythromycin on gastric emptying is modified by physiological changes in the blood glucose concentration. Am J Gastroenterol 1999;94(8):2074–9.

[38] Schvarcz E, Palmer M, Aman J, et al. Physiological hyperglycemia slows gastric emptying in normal subjects and patients with insulin-dependent diabetes mellitus. Gastroenterology 1997;113(1):60–6.

[39] Fraser RJ, Horowitz M, Maddox AF, et al. Hyperglycaemia slows gastric emptying in type 1 (insulin-dependent) diabetes mellitus. Diabetologia 1990;33(11):675–80.

[40] Samsom M, Akkermans LM, Jebbink RJ, et al. Gastrointestinal motor mechanisms in hyperglycaemia induced delayed gastric emptying in type I diabetes mellitus. Gut 1997; 40(5):641–6.

[41] Russo A, Stevens JE, Chen R, et al. Insulin-induced hypoglycemia accelerates gastric emptying of solids and liquids in long-standing type 1 diabetes. J Clin Endocrinol Metab 2005;90(8):4489–95.

[42] Takahashi T, Matsuda K, Kono T, et al. Inhibitory effects of hyperglycemia on neural activity of the vagus in rats. Intensive Care Med 2003;29(2):309–11.

[43] Mizuno Y, Oomura Y. Glucose responding neurons in the nucleus tractus solitarius of the rat: in vitro study. Brain Res 1984;307(1–2):109–16.

[44] Liu M, Seino S, Kirchgessner AL. Identification and characterization of glucoresponsive neurons in the enteric nervous system. J Neurosci 1999;19(23):10305–17.

[45] Yeap BB, Russo A, Fraser RJ, et al. Hyperglycemia affects cardiovascular autonomic nerve function in normal subjects. Diabetes Care 1996;19(8):880–2.
[46] Kong MF, King P, Macdonald IA, et al. Euglycaemic hyperinsulinaemia does not affect gastric emptying in type I and type II diabetes mellitus. Diabetologia 1999;42(3): 365–72.
[47] Nathan DM, Cleary PA, Backlund JY, et al. Intensive diabetes treatment and cardiovascular disease in patients with type 1 diabetes. N Engl J Med 2005;353(25): 2643–53.
[48] The Diabetes Control and Complications Trial [DCCT] Research Group. The effect of intensive treatment of diabetes on the development and progression of long-term complications in insulin-dependent diabetes mellitus. The diabetes control and complications trial research group. N Engl J Med 1993;329(14):977–86.
[49] UK Prospective Diabetes Study [UKPDS] Group. Intensive blood-glucose control with sulphonylureas or insulin compared with conventional treatment and risk of complications in patients with type 2 diabetes (UKPDS 33). UK Prospective Diabetes Study (UKPDS) Group. Lancet 1998;352(9131):837–53.
[50] Rayner CK, Horowitz M. Gastrointestinal motility and glycemic control in diabetes: the chicken and the egg revisited? J Clin Invest 2006;116(2):299–302.
[51] Monnier L, Lapinski H, Colette C. Contributions of fasting and postprandial plasma glucose increments to the overall diurnal hyperglycemia of type 2 diabetic patients: variations with increasing levels of HbA(1c). Diabetes Care 2003;26(3):881–5.
[52] Beisswenger P, Heine RJ, Leiter LA, et al. Prandial glucose regulation in the glucose triad: emerging evidence and insights. Endocrine 2004;25(3):195–202.
[53] Gerich JE. Clinical significance, pathogenesis, and management of postprandial hyperglycemia. Arch Intern Med 2003;163(11):1306–16.
[54] Bastyr EJ 3rd, Stuart CA, Brodows RG, et al. Therapy focused on lowering postprandial glucose, not fasting glucose, may be superior for lowering HbA1c. IOEZ Study Group. Diabetes Care 2000;23(9):1236–41.
[55] Jones KL, MacIntosh C, Su YC, et al. Guar gum reduces postprandial hypotension in older people. J Am Geriatr Soc 2001;49(2):162–7.
[56] Horowitz M, Jones KL, Rayner CK, et al. 'Gastric' hypoglycaemia—an important concept in diabetes management. Neurogastroenterol Motil 2006;18(6):405–7.
[57] Chandalia M, Garg A, Lutjohann D, et al. Beneficial effects of high dietary fiber intake in patients with type 2 diabetes mellitus. N Engl J Med 2000;342(19):1392–8.
[58] Gentilcore D, Chaikomin R, Jones KL, et al. Effects of fat on gastric emptying of, and the glycemic, insulin and incretin responses to, a carbohydrate meal in type 2 diabetes. J Clin Endocrinol Metab 2006;91(6):2062–7.
[59] Egan JM, Clocquet AR, Elahi D. The insulinotropic effect of acute exendin-4 administered to humans: comparison of nondiabetic state to type 2 diabetes. J Clin Endocrinol Metab 2002;87(3):1282–90.
[60] Nauck M. Therapeutic potential of glucagon-like peptide 1 in type 2 diabetes. Diabet Med 1996;13(9 Suppl 5):S39–43.
[61] Nauck MA, Meier JJ. Glucagon-like peptide 1 and its derivatives in the treatment of diabetes. Regul Pept 2005;128(2):135–48.
[62] Thompson RG, Gottlieb A, Organ K, et al. Pramlintide: a human amylin analogue reduced postprandial plasma glucose, insulin, and C-peptide concentrations in patients with type 2 diabetes. Diabet Med 1997;14(7):547–55.
[63] Schwartz JG, Guan D, Green GM, et al. Treatment with an oral proteinase inhibitor slows gastric emptying and acutely reduces glucose and insulin levels after a liquid meal in type II diabetic patients. Diabetes Care 1994;17(4):255–62.
[64] Phillips WT, Schwartz JG, McMahan CA. Reduced postprandial blood glucose levels in recently diagnosed non-insulin-dependent diabetics secondary to pharmacologically induced delayed gastric emptying. Dig Dis Sci 1993;38(1):51–8.

[65] Gonlachanvit S, Hsu CW, Boden GH, et al. Effect of altering gastric emptying on postprandial plasma glucose concentrations following a physiologic meal in type-II diabetic patients. Dig Dis Sci 2003;48(3):488–97.

[66] Firth M, Prather CM. Gastrointestinal motility problems in the elderly patient. Gastroenterology 2002;122(6):1688–700.

[67] Kupfer RM, Heppell M, Haggith JW, et al. Gastric emptying and small-bowel transit rate in the elderly. J Am Geriatr Soc 1985;33(5):340–3.

[68] Madsen JL, Graff J. Effects of ageing on gastrointestinal motor function. Age Ageing 2004; 33(2):154–9.

[69] Brogna A, Ferrara R, Bucceri AM, et al. Influence of aging on gastrointestinal transit time. An ultrasonographic and radiologic study. Invest Radiol 1999;34(5):357–9.

[70] Horowitz M, Maddern GJ, Chatterton BE, et al. Changes in gastric emptying rates with age. Clin Sci (Lond) 1984;67(2):213–8.

[71] Clarkston WK, Pantano MM, Morley JE, et al. Evidence for the anorexia of aging: gastrointestinal transit and hunger in healthy elderly vs. young adults. Am J Physiol 1997;272(1 Pt 2):R243–8.

[72] Evans MA, Triggs EJ, Cheung M, et al. Gastric emptying rate in the elderly: implications for drug therapy. J Am Geriatr Soc 1981;29(5):201–5.

[73] Nakae Y, Onouchi H, Kagaya M, et al. Effects of aging and gastric lipolysis on gastric emptying of lipid in liquid meal. J Gastroenterol 1999;34(4):445–9.

[74] Chassagne P, Capet C, Verdonck A, et al. Does age influence the gastric emptying of solids? Am J Gastroenterol 2003;98(7):1659–61.

[75] Kao CH, Lai TL, Wang SJ, et al. Influence of age on gastric emptying in healthy Chinese. Clin Nucl Med 1994;19(5):401–4.

[76] Moore JG, Tweedy C, Christian PE, et al. Effect of age on gastric emptying of liquid–solid meals in man. Dig Dis Sci 1983;28(4):340–4.

[77] O'Donovan D, Hausken T, Lei Y, et al. Effect of aging on transpyloric flow, gastric emptying, and intragastric distribution in healthy humans—impact on glycemia. Dig Dis Sci 2005;50(4):671–6.

[78] Cook CG, Andrews JM, Jones KL, et al. Effects of small intestinal nutrient infusion on appetite and pyloric motility are modified by age. Am J Physiol 1997;273(2 Pt 2):R755–61.

[79] MacIntosh CG, Andrews JM, Jones KL, et al. Effects of age on concentrations of plasma cholecystokinin, glucagon-like peptide 1, and peptide YY and their relation to appetite and pyloric motility. Am J Clin Nutr 1999;69(5):999–1006.

[80] Shimamoto C, Hirata I, Hiraike Y, et al. Evaluation of gastric motor activity in the elderly by electrogastrography and the (13)C-acetate breath test. Gerontology 2002;48(6):381–6.

[81] MacIntosh CG, Horowitz M, Verhagen MA, et al. Effect of small intestinal nutrient infusion on appetite, gastrointestinal hormone release, and gastric myoelectrical activity in young and older men. Am J Gastroenterol 2001;96(4):997–1007.

[82] Levanon D, Zhang M, Chen JD. Efficiency and efficacy of the electrogastrogram. Dig Dis Sci 1998;43(5):1023–30.

[83] Pfaffenbach B, Adamek RJ, Kuhn K, et al. Electrogastrography in healthy subjects. Evaluation of normal values, influence of age and gender. Dig Dis Sci 1995;40(7):1445–50.

[84] Sturm K, Parker B, Wishart J, et al. Energy intake and appetite are related to antral area in healthy young and older subjects. Am J Clin Nutr 2004;80(3):656–67.

[85] MacIntosh CG, Morley JE, Wishart J, et al. Effect of exogenous cholecystokinin (CCK)-8 on food intake and plasma CCK, leptin, and insulin concentrations in older and young adults: evidence for increased CCK activity as a cause of the anorexia of aging. J Clin Endocrinol Metab 2001;86(12):5830–7.

[86] Sturm K, MacIntosh CG, Parker BA, et al. Appetite, food intake, and plasma concentrations of cholecystokinin, ghrelin, and other gastrointestinal hormones in undernourished older women and well-nourished young and older women. J Clin Endocrinol Metab 2003;88(8):3747–55.

[87] Rayner CK, MacIntosh CG, Chapman IM, et al. Effects of age on proximal gastric motor and sensory function. Scand J Gastroenterol 2000;35(10):1041–7.

[88] Mitsukawa T, Takemura J, Nakazato M, et al. Effects of aging on plasma islet amyloid polypeptide basal level and response to oral glucose load. Diabetes Res Clin Pract 1992; 15(2):131–4.

[89] Rigamonti AE, Pincelli AI, Corra B, et al. Plasma ghrelin concentrations in elderly subjects: comparison with anorexic and obese patients. J Endocrinol 2002;175(1):R1–5.

[90] Parker BA, Chapman IM. Food intake and ageing—the role of the gut. Mech Ageing Dev 2004;125(12):859–66.

[91] Purnell JQ, Weigle DS, Breen P, et al. Ghrelin levels correlate with insulin levels, insulin resistance, and high-density lipoprotein cholesterol, but not with gender, menopausal status, or cortisol levels in humans. J Clin Endocrinol Metab 2003;88(12):5747–52.

[92] Cryer B, Redfern JS, Goldschmiedt M, et al. Effect of aging on gastric and duodenal mucosal prostaglandin concentrations in humans. Gastroenterology 1992;102(4 Pt 1): 1118–23.

[93] Feldman M, Cryer B. Effects of age on gastric alkaline and nonparietal fluid secretion in humans. Gerontology 1998;44(4):222–7.

[94] Feldman M, Cryer B, McArthur KE, et al. Effects of aging and gastritis on gastric acid and pepsin secretion in humans: a prospective study. Gastroenterology 1996;110(4):1043–52.

[95] Farinati F, Formentini S, Della Libera G, et al. Changes in parietal and mucous cell mass in the gastric mucosa of normal subjects with age: a morphometric study. Gerontology 1993; 39(3):146–51.

[96] Hackelsberger A, Platzer U, Nilius M, et al. Age and Helicobacter pylori decrease gastric mucosal surface hydrophobicity independently. Gut 1998;43(4):465–9.

[97] Lee M, Hardman WE, Cameron I. Age-related changes in gastric mucosal repair and proliferative activities in rats exposed acutely to aspirin. Gerontology 1998;44(4): 198–203.

[98] Lee M. Age-related changes in gastric blood flow in rats. Gerontology 1996;42(5):289–93.

[99] Goldschmiedt M, Barnett CC, Schwarz BE, et al. Effect of age on gastric acid secretion and serum gastrin concentrations in healthy men and women. Gastroenterology 1991;101(4): 977–90.

[100] Baron JH. Studies of basal and peak acid output with an augmented histamine test. Gut 1963;4:136–44.

[101] Blackman AH, Lambert DL, Thayer WR, et al. Computed normal values for peak acid output based on age, sex and body weight. Am J Dig Dis 1970;15(9):783–9.

[102] Grossman MI, Kirsner JB, Gillespie IE. Basal and histalog-stimulated gastric secretion in control subjects and in patients with peptic ulcer or gastric cancer. Gastroenterology 1963; 45:14–26.

[103] Kinoshita Y, Kawanami C, Kishi K, et al. Helicobacter pylori independent chronological change in gastric acid secretion in the Japanese. Gut 1997;41(4):452–8.

[104] Collen MJ, Abdulian JD, Chen YK. Age does not affect basal gastric acid secretion in normal subjects or in patients with acid-peptic disease. Am J Gastroenterol 1994;89(5): 712–6.

[105] Katelaris PH, Seow F, Lin BP, et al. Effect of age, Helicobacter pylori infection, and gastritis with atrophy on serum gastrin and gastric acid secretion in healthy men. Gut 1993;34(8):1032–7.

[106] Haruma K, Kamada T, Kawaguchi H, et al. Effect of age and Helicobacter pylori infection on gastric acid secretion. J Gastroenterol Hepatol 2000;15(3):277–83.

[107] Saltzman JR, Kowdley KV, Perrone G, et al. Changes in small-intestine permeability with aging. J Am Geriatr Soc 1995;43(2):160–4.

[108] Meciano Filho J, Carvalho VC, de Souza RR. Nerve cell loss in the myenteric plexus of the human esophagus in relation to age: a preliminary investigation. Gerontology 41(1):18–21.

[109] de Souza RR, Moratelli HB, Borges N, et al. Age-induced nerve cell loss in the myenteric plexus of the small intestine in man. Gerontology 1993;39(4):183–8.

[110] Gomes OA, de Souza RR, Liberti EA. A preliminary investigation of the effects of aging on the nerve cell number in the myenteric ganglia of the human colon. Gerontology 1997;43(4): 210–7.

[111] Saffrey MJ. Ageing of the enteric nervous system. Mech Ageing Dev 2004;125(12):899–906.

[112] Phillips RJ, Powley TL. As the gut ages: timetables for aging of innervation vary by organ in the Fischer 344 rat. J Comp Neurol 2001;434(3):358–77.

[113] Wiley JW. Aging and neural control of the GI tract: III. Senescent enteric nervous system: lessons from extraintestinal sites and nonmammalian species. Am J Physiol Gastrointest Liver Physiol 2002;283(5):G1020–6.

[114] Smits GJ, Lefebvre RA. Influence of age on responsiveness of rat gastric fundus to agonists and to stimulation of intrinsic nerves. Eur J Pharmacol 1992;223(1):97–102.

[115] Moller N, Gormsen L, Fuglsang J, et al. Effects of aging on insulin secretion and action. Horm Res 2003;60(Suppl 1):102–4.

[116] Meneilly GS, Ryan AS, Veldhuis JD, et al. Increased disorderliness of basal insulin release, attenuated insulin secretory burst mass, and reduced ultradian rhythmicity of insulin secretion in older individuals. J Clin Endocrinol Metab 1997;82(12):4088–93.

[117] Chang AM, Halter JB. Aging and insulin secretion. Am J Physiol Endocrinol Metab 2003; 284(1):E7–12.

[118] Chen M, Bergman RN, Pacini G, et al. Pathogenesis of age-related glucose intolerance in man: insulin resistance and decreased beta-cell function. J Clin Endocrinol Metab 1985; 60(1):13–20.

[119] Roder ME, Schwartz RS, Prigeon RL, et al. Reduced pancreatic B cell compensation to the insulin resistance of aging: impact on proinsulin and insulin levels. J Clin Endocrinol Metab 2000;85(6):2275–80.

[120] Jackson RA, Hawa MI, Roshania RD, et al. Influence of aging on hepatic and peripheral glucose metabolism in humans. Diabetes 1988;37(1):119–29.

[121] American Diabetes Association. Standards in Medical Care in Diabetes-2006. 2006.

[122] Bruce DG, Davis WA, Davis TM. Glycemic control in older subjects with type 2 diabetes mellitus in the Fremantle Diabetes Study. J Am Geriatr Soc 2000;48(11):1449–53.

[123] Porksen N. The in vivo regulation of pulsatile insulin secretion. Diabetologia 2002;45(1): 3–20.

[124] Ahren B, Pacini G. Age-related reduction in glucose elimination is accompanied by reduced glucose effectiveness and increased hepatic insulin extraction in man. J Clin Endocrinol Metab 1998;83(9):3350–6.

[125] Pacini G, Beccaro F, Valerio A, et al. Reduced beta-cell secretion and insulin hepatic extraction in healthy elderly subjects. J Am Geriatr Soc 1990;38(12):1283–9.

[126] Dechenes CJ, Verchere CB, Andrikopoulos S, et al. Human aging is associated with parallel reductions in insulin and amylin release. Am J Physiol 1998;275(5 Pt 1):E785–91.

[127] Fritsche A, Madaus A, Stefan N, et al. Relationships among age, proinsulin conversion, and beta-cell function in nondiabetic humans. Diabetes 2002;51(Suppl 1):S234–9.

[128] Gumbiner B, Polonsky KS, Beltz WF, et al. Effects of aging on insulin secretion. Diabetes 1989;38(12):1549–56.

[129] Scheen AJ, Sturis J, Polonsky KS, et al. Alterations in the ultradian oscillations of insulin secretion and plasma glucose in aging. Diabetologia 1996;39(5):564–72.

[130] Chiu KC, Lee NP, Cohan P, et al. Beta cell function declines with age in glucose tolerant Caucasians. Clin Endocrinol (Oxf) 2000;53(5):569–75.

[131] Meneilly GS, Veldhuis JD, Elahi D. Deconvolution analysis of rapid insulin pulses before and after six weeks of continuous subcutaneous administration of glucagon-like peptide-1 in elderly patients with type 2 diabetes. J Clin Endocrinol Metab 2005; 90(11):6251–6.

[132] Meneilly GS, Ryan AS, Minaker KL, et al. The effect of age and glycemic level on the response of the beta-cell to glucose-dependent insulinotropic polypeptide and peripheral tissue sensitivity to endogenously released insulin. J Clin Endocrinol Metab 1998;83(8): 2925–32.

[133] Meneilly GS, Demuth HU, McIntosh CH, et al. Effect of ageing and diabetes on glucose-dependent insulinotropic polypeptide and dipeptidyl peptidase IV responses to oral glucose. Diabet Med 2000;17(5):346–50.

[134] Elahi D, Andersen DK, Muller DC, et al. The enteric enhancement of glucose-stimulated insulin release. The role of GIP in aging, obesity, and non-insulin-dependent diabetes mellitus. Diabetes 1984;33(10):950–7.

[135] O'Meara NM, Sturis J, Van Cauter E, et al. Lack of control by glucose of ultradian insulin secretory oscillations in impaired glucose tolerance and in non-insulin-dependent diabetes mellitus. J Clin Invest 1993;92(1):262–71.

[136] Ferrannini E, Vichi S, Beck-Nielsen H, et al. Insulin action and age. European Group for the Study of Insulin Resistance (EGIR). Diabetes 1996;45(7):947–53.

[137] O'Shaughnessy IM, Kasdorf GM, Hoffmann RG, et al. Does aging intensify the insulin resistance of human obesity? J Clin Endocrinol Metab 1992;74(5):1075–81.

[138] Basu R, Breda E, Oberg AL, et al. Mechanisms of the age-associated deterioration in glucose tolerance: contribution of alterations in insulin secretion, action, and clearance. Diabetes 2003;52(7):1738–48.

[139] Pacini G, Valerio A, Beccaro F, et al. Insulin sensitivity and beta-cell responsivity are not decreased in elderly subjects with normal OGTT. J Am Geriatr Soc 1988;36(4):317–23.

[140] Boden G, Chen X, DeSantis RA, et al. Effects of age and body fat on insulin resistance in healthy men. Diabetes Care 1993;16(5):728–33.

[141] Coon PJ, Rogus EM, Drinkwater D, et al. Role of body fat distribution in the decline in insulin sensitivity and glucose tolerance with age. J Clin Endocrinol Metab 1992;75(4): 1125–32.

[142] Carey DG, Jenkins AB, Campbell LV, et al. Abdominal fat and insulin resistance in normal and overweight women: Direct measurements reveal a strong relationship in subjects at both low and high risk of NIDDM. Diabetes 1996;45(5):633–8.

[143] O'Shaughnessy IM, Myers TJ, Stepniakowski K, et al. Glucose metabolism in abdominally obese hypertensive and normotensive subjects. Hypertension 1995;26(1):186–92.

[144] Cefalu WT, Wang ZQ, Werbel S, et al. Contribution of visceral fat mass to the insulin resistance of aging. Metabolism 1995;44(7):954–9.

[145] Utzschneider KM, Carr DB, Hull RL, et al. Impact of intra-abdominal fat and age on insulin sensitivity and beta-cell function. Diabetes 2004;53(11):2867–72.

[146] Gabriely I, Ma XH, Yang XM, et al. Removal of visceral fat prevents insulin resistance and glucose intolerance of aging: an adipokine-mediated process? Diabetes 2002;51(10): 2951–8.

[147] Colombo M, Kruhoeffer M, Gregersen S, et al. Energy restriction prevents the development of type 2 diabetes in Zucker diabetic fatty rats: coordinated patterns of gene expression for energy metabolism in insulin-sensitive tissues and pancreatic islets determined by oligonucleotide microarray analysis. Metabolism 2006;55(1):43–52.

[148] Meneilly GS, Elahi D, Minaker KL, et al. Impairment of noninsulin-mediated glucose disposal in the elderly. J Clin Endocrinol Metab 1989;68(3):566–71.

[149] Petersen KF, Befroy D, Dufour S, et al. Mitochondrial dysfunction in the elderly: possible role in insulin resistance. Science 2003;300(5622):1140–2.

[150] Fulop T Jr, Nagy JT, Worum I, et al. Glucose intolerance and insulin resistance with aging—studies on insulin receptors and post-receptor events. Arch Gerontol Geriatr 1987; 6(2):107–15.

[151] Bunout D, Barrera G, de la Maza P, et al. Seasonal variation in insulin sensitivity in healthy elderly people. Nutrition 2003;19(4):310–6.

[152] Gravholt CH, Holck P, Nyholm B, et al. No seasonal variation of insulin sensitivity and glucose effectiveness in men. Metabolism 2000;49(1):32–8.

[153] Chiu KC, Chu A, Go VL, et al. Hypovitaminosis D is associated with insulin resistance and beta cell dysfunction. Am J Clin Nutr 2004;79(5):820–5.

[154] Meneilly GS, Elahi D. Metabolic alterations in middle-aged and elderly lean patients with type 2 diabetes. Diabetes Care 2005;28(6):1498–9.

[155] Meneilly GS, Elliott T, Tessier D, et al. NIDDM in the elderly. Diabetes Care 1996;19(12): 1320–5.

[156] Kim J, Choi S, Kong B, et al. Insulin secretion and sensitivity during oral glucose tolerance test in Korean lean elderly women. J Korean Med Sci 2001;16(5):592–7.

[157] Juneja R, Palmer JP. Type 1 1/2 diabetes: myth or reality? Autoimmunity 1999;29(1):65–83.

[158] Arner P, Pollare T, Lithell H. Different aetiologies of type 2 (non-insulin-dependent) diabetes mellitus in obese and non-obese subjects. Diabetologia 1991;34(7):483–7.

[159] Chan WB, Tong PC, Chow CC, et al. The associations of body mass index, C-peptide and metabolic status in Chinese Type 2 diabetic patients. Diabet Med 2004;21(4):349–53.

[160] Tentolouris N, Grapsas E, Stambulis E, et al. Impact of body mass on autonomic function in persons with type 2 diabetes. Diabetes Res Clin Pract 1999;46(1):29–33.

[161] Straub RH, Thum M, Hollerbach C, et al. Impact of obesity on neuropathic late complications in NIDDM. Diabetes Care 1994;17(11):1290–4.

[162] Arvanitakis Z, Wilson RS, Li Y, et al. Diabetes and function in different cognitive systems in older individuals without dementia. Diabetes Care 2006;29(3):560–5.

[163] Hassing LB, Hofer SM, Nilsson SE, et al. Comorbid type 2 diabetes mellitus and hypertension exacerbates cognitive decline: evidence from a longitudinal study. Age Ageing 2004;33(4):355–61.

[164] Peila R, Rodriguez BL, Launer LJ. Type 2 diabetes, APOE gene, and the risk for dementia and related pathologies: The Honolulu-Asia Aging Study. Diabetes 2002;51(4):1256–62.

[165] Messier C. Impact of impaired glucose tolerance and type 2 diabetes on cognitive aging. Neurobiol Aging 2005;26(Suppl 1):26–30.

[166] Wu JH, Haan MN, Liang J, et al. Impact of antidiabetic medications on physical and cognitive functioning of older Mexican Americans with diabetes mellitus: a population-based cohort study. Ann Epidemiol 2003;13(5):369–76.

[167] Messier C, Desrochers A, Gagnon M. Effect of glucose, glucose regulation, and word imagery value on human memory. Behav Neurosci 1999;113(3):431–8.

[168] Gradman TJ, Laws A, Thompson LW, et al. Verbal learning and/or memory improves with glycemic control in older subjects with non-insulin-dependent diabetes mellitus. J Am Geriatr Soc 1993;41(12):1305–12.

[169] Meneilly GS, Cheung E, Tessier D, et al. The effect of improved glycemic control on cognitive functions in the elderly patient with diabetes. J Gerontol 1993;48(4): M117–21.

[170] Mussell M, Hewer W, Kulzer B, et al. Effects of improved glycaemic control maintained for 3 months on cognitive function in patients with Type 2 diabetes. Diabet Med 2004;21(11): 1253–6.

[171] Abbatecola AM, Rizzo MR, Barbieri M, et al. Postprandial plasma glucose excursions and cognitive functioning in aged type 2 diabetics. Neurology 2006;67(2):235–40.

[172] Araki Y, Nomura M, Tanaka H, et al. MRI of the brain in diabetes mellitus. Neuroradiology 1994;36(2):101–3.

[173] den Heijer T, Vermeer SE, van Dijk EJ, et al. Type 2 diabetes and atrophy of medial temporal lobe structures on brain MRI. Diabetologia 2003;46(12):1604–10.

[174] Park SW, Goodpaster BH, Strotmeyer ES, et al. Decreased muscle strength and quality in older adults with type 2 diabetes: the health, aging, and body composition study. Diabetes 2006;55(6):1813–8.

[175] Nimmo WS. Drugs, diseases and altered gastric emptying. Clin Pharmacokinet 1976;1(3): 189–203.

[176] Lamy PP. Comparative pharmacokinetic changes and drug therapy in an older population. J Am Geriatr Soc 1982;30(Suppl 11):S11–9.

[177] Groop LC, Luzi L, DeFronzo RA, et al. Hyperglycaemia and absorption of sulphonylurea drugs. Lancet 1989;2(8655):129–30.

[178] Nimmo WS, Heading RC, Wilson J, et al. Inhibition of gastric emptying and drug absorption by narcotic analgesics. Br J Clin Pharmacol 1975;2(6):509–13.

[179] Gainsborough N, Maskrey VL, Nelson ML, et al. The association of age with gastric emptying. Age Ageing 1993;22(1):37–40.

[180] Divoll M, Ameer B, Abernethy DR, et al. Age does not alter acetaminophen absorption. J Am Geriatr Soc 1982;30(4):240–4.

[181] Divoll M, Greenblatt DJ, Ameer B, et al. Effect of food on acetaminophen absorption in young and elderly subjects. J Clin Pharmacol 1982;22(11–12):571–6.

[182] Kay L. Prevalence, incidence and prognosis of gastrointestinal symptoms in a random sample of an elderly population. Age Ageing 1994;23(2):146–9.

[183] Talley NJ, Evans JM, Fleming KC, et al. Nonsteroidal antiinflammatory drugs and dyspepsia in the elderly. Dig Dis Sci 1995;40(6):1345–50.

[184] O'Riordan TG, Tobin A, O'Morain C. Helicobacter pylori infection in elderly dyspeptic patients. Age Ageing 1991;20(3):189–92.

[185] Merle L, Laroche ML, Dantoine T, et al. Predicting and preventing adverse drug reactions in the very old. Drugs Aging 2005;22(5):375–92.

[186] Chiasson JL, Josse RG, Gomis R, et al. Acarbose for prevention of type 2 diabetes mellitus: the STOP-NIDDM randomised trial. Lancet 2002;359(9323):2072–7.

[187] Knowler WC, Barrett-Connor E, Fowler SE, et al. Reduction in the incidence of type 2 diabetes with lifestyle intervention or metformin. N Engl J Med 2002; 346(6):393–403.

[188] Meyer KA, Kushi LH, Jacobs DR Jr, et al. Carbohydrates, dietary fiber, and incident type 2 diabetes in older women. Am J Clin Nutr 2000;71(4):921–30.

[189] Kim HJ, Lee JS, Kim CK. Effect of exercise training on muscle glucose transporter 4 protein and intramuscular lipid content in elderly men with impaired glucose tolerance. Eur J Appl Physiol 2004;93(3):353–8.

[190] Franz MJ, Bantle JP, Beebe CA, et al. Evidence-based nutrition principles and recommendations for the treatment and prevention of diabetes and related complications. Diabetes Care 2002;25(1):148–98.

[191] Sigal RJ, Kenny GP, Wasserman DH, et al. Physical activity/exercise and type 2 diabetes: a consensus statement from the American Diabetes Association. Diabetes Care 2006;29(6): 1433–8.

[192] Pontiroli AE, Calderara A, Pacchioni M, et al. Insulin requirement in elderly patients with non-insulin dependent diabetes mellitus (NIDDM). Aging (Milano) 1989;1(2):147–52.

[193] Schwartz AV, Hillier TA, Sellmeyer DE, et al. Older women with diabetes have a higher risk of falls: a prospective study. Diabetes Care 2002;25(10):1749–54.

[194] Schwartz AV, Sellmeyer DE, Ensrud KE, et al. Older women with diabetes have an increased risk of fracture: a prospective study. J Clin Endocrinol Metab 2001;86(1): 32–8.

[195] Matyka K, Evans M, Lomas J, et al. Altered hierarchy of protective responses against severe hypoglycemia in normal aging in healthy men. Diabetes Care 1997;20(2): 135–41.

[196] Oiknine R, Mooradian AD. Drug therapy of diabetes in the elderly. Biomed Pharmacother 2003;57(5–6):231–9.

[197] Meneilly GS, Greig N, Tildesley H, et al. Effects of 3 months of continuous subcutaneous administration of glucagon-like peptide 1 in elderly patients with type 2 diabetes. Diabetes Care 2003;26(10):2835–41.

[198] Meneilly GS, McIntosh CH, Pederson RA, et al. Glucagon-like peptide-1 (7–37) augments insulin release in elderly patients with diabetes. Diabetes Care 2001;24(5):964–5.

[199] Meneilly GS, McIntosh CH, Pederson RA, et al. Effect of glucagon-like peptide 1 on non-insulin-mediated glucose uptake in the elderly patient with diabetes. Diabetes Care 2001;24(11):1951–6.

[200] Edwards CM, Stanley SA, Davis R, et al. Exendin-4 reduces fasting and postprandial glucose and decreases energy intake in healthy volunteers. Am J Physiol Endocrinol Metab 2001;281(1):E155–61.

[201] Kolterman OG, Buse JB, Fineman MS, et al. Synthetic exendin-4 (exenatide) significantly reduces postprandial and fasting plasma glucose in subjects with type 2 diabetes. J Clin Endocrinol Metab 2003;88(7):3082–9.

[202] Meneilly GS, McIntosh CH, Pederson RA, et al. Glucagon-like peptide-1 (7–37) augments insulin-mediated glucose uptake in elderly patients with diabetes. J Gerontol A Biol Sci Med Sci 2001;56(11):M681–5.

[203] Knop FK, Vilsboll T, Larsen S, et al. No hypoglycemia after subcutaneous administration of glucagon-like peptide-1 in lean type 2 diabetic patients and in patients with diabetes secondary to chronic pancreatitis. Diabetes Care 2003;26(9):2581–7.

[204] Linnebjerg H, Kothare PA, Skrivanek Z, et al. Exenatide: effect of injection time on postprandial glucose in patients with Type 2 diabetes. Diabet Med 2006;23(3):240–5.

[205] Nauck MA, Niedereichholz U, Ettler R, et al. Glucagon-like peptide 1 inhibition of gastric emptying outweighs its insulinotropic effects in healthy humans. Am J Physiol 1997; 273(5 Pt 1):E981–8.

[206] O'Donovan D, Feinle-Bisset C, Jones K, et al. Idiopathic and Diabetic Gastroparesis. Curr Treat Options Gastroenterol 2003;6(4):299–309.

[207] Crowell MD, Mathis C, Schettler VA, et al. The effects of tegaserod, a 5-HT receptor agonist, on gastric emptying in a murine model of diabetes mellitus. Neurogastroenterol Motil 2005;17(5):738–43.

[208] Asakawa H, Hayashi I, Fukui T, et al. Effect of mosapride on glycemic control and gastric emptying in type 2 diabetes mellitus patients with gastropathy. Diabetes Res Clin Pract 2003;61(3):175–82.

[209] Murray CD, Martin NM, Patterson M, et al. Ghrelin enhances gastric emptying in diabetic gastroparesis: a double blind, placebo controlled, crossover study. Gut 2005;54(12):1693–8.

[210] Mansi C, Savarino V, Vigneri S, et al. Gastrokinetic effects of levosulpiride in dyspeptic patients with diabetic gastroparesis. Am J Gastroenterol 1995;90(11):1989–93.

[211] Melga P, Mansi C, Ciuchi E, et al. Chronic administration of levosulpiride and glycemic control in IDDM patients with gastroparesis. Diabetes Care 1997;20(1):55–8.

[212] Bromer MQ, Friedenberg F, Miller LS, et al. Endoscopic pyloric injection of botulinum toxin A for the treatment of refractory gastroparesis. Gastrointest Endosc 2005;61(7):833–9.

[213] Forster J, Sarosiek I, Lin Z, et al. Further experience with gastric stimulation to treat drug refractory gastroparesis. Am J Surg 2003;186(6):690–5.

[214] Lin Z, Forster J, Sarosiek I, et al. Treatment of diabetic gastroparesis by high-frequency gastric electrical stimulation. Diabetes Care 2004;27(5):1071–6.

[215] Lin Z, Sarosiek I, Forster J, et al. Symptom responses, long-term outcomes and adverse events beyond 3 years of high-frequency gastric electrical stimulation for gastroparesis. Neurogastroenterol Motil 2006;18(1):18–27.

[216] van der Voort IR, Becker JC, Dietl KH, et al. Gastric electrical stimulation results in improved metabolic control in diabetic patients suffering from gastroparesis. Exp Clin Endocrinol Diabetes 2005;113(1):38–42.

[217] Tonini M, De Ponti F, Di Nucci A, et al. Review article: cardiac adverse effects of gastrointestinal prokinetics. Aliment Pharmacol Ther 1999;13(12):1585–91.

[218] Edelbroek MA, Horowitz M, Wishart JM, et al. Effects of erythromycin on gastric emptying, alcohol absorption and small intestinal transit in normal subjects. J Nucl Med 1993;34(4):582–8.

CLINICS IN
GERIATRIC
MEDICINE

ELSEVIER
SAUNDERS

Clin Geriatr Med 23 (2007) 809–821

Inflammatory Bowel Diseases in the Elderly

Prabhakar P. Swaroop, MD

*Division of Digestive and Liver Diseases, Department of Internal Medicine,
UT Southwestern Medical Center, 5323 Harry Hines Boulevard,
Dallas, TX 75390-8887, USA*

Epidemiology

Although inflammatory bowel diseases (IBDs) were initially described in young adults, experts now know that elderly individuals are also at risk for developing this disorder for the first time in their 60s and 70s. Several population-based studies worldwide describe incidence, prevalence, and other demographic factors associated with this risk, including age, gender, race, and geographic distribution [1–6]. As the current population of patients who have IBD is aging, the population of elderly who have IBD is expected to increase. This population increase is in addition to the individuals who are diagnosed with IBD for the first time as they grow old. Bimodal distribution of this disease has been commonly reported, but several studies have failed to show this pattern. Studies have shown that 10% to 15% of cases of IBD are diagnosed in patients aged 60 years or older [7].

In several recent epidemiologic studies, the traditional bimodal distribution of IBD was not uniformly seen. Gender-related differences in late-onset disease was apparent, with men having a higher risk for diagnosis in the fifth and sixth decades of life. Several recent studies have described alterations in gut flora in elderly individuals, which was especially apparent with reduction in putatively protective bifidobacteria [8,9]. A higher proportion of enterobacteria was also described in the flora of elderly volunteers irrespective of geographic location [10]. In other studies examining the bacterial flora in patients who have Crohn's disease, enterobacteria were found to be significantly increased in active and quiescent Crohn's disease [11,12].

E-mail address: prabhakar.swaroop@utsouthwestern.edu

0749-0690/07/$ - see front matter. Published by Elsevier Inc.
doi:10.1016/j.cger.2007.06.007   *geriatric.theclinics.com*

Clinical manifestations

Although ulcerative colitis and Crohn's disease are generally accepted as two distinct clinical syndromes, these conditions in fact represent a spectrum of diseases. Currently, no diagnostic test, including histopathology, serology, and clinical behavior, has been established as a gold standard. The behavior of ulcerative colitis and Crohn's disease in the elderly population is similar to that observed in younger populations. A recent publication from Japan described a change in clinical characteristic of ulcerative colitis based on analysis of 844 hospital-based patients from 1981 to 2000. The proportion of mild colitis and proctitis was significantly larger in patients who experienced onset at older than 60 years, relative to those who experienced onset at younger than 30 years ($P<.016$). The proportion of patients who experienced onset at older age ($P = .09$); were male ($P<.01$); had mild colitis ($P<.01$), proctitis ($P<.01$), or one-attack-only type ($P<.01$); and were not treated with corticosteroid ($P<.01$) showed a chronologic increase from 1981 to 2000 [13]. As with younger population, the full clinical spectrum of ulcerative colitis can be seen in the elderly, including extraintestinal manifestations. Because elderly people may have coexisting conditions that may mask or mimic the clinical symptoms of ulcerative colitis (eg, ischemic colitis, diverticular bleeding, diverticulitis) and increased incidence of infections such as *Clostridium difficile* colitis, care must be taken to make a correct diagnosis. In patients who have longstanding colonic inflammation caused by ulcerative colitis, Crohn's disease, or indeterminate colitis, a lower prevalence of colonic diverticuli has also been noticed [14].

Differential diagnosis

Because elderly individuals tend to have additional comorbid conditions, several other causes of gastrointestinal symptoms should be considered and ruled out. Infections (eg, shigella, salmonella, clostridium, *Yersinia enterocolitica*, viruses such as cytomegalovirus and parasites, *Escherichia coli* O157:H7, *Klebsiella oxytoca*), diverticular diseases, radiation-induced colitis, nonsteroidal anti-inflammatory drug–induced colitis, other drug-induced colitis (eg, gold compounds, estrogens, 5-flucytosine, methyldopa, ticlopidine, sodium phosphate enemas, penicillamine, sulfasalazine), ischemic colitis, and colorectal cancer should be included in the differential diagnosis.

Workup of patients presenting with signs and symptoms of IBD should begin with a careful history, including family history of IBD, comorbid conditions, drug history, and history of prior radiation therapy. Stool culture and fecal analysis of *C difficile* toxin, specific assays for *E coli* O157:H7, and serologic testing for amoeba should be requested when clinical suspicion is high.

Endoscopic examination (proctosigmoidoscopy or colonoscopy) will show changes characteristic of IBD, including erythema, ulcerations, loss of vascularity, granulation, or pseudopolyp formation. Biopsies obtained from these examinations can be used in conjunction with clinical features to establish diagnosis [15]. Other diagnostic modalities include capsule enteroscopy, radiologic evaluation (eg, small bowel series, endoscopic ultrasound, CT enterography, MRI), and serology (eg, ASCA, Anti-Saccharomyces Cerevisiae Antibody; OmpC, Outer membrane porin Protein C; CBir1, Anti-flagellin antibody; pANCA, Perinuclear anti-neutrophil cytoplasmic antibody).

Treatment options

Treatment options for the elderly are essentially the same as those for the younger population, and may involve the use of high-dose steroids, amino-salicylates in various formulations, immunomodulators (eg, azathioprine, 6-mercaptopurine, methotrexate, cyclosporine), various biologic agents, and surgery.

The choice of specific agents depends on several factors, including

- Location of inflammation (terminal ileum, rest of the small bowel, colonic or inflammation involving both small bowel and the colon)
- Disease behavior (inflammation, stricture, penetrating)
- Degree of inflammatory response
- Extraintestinal manifestations
- Comorbid conditions
- Use of the other concomitant medications
- Symptoms of the patients

Advancements in understanding the pathophysiology of IBD have recently made interrupting the inflammatory cascade possible.

The goal of treatment should include

- Induction of remission
- Maintenance of remission
- Prevention of recurrence
- Improvement of quality of life
- Avoidance of complications from the disease and treatment

With these in mind, treatment plans should be individually tailored. The following sections summarize the treatment options available.

Corticosteroids

Corticosteroids as oral, parenteral, and topical agents have been used for several decades to treat IBD [16,17]. Budesonide, a poorly absorbed cortico-steroid that has high first-pass metabolism was recently approved to treat ileocecal and right colonic Crohn's disease (grade A) [18,19]. Use of oral ste-roids such as prednisone is reserved for patients who have undergone failed therapy with mesalamine or budesonide. Corticosteroids are effective in controlling the inflammatory response seen in Crohn's disease and ulcerative colitis (grade A); however, their efficacy is inadequate in patients who have fistulizing disease and therefore they should not be used in patients who have fistulae (grade B) [20–23].

Intravenous corticosteroids can be used in hospitalized patients whose disease does not respond to oral corticosteroids. Corticosteroids are not effective in maintaining remission in patients who have ulcerative colitis and Crohn's disease (grade A). In some patients who have mild to moderate ileocolonic Crohn's disease, budesonide may be used for maintenance up to 3 months (grade A) [19].

When patients are treated with corticosteroids, care must be taken to minimize the potential of adverse effects, namely loss of bone mineral density, hyperglycemia, infectious complications, adrenal suppression, and hypertension (grade B) [24–26]. Elderly patients are vulnerable to accelerated bone loss and changes in mental status, and therefore corticosteroids should be tapered as quickly as possible, ideally within 8 to 10 weeks.

Elderly patients taking long-term corticosteroids should undergo baseline assessment of bone density (grade A) [27], and use of bisphosphonate should be considered (grade A) [28,29] along with vitamin D and calcium supplementation.

Azathioprine and 6-mercaptopurine

Azathioprine (AZA) and 6-mercaptopurine (6MP) are thiopurine analogs and should be considered for patients who are corticosteroid-dependent or have required frequent treatment with corticosteroids. A recent study also showed that these agents reduced the risk for postsurgical recurrence of Cohn's disease [30]. Before initiating therapy with these agents, thiopurine methyltransferase genotype or enzyme activity should be measured to detect patients who have either intermediate or null activity of this enzyme (grade B) [31–34]. Patients who are heterozygotes (or have full enzyme activity) should be considered for therapy with AZA 2.0 to 3.0 mg/kg/d or 6MP 1.0 to 1.5 mg/kg/d. Patients who experience intermediate activity should be started on half the dosage, and patients who experience low or no activity should not be started on AZA or 6MP (grade B). When initiating therapy or during dosage adjustment, complete blood count and liver function tests should be performed at least every 2 weeks and then at least every 3 months (grade B) when the patient is on stable dosage of medication [35–37]. Combining immunomodulators with infliximab can be an effective option in patients who have required frequent introduction of corticosteroids (grade A) [37,38].

Thiopurine metabolites should also be monitored. 6-Thioguanine and 6-methyl mercaptopurine can be measured to ensure compliance, optimize the dosage, or predict either hepatotoxicity or myelosuppression. Elevated levels of 6-thioguanine has been associated with the likelihood of response and myelotoxicity. Elevated levels of 6-methyl mercaptopurine are associated with the risk for abnormal liver function tests (grade B) [35].

Methotrexate

Methotrexate is another immunosuppressive agent, which can be administered intramuscularly or subcutaneously. In 2000, Feagan and colleagues [39] reported its efficacy in inducing remission in patients who had steroid-dependent and steroid-refractory Crohn's disease. Parenteral methotrexate is recommended to induce and maintain remission of active Crohn's disease (grade B) [40,41]. Its role in the management of ulcerative colitis is unclear because of the lack of evidence showing its efficacy [42]. Again, routine monitoring of complete blood count and liver function tests are recommended (grade B).

5-Aminosalicylates

5-Aminosalicylates are used in patients who have mild to moderate disease activity and are available in both oral and topical formulations. However, oral formulations are essentially topical in nature, because through varying the mechanism of delivery, specific portions of small bowel and colon can be reached. Commonly used aminosalicylates include sulfasalazine, olsalazine, mesalamine, and balsalazide. The decision to use one formulation depends on the extent of disease and tolerability. In patients whose extent of inflammation is limited to the rectum or sigmoid region, topical therapy with mesalamine enema may be able to induce remission. Good evidence shows a role for 5- aminosalicylate compounds in the induction and maintenance of remission of ulcerative colitis, and the response seems to be dose-dependent (grade A) [43–46].

A new formulation of mesalamine with MMX technology was recently approved by the US Food and Drug Administration for the induction of remission in mild to moderate ulcerative colitis (LIALDA mesalamine with MMX technology, Shire Pharmaceuticals Inc., Wayne, Pennsylvania). A significantly greater proportion of patients receiving MMX mesalamine 2.4 g/d given once daily (40.5%; $P = .01$) and 4.8 g/d given once daily (41.2%; $P = .007$) experienced clinical and endoscopic remission at week 8 compared with those receiving placebo (22.1%) [47]. This formulation offers a convenient once-a-day dosage, possibly enhancing patient adherence (Table 1). Topical mesalamine preparations include Canasa suppositories (Axcan Pharma, Birmingham, Alabama) and mesalamine enemas.

In the treatment of postoperative Crohn's disease, mesalamine has not been consistently effective and its overall benefit has been minimal. A meta-analysis of 15 studies performed in 1997 showed that therapy with mesalamine significantly reduced the risk for symptomatic relapse (pooled risk

Table 1
Formulations of oral 5-aminosalicylates

Formulation	Dosage
Azulfidine (sulfasalazine)	3–6 g/d in three to six doses
Asacol (mesalamine)	Two 400-mg tablets tid
Pentasa (mesalamine)	1 g qid
Colazal (balsalazide)	Three 750-mg capsules tid
Dipentum (olsalazine)	1 g bid
Lialda (mesalamine)	Two to four 1.2-g tablets sid

difference, -6.3%; 95% CI, -10.4% to -2.1%). The pooled risk difference was significant in the postsurgical setting (-13.1%; 95% CI, -21.8% to -4.5%) but not the medical setting (-4.7%; 95% CI, -9.6% to 2.8%) [48]. In another study, oral mesalamine at 4 g/d for postoperative maintenance showed no efficacy [49]. Several other studies have shown small differences between placebo and mesalamine in reducing Crohn's disease activity index [50,51]. Based on these and several other studies, the role of mesalamine in inducing and maintaining remission of Crohn's disease is minimal (grade A).

Antibiotics

Commonly used antibiotics in the treatment of Crohn's disease are metronidazole, ciprofloxacin, clarithromycin, and rifaximin. The role of antibiotics in treating ulcerative colitis is very minimal except in the setting of infectious complications [52]. However, a recent long-term follow-up study showed that a 2-week antibiotic combination therapy against *Fusobacterium varium* was effective and safe in patients who had chronic active ulcerative colitis [53]. The role of antibiotics in Crohn's disease has been established in fistulizing manifestation, but controlled trials do not consistently show efficacy in mildly to moderately and severely active disease. In a controlled trial to prevent recurrence after ileal resection, metronidazole therapy statistically reduced the clinical recurrence rates at 1 year (4% versus 25%). Reductions at 2 years (26% versus 43%) and 3 years (30% versus 50%) were not significant [54].

Although antibiotics are traditionally used to treat perianal Crohn's disease, no randomized controlled trials examine the effects of ciprofloxacin and metronidazole. The recommendation is based on reports of case series (grade B) [55–57]. Rifaximin, a novel nonabsorbable antibiotic, was also studied in a recently published multicenter, double-blind, randomized, placebo-controlled trial in mildly to moderately active Crohn's disease. Although the difference between the placebo and rifaximin arms did not reach statistical difference, more patients in the placebo group underwent failed treatment than those who received rifaximin 800 mg twice a day [58].

Infliximab

Infliximab is a chimeric monoclonal antibody to human tumor necrosis factor (TNF) α and is approved for use in Crohn's disease and ulcerative colitis. It is recommended for patients who have Crohn's disease who have not experienced satisfactory clinical response from adequate therapy with conventional agents and for those who have fistulizing Crohn's disease. Those who respond to induction therapy should undergo maintenance therapy (grade A) [37,38,59–62]. Patients who have active ulcerative colitis who have not achieved satisfactory clinical response to conventional therapy and maintenance should be considered for treatment with infliximab (grade A) [63–65].

For induction, infliximab is recommended to be started as an intravenous infusion over 2 hours at the dosage of 5 mg per kilogram of body weight, and three induction dosages should be administered at weeks 0, 2, and 6. This treatment should be followed by a maintenance therapy of infliximab at 5 mg per kg of body weight every 8 weeks. In patients who lose response, the dosage should be increased to 10 mg per kilogram of body weight or the interval reduced to every 6 weeks, depending on the clinical response.

For patients who have fistulizing Crohn's disease, care must be taken to exclude abscess. Screening for latent and active tuberculosis should be performed before the outset of therapy and repeated every year. Infliximab should be avoided in patients who have active infections, demyelinating disorders, known hypersensitivity to infliximab, severe congestive heart failure, or current or recent malignancy.

Adalimumab

Adalimumab is a recombinant, fully human immunoglobulin G1 monoclonal antibody targeting TNF. Several recent studies examined its role in induction and maintenance of remission. It seems to be well tolerated and to be a clinically beneficial option for patients who have Crohn's disease who have previously lost their response to or cannot tolerate infliximab [66]. It also seems to induce and maintain remission more effectively than placebo in patients who have Crohn's disease [67–69].

Certolizumab

Certolizumab is a polyethylene glycolated Fab fragment of humanized anti–TNF monoclonal antibody. It has also undergone several trials, but its efficacy may have been masked by high response rates in the placebo group. Post hoc analysis of patients who had C-reactive protein greater than 10 mg/L showed a clearer separation between active treatment and placebo (week 12 clinical response: certolizumab 400 mg, 53.1%; placebo, 17.9%; $P = .005$) owing to lower placebo response rate than patients who had C-reactive protein levels of less than 10 mg/L [70].

Colorectal cancer

Longstanding IBD increases the risk for gastrointestinal malignancies, especially colorectal cancer. Colorectal cancer associated with IBD accounts for 1% to 2% of all cases of colorectal cancer but is responsible for up to 15% of deaths in patients who have IBD [71]. Risk factors for colorectal cancer in patients who have IBD have been traditionally described to be extent of inflammation and duration of disease. In a Veteran's Administration (VA) hospital–based study, occurrence of colorectal cancer in patients who had IBD was found to be influenced by age (odds ratio [OR], 1.45; 95% CI, 1.35–1.57), sclerosing cholangitis (OR, 3.41; 95% CI, 2.03–5.73), and history of a disease associated with consumption of nonsteroidal anti-inflammatory drugs (OR, 0.84; 95% CI, 0.65–1.09). Presence of IBD was not associated with a significant influence on colorectal cancer mortality [72]. Retrospective correlative studies have suggested that 5-aminosalicylate and folic acid may reduce the risk for colorectal cancer in patients who have longstanding IBD [73–75].

Although patients who have IBD have a similar colorectal cancer prognosis to patients who have sporadic colorectal cancers [76], a recent study by Larsen and colleagues [77] showed that Crohn's disease may worsen the prognosis of colorectal cancer, particularly when regional spread is present.

Newer modalities, including chromoendoscopy with indigo carmine or methylene blue, high-magnification chromoscopic colonoscopy, narrow-band imaging, and confocal endomicroscopy, are promising to enhance detection of dysplastic lesions, especially flat low-grade dysplasia [78,79]. Regardless of these new technologies, the current recommendation is to perform annual colonoscopies with random biopsies after 8 to 10 years of ulcerative colitis (grade B). Multiple biopsies should be obtained from every 10 cm, except in the rectosigmoid region where they should be obtained from every 5 cm (grade B) [80–82].

If colorectal cancer is found, colectomy is recommended. Dysplasia in ulcerative colitis may be classified as flat or elevated (dysplasia-associated lesion or mass). Findings of high-grade dysplasia in flat mucosa often indicate concurrent or future risk for cancer. In these cases, total colectomy can be recommended (grade B). A meta-analysis examining the outcomes showed that when low-grade dysplasia is detected on surveillance, patients have a 9-fold risk for developing cancer (OR, 9.0; 95% CI, 4.0–20.5) and 12-fold risk for developing any advanced lesion (OR, 11.9; 95% CI, 5.2–27) [83]. Because of the high risk for flat low-grade dysplasia to progress into advanced neoplasia, total colectomy should also be considered in these patients (grade B) [84]. The clinical distinction between polypoid dysplastic lesions associated with chronic ulcerative colitis and sporadic adenomas is important, because the former is an indication for colectomy, whereas the latter is usually treated with simple polypectomy. Recent data suggest that adenoma-like lesions, regardless of the grade of dysplasia or the location of the lesion (eg, inside or outside areas of established colitis), may be treated adequately with polypectomy if the patient has no other areas of flat dysplasia [85–87].

In a study examining predominantly male patients older than 50 years at VA hospitals who required surgery for ulcerative colitis, the mean duration of disease was 23 years, with indications for elective surgery being intractability (59%), mass or stricture (27%), and dysplasia (14%) [88]. Elderly patients who have IBD have an increased rate of postoperative complications along with increased hospital stay and operating room time. This effect of age persisted when adjusted for comorbidity and immunosuppressive therapy. Complications are most dependent on surgical indications, with obstruction being the least and bleeding the worst predictive factors [89], whereas a few other studies did not find age to be a particular risk factor for mortality, postsurgical anastomotic leaks, or intra-abdominal sepsis [90,91].

References

[1] Halme L, von Smitten K, Husa A. The incidence of Crohn's disease in the Helsinki metropolitan area during 1975–1985. Ann Chir Gynaecol 1989;78:115–9.
[2] Gower-Rousseau C, Salomez JL, Dupas JL, et al. Incidence of inflammatory bowel disease in northern France (1988–1990). Gut 1994;35:1433–8.
[3] Abdul-Baki H, Elhajj I, El-Zahabi LM, et al. Clinical epidemiology of inflammatory bowel disease in Lebanon. Inflamm Bowel Dis 2007 Apr;13(4):475–80.
[4] Jess T, Riis L, Vind I, et al. Changes in clinical characteristics, course, and prognosis of inflammatory bowel disease during the last 5 decades: a population-based study from Copenhagen, Denmark. Inflamm Bowel Dis 2007 Apr;13(4):481–9.
[5] Lakatos PL. Recent trends in the epidemiology of inflammatory bowel diseases: up or down? World J Gastroenterol 2006;12(38):6102–8.
[6] Hanauer SB. Inflammatory bowel disease: epidemiology, pathogenesis, and therapeutic opportunities. Inflamm Bowel Dis 2006;12(Suppl 1):S3–9.
[7] Softley A, Myren J, Clamp SE, et al. Inflammatory bowel disease in the elderly patient. Scand J Gastroenterol Suppl 1988;144:27–30.
[8] Hopkins MJ, Sharp R, Macfarlane GT. Age and disease related changes in intestinal bacterial populations assessed by cell culture, 16S rRNA abundance, and community cellular fatty acid profiles. Gut 2001;48(2):198–205.
[9] Bartosch S, Woodmansey EJ, Paterson JC, et al. Microbiological effects of consuming a synbiotic containing Bifidobacterium bifidum, Bifidobacterium lactis, and oligofructose in elderly persons, determined by real-time polymerase chain reaction and counting of viable bacteria. Clin Infect Dis 2005;40(1):28–37.
[10] Mueller S, Saunier K, Hanisch C, et al. Differences in fecal microbiota in different European study populations in relation to age, gender, and country: a cross-sectional study. Appl Environ Microbiol 2006;72(2):1027–33.
[11] Seksik P, Rigottier-Gois L, Gramet G, et al. Alterations of the dominant faecal bacterial groups in patients with Crohn's disease of the colon. Gut 2003;52(2):237–42.
[12] Falconieri P, Borrelli O, Cucchiara S. Gut-associated bacterial microbiota in paediatric patients with inflammatory bowel disease. Gut 2006;55(12):1760–7.

[13] Fujimoto T, Kato J, Nasu J, et al. Change of clinical characteristics of ulcerative colitis in Japan: analysis of 844 hospital-based patients from 1981 to 2000. Eur J Gastroenterol Hepatol 2007;19(3):229–35.

[14] Lahat A, Avidan B, Bar-Meir S, et al. Long-standing colonic inflammation is associated with a low prevalence of diverticuli in inflammatory bowel disease patients. Inflamm Bowel Dis 2007;13(6):733–6.

[15] Yantiss RK, Odze RD. Diagnostic difficulties in inflammatory bowel pathology. Histopathology 2006;48(2):116–32.

[16] Truelove SC, Witts LJ. Cortisone in ulcerative colitis: preliminary report on a therapeutic trial. Br Med J 1954;4884:375–8.

[17] Truelove SC, Witts LJ. Cortisone in ulcerative colitis: final report on therapeutic trial. Br Med J 1955;4947:1041–8.

[18] Lofberg R, Rutgeerts P, Malchow H, et al. Budesonide prolongs time to relapse in ileal and ileocaecal Crohn's disease. A placebo controlled one year study. Gut 1996;39:82–6.

[19] Sandborn WJ, Lofberg R, Feagan BG, et al. Budesonide for maintenance of remission in patients with Crohn's disease in medically induced remission: a predetermined pooled analysis of four randomized, double blind, placebo-controlled trials. Am J Gastroenterol 2005;100:1780–7.

[20] Meyers S, Sachar DB, Goldberg JD, et al. Corticotropin versus hydrocortisone in the intravenous treatment of ulcerative colitis. A prospective, randomized, double blind clinical trial. Gastroenterology 1983;85:351–7.

[21] Jarnerot G, Rolny P, Sandberg-Gertzen H. Intensive intravenous treatment of ulcerative colitis. Gastroenterology 1985;89:1005–13.

[22] Shepherd HA, Barr GD, Jewell DP. Use of an intravenous steroid regimen in the treatment of acute Crohn's disease. J Clin Gastroenterol 1986;8:154–9.

[23] Chun A, Chadi RM, Korelitz BI, et al. Intravenous corticotropin vs. hydrocortisone in the treatment of hospitalized patients with Crohn's disease: a randomized double blind study and follow-up. Inflamm Bowel Dis 1998;4:177–81.

[24] Thomas TPL. The complications of systemic corticosteroid treatment in the elderly. Gerontology 1984;30:60–5.

[25] Akerkar GA, Peppercorn MA, Hamel MB, et al. Corticosteroid-associated complications in the elderly Crohn's disease patients. Am J Gastroenterol 1997;92:461–4.

[26] Aberra FN, Lewis JD, Hass D, et al. Corticosteroids and immunomodulators: postoperative infectious complication risk in inflammatory bowel disease patients. Gastroenterology 2003;125:320–7.

[27] Bernstein CN, Leslie WD, Leboff MS. AGA technical review on osteoporosis in gastrointestinal diseases. Gastroenterology 2003;124:795–841.

[28] Haderslev KV, Tjellesen L, Sorenson HA, et al. Alendronate increases lumbar spine bone density in patients with Crohn's disease. Gastroenterology 2000;119:639–46.

[29] Saag KG, Emkey R, Schnitzer TJ, et al. Alendronate for the prevention and treatment of glucocorticoid-induced osteoporosis. N Engl J Med 1998;339:292–9.

[30] Hanauer SB, Korelitz BI, Rutgeerts P, et al. Postoperative maintenance of Crohn's disease remission with 6-mercaptopurine, mesalamine, or placebo: a 2 year trial. Gastroenterology 2004;127:723–9.

[31] Black AJ, McLeod HL, Capell HA, et al. Thiopurine methyltransferase genotype predicts therapy-limiting severe toxicity from azathioprine. Ann Intern Med 1998;129:716–8.

[32] Dubunsky MC, Lamothe S, Yang HY, et al. Pharmacogenomics and metabolites measurement for 6-mercaptopurine therapy in inflammatory bowel disease. Gastroenterology 2000;118:705–13.

[33] Su C, Lichtenstein GR. Treatment of inflammatory bowel disease with azathioprine and 6-mercaptopurine. Gastroenterol Clin North Am 2004;33:209–34.

[34] Cuffari C, Hunt S, Bayless T. Utilisation of erythrocyte 6-thioguanine metabolite levels to optimize azathioprine therapy in patients in inflammatory bowel disease. Gut 2001;48: 642–6.

[35] Aberra FN, Lichtenstein GR. Review article: monitoring of immunomodulators in inflammatory bowel disease. Aliment Pharmacol Ther 2005;21:307–19.

[36] Dubinsky MC, Reyes E, Ofman J. A Cost-effective analysis of alternative disease management strategies in patients with Crohn's disease treated with azathioprine or 6-mercaptopurine. Am J Gastroenterol 2005;100(10):2239–47.

[37] Hanauer SB, Feagan BG, Lichtenstein GR, et al. Maintenance infliximab for Crohn's disease: ACCENT I randomized trial. Lancet 2002;359:1541–9.

[38] Lemann M, Mary JY, Duclos B, et al. Infliximab plus azathioprine for steroid dependent Crohn's disease patients: A randomized placebo controlled trial. Gastroenterology 2006; 130:1054–61.

[39] Feagan BG, Fedorak RN, Irvine EJ, et al. A comparison of methotrexate with placebo for the maintenance of remission in Crohn's disease. North American Crohn's Study Group Investigators. N Engl J Med 2000;342:1627–32.

[40] Chong TY, Hanauer SB, Cohen RD. Efficacy of parenteral methotrexate in refractory Crohn's disease. Aliment Pharmacol Ther 2001;15:35–44.

[41] Feagan BG, Rochon J, Fedorak RN, et al. Methotrexate for the treatment of Crohn's disease. The North American Crohn's Study Group Investigators. N Engl J Med 1995; 332:292–7.

[42] Fraser G, Ben Bassat O, Segal N, et al. Parenteral methotrexate is not effective treatment for refractory ulcerative colitis. Gastroenterology 2003;124(Suppl 1):A525.

[43] Misiewicz J, Lennard-Jones J, Connell A, et al. Controlled trial of sulphasalazine in maintenance therapy for ulcerative colitis. Lancet 1965;1:185–8.

[44] Prakash A, Spencer CM. Balsalazide. Drugs 1998;56:83–9.

[45] Vecchi M, Meucci G, Gionchetti P, et al. Oral versus combination mesalazine therapy in active ulcerative colitis: a double-blind, double dummy, randomized multicentre study. Aliment Pharmacol Ther 2001;15:251–6.

[46] Marshall J, Irvine E. Rectal aminosalicylate therapy for distal ulcerative colitis: a meta-analysis. Aliment Pharmacol Ther 1995;9:293–300.

[47] Kamm MA, Sandborn WJ, Gassull M, et al. Once daily high concentration MMX mesalamine in active ulcerative colitis. Gastroenterology 2007;132(1):66–75.

[48] Camma C, Guinta M, Rosselli M, et al. Mesalamine in the maintenance treatment of Crohn's disease: a meta-analysis adjusted for confounding variables. Gastroenterology 1997;113:1465–73.

[49] Lochs H, Mayer M, Fleig WE, et al. Prophylaxis of postoperative relapse in Crohn's disease with mesalamine: European Cooperative Crohn's Disease Study VI. Gastroenterology 2000; 118:264–73.

[50] Summers RW, Switz DM, Sessions JT Jr, et al. National Cooperative Crohn's Disease Study: results of drug treatment. Gastroenterology 1979;77:847–69.

[51] Singleton JW, Hanauer SB, Gitnick GL, et al. Mesalamine capsules for the treatment of active Crohn's disease: results of a 16 week trial. Pentasa Crohn's Disease Study Group. Gastroenterology 1993;104:1293–301.

[52] Thukral C, Travassos WJ, Peppercorn MA. The role of antibiotics in inflammatory bowel disease. Curr Treat Options Gastroenterol 2005;8(3):223–8.

[53] Ohkusa T, Nomura T, Terai T. Effectiveness of antibiotic combination therapy in patients with active ulcerative colitis: a randomized, controlled pilot trial with long term follow up. Scand J Gastroenterol 2005;40(11):1334–42.

[54] Rutgeerts P, Hiele M, Gebos K, et al. Controlled trial of metronidazole treatment for prevention of Crohn's recurrence after ileal resection. Gastroenterology 1995;108(6):1617–21.

[55] Solomon MJ, McLeod RS, O'Connor BI, et al. Combination ciprofloxacin and metronidazole in severe perianal Crohn's disease. Can J Gastroenterol 1993;7:571–3.

[56] Brandt LJ, Berstein LH, Boley SJ, et al. Metronidazole therapy for perineal Crohn's disease: a follow up study. Gastroenterology 1982;83:383–7.

[57] Berstein LH, Frank MS, Brandt LJ, et al. Healing of perianal Crohn's disease with metronidazole. Gastroenterology 1980;79:357–65.

[58] Prantera C, Lochs H, Campieri M, et al. Antibiotic treatment of Crohn's disease: results of a multicentre, double blind, randomized, placebo-controlled trial with rifaximin. Aliment Pharmacol Ther 2006;23(8):1117–25.

[59] Rutgeerts P, D'Haens G, Targan S, et al. Efficacy and safety of retreatment with anti-tumor necrosis factor antibody (infliximab) to maintain remission in Crohn's disease. Gastroenterology 1999;117:761–9.

[60] Hanauer SB, Wagner CL, Bala M, et al. Incidence and importance of antibody responses to infliximab after maintenance or episodic treatment in Crohn's disease. Clin Gastroenterol Hepatol 2004;2:542–53.

[61] Rutgeerts P, Feagan BG, Lichtenstein GR, et al. Comparison of scheduled and episodic treatment strategies of infliximab in Crohn's disease. Gastroenterology 2004;126:402–13.

[62] Present DH, Rutgeerts P, Targan S, et al. Infliximab for the treatment of fistulas in patients with Crohn's disease. N Engl J Med 1999;340:1398–405.

[63] Sands BE, Tremains WJ, Sandborn WJ, et al. Infliximab in the treatment of severe steroid refractory ulcerative colitis: a pilot study. Inflamm Bowel Dis 2001;7:83–8.

[64] Rutgeerts P, Feagan B, Olson A, et al. A randomized placebo controlled trial of infliximab therapy for active ulcerative colitis: act I trial [abstract]. Gastroenterology 2005;128:A689.

[65] Sandborn W, Rachmilewith D, Hanauer S, et al. Infliximab induction and maintenance therapy for ulcerative colitis: the act 2 trial [abstract]. Gastroenterology 2005;128(Suppl 2):A688.

[66] Sandborn WJ, Hanauer S, Loftus EV Jr, et al. An open label study of the human anti-TNF monoclonal antibody adalimumab in subjects with prior loss of response or intolerance to infliximab for Crohn's disease. Am J Gastroenterol 2004;99(10):1984–9.

[67] Sandborn WJ, Hanauer SB, Rutgeerts PJ, et al. Adalimumab for maintenance treatment of Crohn's disease: results of the CLASSIC II trial. Gut 2007.

[68] Colomber JF, Sandborn WJ, Rutgeerts P, et al. Adalimumab for the maintenance of clinical response and remission in patients with Crohn's disease: the CHARM trial. Gastroenterology 2007;132(1):52–65.

[69] Hanauer SB, Sandborn WJ, Rutgeerts P, et al. Human anti-tumor necrosis factor monoclonal antibody (adalimumab) in Crohn's disease: the CLASSIC-I trial. Gastroenterology 2006;130(2):323–33.

[70] Schreiber S, Rutgeerts P, Fedorak RN, et al. A randomized, placebo-controlled trial of certolizumab pegol (CDP 870) for treatment of Crohn's disease. Gastroenterology 2005;129(3):807–18.

[71] Munkholm P. Review article: the incidence and prevalence of colorectal cancer in inflammatory bowel disease. Aliment Pharmacol Ther 2003;18(Suppl 2):1–5.

[72] Bansal P, Sonnenberg A. Risk factors of colorectal cancer in inflammatory bowel disease. Am J Gastroenterol 1996;91(1):44–8.

[73] Rubin DT, LoSavio A, Yadron N, et al. Aminosalicylate therapy in the prevention of dysplasia and colorectal cancer in ulcerative colitis. Clin Gastroenterol Hepatol 2006;4(11):1346–50.

[74] Velayos FS, Terdiman JP, Walsh JM. Effect of 5-aminosalicylate use on colorectal cancer and dysplasia risk: a systematic review and metaanalysis of observational studies. Am J Gastroenterol 2005;100(6):1354–6.

[75] Lashner BA, Heidenreich PA, Su GL, et al. Effect of folate supplementation on the incidence of dysplasia and cancer in chronic ulcerative colitis. A case-control study. Gastroenterology 1989;97(2):255–9.

[76] Delaunoit T, Limburg PJ, Goldberg RM, et al. Colorectal cancer prognosis among patients with inflammatory bowel disease. Clin Gastroenterol Hepatol 2006;4(3):335–42.

[77] Larsen M, Mose H, Gilsum M, et al. Survival after colorectal cancer in patients with Crohn's disease: a nationwide population based Danish follow-up study. Am J Gastroenterol 2007; 102(1):163–7.

[78] Kiesslich R, Neurath MF. Chromoendoscopy and other novel imaging techniques. Gastroenterol Clin North Am 2006;35(3):605–19.

[79] Hirata M, Tanaka S, Oka S, et al. Magnifying endoscopy with narrow band imaging for diagnosis of colorectal tumors. Gastrointest Endosc 2007.

[80] Greenstein AJ, Slater G, Heimann TM, et al. Comparison of multiple synchronous colorectal cancers in ulcerative colitis, familial polyposis coli, and de novo cancer. Ann Surg 1986; 203:123–8.

[81] Connell WR, Lennard-Jones JE, Williams CB, et al. Factors affecting the outcome of endoscopic surveillance for cancer in ulcerative colitis. Gastroenterology 1994;107:934–44.

[82] Lashner BA, Silverstein MD, Hanauer SB. Hazard rates for dysplasia and cancer in ulcerative colitis. Results from a surveillance program. Dig Dis Sci 1989;10:1536–41.

[83] Thomas T, Abrams KA, Robinson RJ, et al. Meta-analysis: cancer risk of low grade dysplasia in chronic ulcerative colitis. Aliment Pharmacol Ther 2007;25(6):657–68.

[84] Ullman T, Croog V, Harpaz N, et al. Progression of flat low-grade dysplasia to advanced neoplasia in patients with ulcerative colitis. Gastroenterology 2003;125(5):1311–9.

[85] Blackstone M, Ridell RW, Rogers BHG, et al. Dysplasia associated lesion or mass (DALM) detected by colonoscopy in longstanding ulcerative colitis: an indication for colectomy. Gastroenterology 1981;80:366–74.

[86] Odze R. Diagnostic problems and advances in inflammatory bowel disease. Mod Pathol 2003;16(4):347–58.

[87] Odze RD. Adenomas and adenoma-like DALMs in chronic ulcerative colitis: a clinical, pathological, and molecular review. Am J Gastroenterol 1999;94(7):1746–50.

[88] Longo WE, Virgo KS, Bahadursingh AN, et al. Patterns of disease and surgical treatment among United States veterans more than 50 years of age with ulcerative colitis. Am J Surg 2003;186(5):514–8.

[89] Page MJ, Poritz LS, Kunselman SJ, et al. Factors affecting surgical risk in elderly patients with inflammatory disease. J Gastrointest Surg 2002;6(4):606–13.

[90] Norris B, Solomon MJ, Eyers AA, et al. Abdominal surgery in the older Crohn's population. Aust N Z J Surg 1999;69:199–204.

[91] Yamamoto T, Allan RN, Keighley MR. Risk factors for intra-abdominal sepsis after surgery in Crohn's disease. Dis Colon Rectum 2000;43(8):1141–5.

ELSEVIER
SAUNDERS

CLINICS IN
GERIATRIC
MEDICINE

Clin Geriatr Med 23 (2007) 823–832

Constipation and Irritable Bowel Syndrome in the Elderly

John E. Morley, MB, BCh[a,b,*]

[a]Division of Geriatric Medicine, Saint Louis University Medical Center,
Saint Louis University School of Medicine, 1402 S. Grand Blvd., M238,
St. Louis, MO 63104, USA
[b]Geriatric Research, Education, and Clinical Center,
St. Louis VA Medical Center, Jefferson Barracks Division,
GRECC, #1 Jefferson Barrackes Drive, 11G/JB,
St. Louis, MO 63125, USA

"The intestines tend to become sluggish with age."

–Hippocrates

Constipation has plagued human beings since the beginning of time. The first documented treatment for constipation was by a physician to one of the Egyptian pharaohs, who was tasked with curing the pharaoh's constipation or going to prison. As he pondered this problem on the banks of the Nile, he observed an Ibis take a mouthful of water, bend its long neck around and squirt it up its anus. He took this as a sign from the god, Toth, and rushed back to administer the first enema to the pharaoh. Following the cure of the pharaoh's constipation, he was given the exalted title of "Guardian of the Royal Bowel Movement."

Perhaps the most famous person to suffer from constipation was Martin Luther, who was responsible for creating the reformation and leading vast numbers of Christians away from the Catholic Church. Many of his famous 95 theses of rebellion against the Pope were written while he was "das klo" (on the toilet). Ayurvedic medicine offered a number of cures for constipation, including never wearing tight clothing or belts, having more water and fresh whole milk, and eating three to five prunes each morning.

Constipation is an extraordinarily common problem in the United States of America. It is a problem for over 33 million adults in the United States and

* Division of Geriatric Medicine, Saint Louis University Medical Center, Saint Louis University School of Medicine, 1402 S. Grand Blvd., M238, St. Louis, MO 63104.
E-mail address: morley@slu.edu

0749-0690/07/$ - see front matter © 2007 Elsevier Inc. All rights reserved.
doi:10.1016/j.cger.2007.06.008   geriatric.theclinics.com

accounts for 2.5 million physician visits and 92,000 hospitalizations each year. This high prevalence of constipation and irritable bowel syndrome has led to the United States being characterized as "a nation obsessed with its bowels."

Diagnostic criteria for constipation

Specific criteria for the diagnosis of constipation were created at a consensus conference in Rome and are known as the Rome Criteria [1]. These criteria are:

1. Straining at defecation for at least a quarter of the time.
2. Lumpy or hard stools for at least a quarter of the time.
3. A sensation of incomplete evacuation for at least a quarter of the time.
4. Two or fewer bowel movements per week.

Epidemiology of constipation in older persons

A number of studies in community dwelling older persons have suggested that the perception of constipation occurs in one out of every four older persons [2–7]. However, when the Rome Criteria are used the prevalence of constipation is somewhat less, at 17% [8]. Harari and colleagues [9] reported that regular laxative use increased with aging, with over 30% of females and 25% of males in their eighties using a laxative at least once a month.

Frailty in older persons is very common and is associated with immobility, poor food intake, and dehydration [10,11]. It is, therefore, not surprising that constipation has been reported to be present in 45% of frail elderly persons [12]. Persons living in nursing homes are at a very high risk of being frail and disabled [13]. Anorexia, dehydration, and weight loss are extraordinarily common in this population [14–17]. Three studies have reported that laxative use in the nursing home occurs in 50% to 65% of residents [18–22]. Half of these older persons took a daily laxative, yet only 62% of them met the criteria for constipation. There was minimal concordance between nurses and the nursing home residents as to whether or not they were constipated. Laxative use was more common in those who were immobile, had Parkinson's disease or diabetes mellitus, or took iron supplements, calcium channel antagonists, or antidepressants with anticholinergic activity [18].

In a study of 21,012 persons using the minimum data set in Nursing Homes the prevalence of constipation was 12.5% [19]. The 3-month incidence was 7%. Major risk factors were decreased fluid intake, pneumonia, Parkinson's disease, and allergies. Frank and colleagues [22] have suggested that the economic cost of constipation in nursing homes if $2,253 for each resident with constipation.

Impact of constipation

Constipation in older persons is associated with a decline in quality of life, a decrease in functional ability, increased pain, dysuria and incontinence, fecal incontinence, stercoral ulcers, and fecaloma [23–28]. The major problem associated with constipation is the development of fecal impaction. In one study fecal impaction was responsible for 7.6% of all cases with intestinal obstruction [29].

Delirium is a common reason for hospital admission [30–32]. Constipation is a common cause of delirium [33]. Leonard and colleagues [34] reported that constipation is associated with physical and verbal aggression.

Causes of constipation

There are multiple causes of constipation. They can be categorized into those caused by mechanical obstruction, metabolic causes, neurologic diseases, psychiatric diseases, and medications. Colon cancer, colonic strictures, and anal stenosis are the most common, caused by mechanical obstruction. Diabetes mellitus is associated with autonomic neuropathy and altered gastro-colie transit time [35]. Hypercalcemia and hypomagnesium slow intestinal transit. Hypothyroidism commonly presents with constipation. Amyloidosis and scleroderma are rare causes of constipation. Cancer and terminal illness commonly are associated with constipation [36,37].

Parkinson's disease is commonly associated with constipation. Persons with a stroke develop constipation secondarily to immobility. Autonomic neuropathy is associated with a sluggish intestine. Persons with dementia and depression often have constipation. Olanzapine is associated with an increase in constipation and laxative use [38]. Depression is underdiagnosed and undertreated, particularly in the African-American community, and an atypical presentation of depression can be constipation [39,40].

Older persons tend to be on large numbers of medicines [41] and many of these medications lead to constipation; the best recognized of these are opiates. Iron and calcium supplements are major causes of constipation. With the increased awareness of the dangers of osteoporosis in older persons, there is increasing use of calcium supplements [42,43]. Anemia occurs commonly in older persons and thus use of iron is common [44]. Antidepressants with anticholinergic activity, which include both tricyclics and selective serotonin uptake inhibitors (eg, paroxetine), lead to constipation, as do antipsychotics and antihistamines. Diuretics result in dehydration. Anti-Parkinsonism drugs, such as L-dopa and bromergocriptine, slow intestinal transit. Perhaps the major unrecognized cause of constipation in older persons is calcium channel antagonists.

Red flags in persons with constipation

While most older persons with constipation can be treated symptomatically, persons who have any of the following conditions should have the causes of the constipation looked at more rigorously:

- Acute onset

- Weight loss
- Rectal bleeding
- Iron deficiency anemia
- Family history of colon cancer

Laboratory testing and constipation

If fecal impaction is suspected an abdominal x-ray should be obtained. It is important to remember that fecal impaction can occur with no stool in the rectum. The radiological diagnosis of fecal impaction requires severe fecal retention, associated with either colonic or rectal dilation with or without air-fluid levels. Colonic dilation is present when the maximum diameter is greater than 6 cm, and rectal dilation when it is greater than 4 cm.

Basic tests for anyone with chronic constipation include a complete blood count, serum blood urea nitrogen, serum creatinine, serum sodium, serum calcium, serum magnesium, a thyroid stumulating hormone (TSH) level, and stool for occult blood. Sigmoidoscopy of colonoscopy should be considered for any person with prolonged chronic constipation.

There are a number of special tests that gastroenterologists use in the workup of constipation in the younger population. These include colon transit manometry, colonic manometry, anorectal manometry, balloon expulsion testing, and defecography. These are virtually never needed in older persons.

Management of constipation

The basic management of constipation consists of four components:

- Adequate fluid intake
- Bulking agents (fiber)
- Toileting after eating
- Exercise

Fiber should not be used in persons who are immobile or who are receiving inadequate fluid. An herbal tea, "Smooth Move," has been associated with increased bowel movements in nursing home residents when compared with placebo [45]. Toileting 15 to 30 minutes after eating makes use of the bastrocolic reflex. The gastrocolie reflex results in propagating spikes in the colon and rectum within a half an hour after a meal. It is more prominent in persons who have had a cholecystectomy, suggesting it is associated with fat in the meals and bile salt release into the small intestine. Biofeedback, using either pressure or electromyography, has been used with varying success [46].

Of the medications that are available for constipation, the stool softeners, diocytyl sodium and calcium sulfosuccinate, should never be used. There is no evidence that they are efficacious and, rarely, they can cause lipoid pneumonia [47]. Despite this, they are the most commonly prescribed laxative to older persons in the long-term care setting.

Stimulant laxatives are prescribed approximately 20% of the time. The stimulant laxatives are senna, biscogyl, and castor oil. They are effective when given acutely for short periods [48–51]. They cause melanosis coli and may cause enteric nerve damage when used long term, though the evidence for this is limited.

Osmotic laxatives include lactulose, sorbitol, magnesium citrate or hydroxide, and polyethylene glycol. They are effective and not absorbed [47]. However, they are often underdosed. Most elderly persons require 50 mL to 100 mL, given at night before going to bed. In these doses they are as effective as senna in preventing opiate-associated constipation. Potential side effects of these laxatives are electrolyte imbalance, nausea, and dehydration.

Enemas, such as sodium biphosphate, tap water, saline, or oil, are inconvenient to give. Generally, they are efficacious. As with the osmotic laxatives, they may cause dehydration. Sodium biphosphate may result in hypocalcemia and hyperphosphatemia.

Tegaserod, a serotonin-4 receptor agonist, has been successfully used to treat constipation in younger persons.

Lubiprostone is an orally administered, bicyclic fatty acid which has minimal systemic absorption [52–54]. It works by activating the CIC-2 chloride channel, resulting in a chloride rich intestinal fluid secretion. It does not affect the cystic fibrosis transmembrane conductance regulator (CFTR) chloride channel and thus, does not lead to sodium result in the intestine. By causing an increase in fluid in the intestine, it causes swelling of fecal material, resulting in increased intestinal motility and stool passage. The most efficacious dose is 24 micrograms twice daily. At this dose, in controlled trials, it has been demonstrated to double the number of spontaneous bowel movements over placebo. It also improved stool consistency, decreased bloating, and showed an improvement of the global assessment of constipation severity. Spontaneous bowel movements occurred within 24 hours in 57% of persons receiving lubiprostone, compared with 37% on placebo.

In long term trials for up to 12 months, lubiprostone decreased abdominal bloating, abdominal discomfort, and constipation severity. Over 1400 patients have been treated in trials, with major side effects being rare. Nausea occurs commonly with the first few doses (31.1%). This is less when the drug is given with food and lower in older persons, and resulted in discontinuation of treatment in 8.4% of those treated. Diarrhea occurred in 13.2% of patients, with 2.2% discontinuing treatment. When the drug is discontinued after 4 weeks, the relapse rate was less than half of that for placebo (18.2% versus 44.4%). Anecdotal experience of lubiprostone in nursing home residents with multiple admissions for fecal impaction has been most encouraging.

Protocol for management of constipation in older persons

Any older person who complains of constipation should have depression considered as a diagnosis and should increase fluid, fiber (if mobile), toilet after meals, and increase exercise. Prune juice may also be added. If the person has fecal impaction, fluid intake should be increased and lubiprostone should be tried. If there is no response, then a tap water enema should be given.

In all chronically constipated persons, calcium channel antagonists should be discontinued and a TSH, calcium magnesium, and stool guiac should be obtained. An osmotic laxative, such as sorbitol at dose of 50 cc to 100 cc, should be used in the evening. If the person has weight loss, rectal bleeding, or iron deficiency anemia, a colonoscopy should be obtained. If there is no response to an osmotic laxative, lubiprostone (24 micrograms, twice daily) should be used. Treatment should be continued for 4 weeks and then withdrawn. If there is a relapse, then lubiprostone should be restarted and continued indefinitely. This protocol is summarized in Fig. 1.

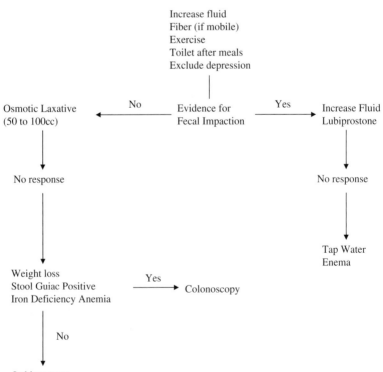

Fig. 1. Simplified protocol for the management of constipation in older persons.

Irritable bowel syndrome in geriatric populations

Irritable bowel syndrome (IBS) occurs in approximately 10% of the older population [55]. Older persons rarely complain of the syndrome to their physician, possibly because they have lived with it most of their life. Only about one in five persons with IBS have the diagnosis made. IBS is associated with a decline in quality of life, increased physician visits, increased hospitalizations, and increased drug use in older persons. It can be associated with decreased food intake and weight loss [56,57].

The prevalence of IBS in nursing home residents is unknown. However, the symptoms of IBS, such as constipation, diarrhea, abdominal pain, and bloating, are very common in long-term care. Physicians appear to have minimal awareness of the problems associated with IBS in older persons and in nursing homes.

IBS is diagnosed by the Rome II Criteria [58]:

- Abdominal pain or discomfort lasting at least 12 weeks (which need not be consecutive) of the preceding 12 months, and including at least two of the three following features:
  - Relief achieved with defecation
  - Onset associated with a change in frequency of stool
  - Onset associated with a change in form (appearance) of stool

The red flags for an in depth workup in older persons are anemia, persistent fever, chronic diarrhea, and family history of colon cancer. The differential diagnosis of IBS includes colon cancer, diverticular disease, ulcerative colitis, regional ileitis, and celiac disease.

The treatment of IBS includes careful explanation of the disease and supportive therapy. Increasing dietary fiber is indicated for many patients, but it can cause adverse events that mimic or exacerbate some IBS symptoms. Targeted food elimination helps some persons.

A number of traditional therapies that generally target a single symptom have been used. These include antispasmodics, anticholinergics, tricyclic antidepressants, anti-diarrheals, and laxatives [59,60]. Recently, selective serotonin receptor reuptake inhibitors, such as citaloprom, have been used with some success. In younger women, alosetron and tegaserod are available and are very successful in some persons [59,61]. In persons where constipation is a major feature, lubiprostone may be tried.

Overall, IBS is an underappreciated condition in older persons. It can cause major problems in quality of life and it should be considered as a diagnosis and treated appropriately when diagnosed.

References

[1] Garrigues V, Galvez C, Ortiz V, et al. Prevalence of constipation: agreement among several criteria and evaluation of the diagnostic accuracy of qualifying symptoms and

self-reported definition in a population-based survey in Spain. Am J Epidemiol 2004;159: 520–6.

[2] Pare P, Ferrazzi S, Thompson WG, et al. An epidemiological survey of constipation in Canada: definitions, rates, and demographics, and predictors of health care seeking. Am J Gastroenterol 2001;96:3130–7.

[3] Thompson WG, Heaton KW. Functional bowel disorders in apparently healthy people. Gastroenterology 1980;79:283–8.

[4] Donald IP, Smith RG, Cruikshank JG, et al. A study of constipation in the elderly living at home. Gerontology 1985;31:112–8.

[5] Whitehead WE, Drinkwater D, Cheskin LJ, et al. Constipation in the elderly living at home. Definition, prevalence, and relationship to lifestyle and health status. J Am Geriatr Soc 1989; 37:423–9.

[6] Campbell AJ, Busby WJ, Horwath CC. Factors associated with constipation in a community based sample of people aged 70 years and over. J Epidemiol Community Health 1993;47: 23–6.

[7] Marfil C, Davies GJ, Dettmar PW. Laxative use and its relationship with straining in a London elderly population: free-living versus institutionalised. J Nutr Health Aging 2005;9: 185–7.

[8] Robson KM, Kiely DK, Lembo T. Development of constipation in nursing home residents. Dis Colon Rectum 2000;43:940–3.

[9] Harari D, Gurwitz JH, Avorn J, et al. How do older persons define constipation? Implications for therapeutic management. J Gen Intern Med 1997;12:63–6.

[10] Morley JE, Kim MJ, Haren MT, et al. Frailty and the aging male. Aging Male 2005;8: 135–40.

[11] Morley JE, Perry HM 3rd, Miller DK. Editorial: something about frailty. J Gerontol A Biol Sci Med Sci 2002;57:M698–704.

[12] Wolfsen CR, Barker JC, Mitteness LS. Constipation in the daily lives of frail elderly people. Arch Fam Med 1993;2:853–8.

[13] Morley JE, Flaherty JH. Putting the "home" back in nursing home. J Gerontol A Biol Sci Med Sci 2002;57:M419–21.

[14] Rolland Y, Kim MJ, Gammack JK, et al. Office management of weight loss in older persons. Am J Med 2006;119:1019–26.

[15] Morley JE, Thomas DR, Wilson MM. Cachexia: pathophysiology and clinical relevance. Am J Clin Nutr 2006;83:735–43.

[16] Wilson MM, Thomas DR, Rubenstein LZ, et al. Appetite assessment: simple appetite questionnaire predicts weight loss in community-dwelling adults and nursing home residents. Am J Clin Nutr 2005;82:1074–81.

[17] Morley JE. Anorexia and weight loss in older persons. J Gerontol A Biol Sci Med Sci 2003; 58:131–7.

[18] Harari D, Gurwitz JH, Avorn J, et al. Correlates of regular laxative use by frail elderly persons. Am J Med 1995;99:513–8.

[19] Harari D, Gurwitz JH, Avorn J, et al. Constipation: assessment and management in an institutionalized elderly population. J Am Geriatr Soc 1994;42:947–52.

[20] Lamy PP, Krug BH. Review of laxative utilization in a skilled nursing facility. J Am Geriatr Soc 1978;26:544–9.

[21] Marfil C, Davies GJ, Dettmar PW. Straining at stool and stool frequency in free-living and institutionalised older adults. J Nutr Health Aging 2005;9:277–80.

[22] Frank L, Schmier J, Kleinman L, et al. Time and economic cost of constipation care in nursing homes. J Am Med Dir Assoc 2002;3:215–23.

[23] Norton C. Constipation in older patients: effects on quality of life. Br J Nurs 2006;15: 188–92.

[24] Tariq SH, Morley JE, Prather CM. Fecal incontinence in the elderly patient. Am J Med 2003; 115:217–27.

[25] Akhtar AJ, Padda M. Fecal incontinence in older patients. J Am Med Dir Assoc 2005;6: 54–60.

[26] Phillips C, Polakoff D, Maue SK, et al. Assessment of constipation management in long-term care patients. J Am Med Dir Assoc 2001;2:149–54.

[27] Rajagopal A, Martin J. Giant fecaloma with idiopathic sigmoid megacolon: report of a case and review of the literature. Dis Colon Rectum 2002;45:833–5.

[28] Potter J, Wagg A. Management of bowel problems in older people: an update. Clin Med 2005;5:289–95.

[29] Sufian S, Matsumoto T. Intestinal obstruction. Am J Surg 1975;130:9–14.

[30] Flaherty JH, Morley JE. Delirium: a call to improve current standards of care. J Gerontol A Biol Sci Med Sci 2004;59:341–3.

[31] Lewis LM, Miller DK, Morley JE, et al. Unrecognized delirium in ED geriatric patients. Am J Emerg Med 1995;13:142–5.

[32] Flaherty JH, Tariq SH, Raghavan S, et al. A model for managing delirious older inpatients. J Am Geriatr Soc 2003;51:1031–5.

[33] Ross DD, Alexander CS. Management of common symptoms in terminally ill patients: part II. Constipation, delirium and dyspnea. Am Fam Physician 2001;64:1019–26.

[34] Leonard R, Tinetti ME, Allore HG, et al. Potentially modifiable resident characteristics that are associated with physical or verbal aggression among nursing home residents with dementia. Arch Intern Med 2006;166:1295–300.

[35] Kim MJ, Rolland Y, Cepeda O, et al. Diabetes mellitus in older men. Aging Male 2006;9: 139–47.

[36] Cartwright JC, Hickman S, Perrin N, et al. Symptom experiences of residents dying in assisted living. J Am Med Dir Assoc 2006;7:219–23.

[37] Cepeda OA, Gammack JK. Cancer in older men: a gender-based review. Aging Male 2006;9: 149–58.

[38] Martin H, Slyk MP, Deymann S, et al. Safety profile assessment of risperidone and olanzapine in long-term care patients with dementia. J Am Med Dir Assoc 2003;4:183–8.

[39] Miller DK, Malmstrom TK, Joshi S, et al. Clinically relevant levels of depressive symptoms in community-dwelling middle-aged African Americans. J Am Geriatr Soc 2004;52:741–8.

[40] Morley JE. The top 10 hot topics in aging. J Gerontol A Biol Sci Med Sci 2004;59: 24–33.

[41] Flaherty JH, Perry HM 3rd, Lynchard GS, et al. Polypharmacy and hospitalization among older home care patients. J Gerontol A Biol Sci Med Sci 2000;55:M552–9.

[42] Kamel HK, Hussain MS, Tariq S, et al. Failure to diagnose and treat osteoporosis in elderly patients hospitalized with hip fracture. Am J Med 2000;109:326–8.

[43] Kamel HK, Perry HM 3rd, Morley JE. Hormone replacement therapy and fractures in older adults. J Am Geriatr Soc 2001;49:179–87.

[44] Tangalos EG, Hoggard JG, Murray AM, et al. Treatment of kidney disease and anemia in elderly, long-term care residents. J Am Med Dir Assoc 2004;5(4 Suppl):H1–6.

[45] Bub S, Brinckmann J, Cicconetti G, et al. Efficacy of an herbal dietary supplement (Smooth Move) in the management of constipation in nursing home residents: a randomized, double-blind, placebo-controlled study. J Am Med Dir Assoc 2006;7:556–61.

[46] Heymen S, Jones KR, Scarlett Y, et al. Biofeedback treatment of constipation: a critical review. Dis Colon Rectum 2003;46:1208–17.

[47] Petticrew M, Watt I, Sheldon T. Systematic review of the effectiveness of laxatives in the elderly. Health Technol Assess 1997;1:1–52, i–iv.

[48] Valverde A, Hay JM, Fingerhut A, et al. Senna vs polyethylene glycol for mechanical preparation the evening before elective colonic or rectal resection: a multicenter controlled trial. French Association for Surgical Research. Arch Surg 1999;134:514–9.

[49] Kinnunen O, Winblad I, Koistinen P, et al. Safety and efficacy of a bulk laxative containing senna versus lactulose in the treatment of chronic constipation in geriatric patients. Pharmacology 1993;47(Suppl 1):253–5.

[50] Agra Y, Sacristan A, Gonzalez M, et al. Efficacy of senna versus lactulose in terminal cancer patients treated with opioids. J Pain Symptom Manage 1998;15:1–7.

[51] Passmore AP, Wilson-Davies K, Stoker C, et al. Chronic constipation in long stay elderly patients: a comparison of lactulose and senna-fibre combination. BMJ 1993;307:769–71.

[52] Schiller LR, Camilleri M. Lubiprostone: viewpoints. Drugs 2006;66:880–1.

[53] Camilleri M, Bharucha AE, Ueno R, et al. Effect of a selective chloride channel activator, lubiprostone, on gastrointestinal transit, gastric sensory, and motor function in healthy volunteers. Am J Physiol Gastrointest Liver Physiol 2006;290:G942–7.

[54] McKeage K, Plosker GL, Siddiqui MA. Lubiprostone. Drugs 2006;66:873–9.

[55] Bharucha AE, Camilleri M. Functional abdominal pain in the elderly. Gastroenterol Clin North Am 2001;30:517–29.

[56] Thomas DR, Ashmen W, Morley JE, et al. Nutritional management in long-term care: development of a clinical guideline. Council for Nutritional Strategies in Long-Term Care. J Gerontol A Biol Sci Med Sci 2000;55:M725–34.

[57] Morley JE. Is weight loss harmful to older men? Aging Male 2006;9:135–7.

[58] Mearin F, Badia X, Balboa A, et al. Irritable bowel syndrome prevalence varies enormously depending on the employed diagnostic criteria: comparison of Rome II versus previous criteria in a general population. Scand J Gastroenterol 2001;36:1155–61.

[59] Heading R, Bardhan K, Hollerbach S, et al. Systematic review: the safety and tolerability of pharmacological agents for treatment of irritable bowel syndrome—a European perspective. Aliment Pharmacol Ther 2006;24:207–36.

[60] Quartero AO, Meineche-Schmidt V, Muris J, et al. Bulking agents, antispasmodic and antidepressant medication for the treatment of irritable bowel syndrome. Cochrane Database Syst Rev 2005;(2):CD003460.

[61] Evans BW, Clark WK, Moore DJ, et al. Tegaserod for the treatment of irritable bowel syndrome. Cochrane Database Syst Rev 2004;(1):CD003960.

ELSEVIER
SAUNDERS

CLINICS IN
GERIATRIC
MEDICINE

Clin Geriatr Med 23 (2007) 833–856

Diarrheal Diseases in the Elderly

Chantri Trinh, MD[a],*,
Kavita Prabhakar, MD, MPH, TM[b]

[a]Division of Geriatric Medicine, Department of Internal Medicine,
Saint Louis University School of Medicine, 1402 South Grand Boulevard #M238,
St. Louis, MO 63104, USA
[b]P.O. Box 687, Brookfield, CT 06804-0687, USA

Diarrheal diseases were important causes of death in the United States in the early 1900s, with the other leading causes including pneumonia, influenza, and tuberculosis [1]. A large proportion of the population did not survive childhood, and most did not live beyond age 65 because of a variety of infectious diseases. By the dawn of the twenty-first century, life expectancy has increased dramatically to 77.8 years for births in the year 2004; heart disease, cancer, and stroke are the leading causes of death. Yet, diarrheal diseases remain a significant cause of morbidity and mortality in the elderly population because of a weakened immune system (immunosenescence), hypochlorhydria, intestinal motility disorders, poor nutritional status, and other underlying chronic medical diseases. For the community-dwelling elderly, diarrhea poses a significant problem, ranging from the burden of incontinence, social embarrassment, and isolation to dehydration, delirium, increased fall and fracture risk, and hospitalization. For the elderly residing in a long-term care facility, diarrhea represents a more serious threat, increasing mortality in those already crippled with multiple medical comorbidities and functional loss. They also have a longer length of hospital stay—7.4 days in patients older than 75 years compared with 4.1 days in those 20 to 49 years of age—and a higher mortality [2]. In a review of national mortality data from 1979 to 1987, death due to diarrhea was greatest in the group aged 74 years and older (51%), followed by adults aged 55 to 74 years (27%), compared with 11% in children younger than 5 years [3].

* Corresponding author.
E-mail address: trinhc@slu.edu (C. Trinh).

Definition

Diarrhea often is a subjective complaint and varies from one patient to the next; the most common features include increased frequency and liquidity of bowel movements. For researchers, diarrhea is defined as increased stool weight, in excess of 200 g/d, and having more than three bowel movements per day. Fecal weight has little clinical significance, however; patients may not be able to estimate weight in grams accurately, and some may have greater stool weight with formed consistency because of a high-fiber diet and not complain of diarrhea. Therefore, a good clinical definition for diarrhea is having more than three loose or watery bowel movements per day compared with individual baseline.

Fecal incontinence presents frequently with loose stools. Some older patients may feel ashamed or embarrassed about fecal accidents and so the symptoms frequently are not volunteered. Some patients complain of diarrhea when they actually have fecal urgency and incontinence. For this reason, evaluation of diarrhea needs to exclude fecal incontinence, especially in the elderly, because it can be a sign of other medical conditions that require a different management strategy.

The chronicity of symptoms helps to distinguish acute from chronic diarrhea and helps to guide the diagnostic approach and treatment strategy. Acute diarrhea usually lasts less than 2 weeks and often is infectious in nature. Diarrhea is considered to be persistent if lasting more than 2 weeks and chronic if lasting more than 4 weeks [4,5].

Because of the physiologic changes of aging, abnormalities in water homeostasis and decreased thirst perception put elderly patients at higher risk for dehydration, especially in the setting of diarrhea. They also are more likely to suffer from complications of volume depletion, such as electrolyte disturbances, delirium, fall and fractures due to orthostatic hypotension, a prolonged infectious course due to immunosenescence, and malnutrition due to associated poor appetite. Therefore, diarrhea in the elderly warrants close monitoring, timely fluid repletion, and prevention of possible complications to minimize delirium, malnutrition, function loss, and most important of all, death. Despite significant associated complications, diarrhea in the elderly has received little attention in the literature and continues to cause significant morbidity and mortality in this frail elderly.

Acute diarrhea

Diarrhea in adults aged 20 years and older usually is coded as gastroenteritis of unknown etiology; it accounted for 77.8% of all discharges according to data from the National Hospital Discharge Survey for the years 1979 through 1995 [2]. The high proportion of unknown cases may be due to the fact that in most cases, diagnostic tests were not performed, especially in outbreak situations and in cases when the disease resolved spontaneously. Furthermore, diagnostics are limited and so not every cause was identifiable. For the known causes of gastroenteritis, bacterial and viral etiologies result in significantly increased hospitalization rates in people aged 65 years and older [2]. Protozoan infections are much less common causes of diarrhea in this age group. Other common noninfectious causes include an adverse drug reaction or the use of laxatives or antacids. Carcinoid tumors, ischemic colitis, diabetes, and thyrotoxicosis are other less common causes of acute diarrhea in the aged. For hospitalized patients and residents of long-term care facilities, acute diarrhea more commonly is due to *Clostridium difficile* infection and is one infection that produces high morbidity and mortality. Other common causes of acute diarrhea in this population include osmotic laxatives use, tube feeding, ischemic colitis, and fecal impaction with overflow diarrhea [6].

In a retrospective analysis of hospital discharges for a period of 16 years in the United States (1979–1995), acute diarrhea accounted for 1.5% of adult hospitalizations annually, 78% of which had no etiology identified [2]. In most cases, symptoms resolved spontaneously over days to weeks. But for the fatal cases in which gastroenteritis was listed in the top three diagnoses, 85% of diarrheal deaths were found in patients aged 60 years and older [7]. This evidence further emphasizes the importance of evaluation and timely management of diarrhea in the elderly to minimize morbidity and mortality risks.

Acute infectious diarrhea

Most cases of acute infectious diarrhea are viral, because of the general short duration and low severity of disease and the low yield of bacterial isolates from stool cultures. Viruses are mostly responsible for gastroenteritis that occurs sporadically and outbreaks in the community or in hospitals and long-term care facilities. Among the diarrheal discharges for the 16-year period (1979–1995), viruses accounted for 13.6%, whereas bacterial causes were identified in 8.7% of cases [2]. Viral gastroenteritis often is self-limiting and lasts for 24 to 48 hours, whereas acute bacterial causes are identified frequently in most cases of severe diarrhea [8]. Diarrhea in the elderly population follows the same trend as that in the general population, but differs in the etiologic agents depending on the location of residence (ie, community living versus long-term care and the hospitalized elderly). In developing countries, bacteria, protozoa, and intestinal parasites were identified as the leading causes of acute gastrointestinal illness because of poor sanitary conditions. In the developed world, caliciviruses, such as the Norwalk, Sapporo, and Norwalk-like viruses, predominate in acute diarrheal illnesses in children and adults, with the exception of rotavirus, which is the most common cause of diarrhea in infants and toddlers [9].

Acute infectious diarrhea with bacterial agents identified also was found in long-term care facilities and hospitals and in the community-living elderly, with *C difficile* being the most common isolate in nursing homes, skilled nursing facilities, and hospitals [10]. Because of a significant mortality risk in patients who have *C difficile* colitis, *C difficile* infection is discussed in detail below.

Clostridium difficile infection and colitis

C difficile–associated disease (CDAD) is the primary cause of antibiotic-related nosocomial diarrhea in much of the developed world, especially with regard to the United States, Canada, and Europe. Since March 2003, escalating rates of CDAD have been reported throughout the United States and Canada [11]. Morbidity and mortality attributable to CDAD have been increasing markedly over the past decade along with a concurrent rise in the percentage of cases that are recurrent or refractory to initial treatment. This is particularly true with respect to the elderly population, including those people who reside in nursing homes or who spend a significant amount of time in hospitals.

C difficile colitis accounts for about 1% of annual hospital admissions in veterans' hospitals in the United States [12]. In recent years, the incidence of *C difficile* infection has doubled from 31/100,000 population in 1996 to 61/100,000 population in 2003, with a disproportionate increase in patients aged 65 years and older [13]. In a regional hospital in Quebec, Canada, there has been a fivefold increase in the incidence of *CDAD* cases, with the most drastic increase occurring in the elderly population together with increases in complication rates and mortality [14]. This disease pattern is similar at other United States hospitals [15–17]. Surgical patients accounted for a significant proportion of the CDAD-affected patients because of perioperative prophylactic antibiotic use [16–19]. Advanced disease with fulminant colitis affects about 4% of patients who have CDAD [20], and the mortality can range from 6% to 30% when pseudomembranous colitis occurs [14,21–25]. In the outpatient setting, the incidence of CDAD is estimated at 7 to 12 cases per 100,000 person-years [26,27].

Transmission

C difficile is a large, obligate, anaerobic, spore-producing gram-positive rod. Person-to-person transmission of the organism has been proven by way of serotyping. Fomites containing *C difficile* spores are varied and include furniture, bedpans, toilets, bathtubs, weighing scales, floors in hospitals, mops, stethoscopes, clothing, and hands. It is possible to culture *C difficile* from various surfaces in about 50% of rooms occupied by patients who have CDAD [28]. Roommates of patients who have CDAD are more likely to acquire *C difficile*–positive stool cultures and diarrhea [29]. Furthermore, transmission of nosocomially acquired CDAD may be facilitated by way of health care workers [29]. This was shown by the reduction in the spread of CDAD cases in hospitals after the institution of contact precautions, with the use of gloves and careful hand-washing techniques after examination of affected patients [30]. Additionally, *C difficile* spores are not eradicated with alcohol-based cleaning solutions. Therefore, hospital rooms occupied by CDAD-infected patients must be cleaned thoroughly with a solution containing bleach to properly disinfect all potentially contaminated environmental surfaces [31].

Clinical presentation

C difficile is responsible for a broad spectrum of enteric conditions, ranging from an asymptomatic carrier state to mild to moderate diarrheal disease to pseudomembranous colitis to fulminant colitis that can include the presence of toxic megacolon or sepsis and may progress to intestinal perforation, peritonitis, sepsis, and death. The typical presentation consists of acute onset of watery diarrhea with lower abdominal cramping relieved by defecation, a low-grade febrile state, and leukocytosis. The incubation period in hospital outbreaks may be as brief as 1 to 2 days or may occur after 5 to 10 days of antibiotic therapy. Moderate to severe CDAD may present with abdominal distention accompanied by pain and profuse watery stools; occasionally it presents with occult colonic bleeding. Systemic symptoms may include generalized malaise, fever, anorexia, and nausea. If the disease is localized to the cecum and ascending colon, the patient may have marked leukocytosis and abdominal pain with little or no diarrhea. It also is possible for patients who have CDAD to have no clinical symptoms while being febrile with an increased white blood cell count. Hypoalbuminemia and anasarca also may occur as a result of prolonged disease course and malnutrition. The incidence of life-threatening CDAD is increasing and may coincide with a decrease in the production of diarrhea secondary to a loss of intestinal muscular tone [32].

Risk factors

There are several risk factors that have been implicated with the development of CDAD. The chief risk factor is exposure to broad-spectrum antibiotics [25]. Any type of antibiotic has the potential to result in CDAD, including macrolides [33] and those used to treat it (metronidazole and vancomycin) [34]. The most likely culprits are clindamycin [35], fluoroquinolones [36–38], and third-generation cephalosporins [39]. The most significant risk factor for the development of CDAD is a history of antibiotic-associated diarrhea; the next most significant are clindamycin therapy [40], diuretic use, and an older age [41]. The longer the duration of antibiotic exposure, the greater the likelihood of acquisition of CDAD; however, CDAD may occur at any time in relation to antimicrobial therapy or even long after the offending antibiotic has been discontinued. In general, the type of patient who usually succumbs to CDAD is geriatric, frail, and hospitalized or possessing a recent history of hospitalization or one who resides in a nursing home or skilled nursing facility.

Additional predisposing factors include the regular use of proton pump inhibitors [42–45] and histamine-2 receptor blockers, gastrointestinal surgery [46], severity of illness at the time of hospital admission [47], ICU stay [41,48], enteral tube feedings [49], and contact with another patient infected with CDAD (eg, roommate [29]). It has been theorized that the use of gastric acid suppressive medications can decrease the acid concentration of the stomach, thereby permitting *C difficile* to pass unharmed into the duodenum and from there into the colon. Also, consumption of nonsteroidal anti-inflammatory agents, but not aspirin, has been linked to an increase in the rate of CDAD; however, this association may have something to do with the patient's comorbidities, all of which may not have been taken into account when the data were analyzed [43,45].

Genetic factors also may play an important role in ascertaining who is predisposed to developing CDAD. One study looked at 125 hospitalized patients and discovered a possibility of a link between genetically determined variations in the production of interleukin-8 and the predisposition to develop CDAD [50]. Also, decreased serum levels of antibody to toxin A have been associated independently with an increased likelihood of acquiring moderate to severe *C difficile* [51].

Diagnosis

The gold standard for the diagnosis of CDAD requires identification of *C difficile* cytotoxins by way of the cytotoxicity assay. This test has a high sensitivity (94%–100%) and specificity (99%) but is expensive and takes 2 to 3 days [52]. Other available tests include enzyme immunoassays (EIAs) that can deliver results in 2 hours. The EIA has a specificity and sensitivity most comparable to that of the cytotoxicity assay and tests for the production of toxins A and B [53,54]. The diagnosis also can be made by visualization of pseudomembranes or raised yellow plaques on sigmoidoscopy or colonoscopy in those with a clinical suspicion for CDAD but with negative stool testing.

Treatment

The first line of therapy for CDAD involves cessation of the suspected offending antibiotic [55]; however, this is not always possible secondary to other comorbidities that may require continuation of said antibiotic. Persistent treatment with potentially offending agents has been linked to nonresolution of CDAD, despite appropriate antimicrobial therapy [56]. In addition to stopping certain antibiotic therapy, supportive measures include oral and intravenous rehydration along with electrolyte replacement. Antiperistaltic agents, such as loperamide, diphenoxylate, and opiates, should be avoided, at least during the initial days of therapy. Strict isolation procedures and contact precaution with gloves and gown should be observed by all health care workers and visitors coming in contact with CDAD-affected patients [57].

Mild CDAD is defined as the absence of any systemic symptoms coupled with mild nonbloody diarrhea. The primary agents used to treat CDAD are metronidazole and vancomycin. Both agents possess equal efficacy; however, metronidazole is the preferred first-line drug [55,58,59]. One of the chief reasons for this, aside from its less expensive cost, is the desire to minimize the emergence of vancomycin-resistant organisms, such as enterococci species. Vancomycin use in mild CDAD is deferred until failure to respond [55,60] or resistance to metronidazole has been documented, the patient is pregnant or unable to tolerate metronidazole (eg, nausea), or if the patient has a documented allergic reaction to metronidazole [55].

Moderate CDAD occurs in the setting of profuse diarrhea that may be accompanied by one or more of the following: marked leukocytosis, generalized diffuse abdominal pain, and increased temperature. Oral vancomycin is preferred in this type of a scenario because of increased intraluminal colonic levels that result from poor absorption in the gut.

Severe CDAD exists with the occurrence of a paralytic ileus or toxic megacolon that may lead to decreased or even no diarrhea being produced. It also can occur in the setting of peritonitis, sepsis, dehydration, and hypotension and eventually may lead to death. This represents a poor prognosis with a high mortality. Emergent subtotal or total colectomy may have to be performed. In one study series, total colectomy was the preferred procedure with a lower mortality compared with a left hemicolectomy [61]. Despite surgical intervention, mortality remained high—between 30% and 60%—for those who underwent surgery [15,17,61,62]. Additionally, intraluminal vancomycin should be given. This can be done in the form of vancomycin retention enemas (500 mg vancomycin dissolved in 100 mL of normal saline) [63]. Intravenous metronidazole also may be considered; however, its role in treating severe CDAD remains to be elucidated.

Relapsed CDAD presents in a similar manner to the initial presentation of CDAD and typically does not result in a progression of disease severity. Approximately 10% to 25% of CDAD cases treated with metronidazole or vancomycin relapse within 2 to 30 days after initiating antibiotic therapy [59,64,65]. Relapsed CDAD refers to new symptoms related to C difficile toxin production after complete resolution of initial CDAD has occurred. Initial relapses should be treated with a repetition of the original medical regimen. For mild relapses, prompt discontinuation of any potentially offending antibiotics should result in resolution of symptoms. If this does not occur and there is evidence of colitis or the patient is debilitated or geriatric, then a repeat course of antimicrobial therapy for 10 to 14 days is warranted. Independent predictors of relapsed disease were age at least 65 years and a hospital stay of at least 16 days after the initial episode occurred [23]. Patients with relapsed disease are at higher risk for developing at least one CDAD-related complication (toxic megacolon, peritonitis, sepsis, shock, hypotension, intestinal perforation, or death within 30 days of diagnosis) [23]. Complicated CDAD recurrent disease has been linked significantly to age, renal failure, and leukocytosis with a white blood count of more than 20,000 cells/μL [13,23,58].

Patients who have experienced one bout of CDAD are at risk for succumbing to future episodes of CDAD after the second round of antimicrobial therapy is completed. For example, in one study involving multiple relapses of CDAD, a relapse rate of 65% was reported in patients who had had one or more episodes of CDAD treated with metronidazole or oral vancomycin [66]. Also, a repeat stool specimen should be tested for the presence of C difficile–associated toxins A or B or perhaps even the newly discovered binary toxin, which has been correlated with increased virulence of C difficile coupled with increased severity of CDAD [67], although the exact role played by the binary toxin remains to be determined. For relapsing CDAD, vancomycin pulse or taper therapy caused a statistically significant reduction in the frequency of recurrence of disease [68].

Asymptomatic carriers usually do not develop CDAD, but may provide a key source of C difficile for transmission to patients who acquire CDAD nosocomially. This group is not to be treated. They are colonized with C difficile but do not exhibit any symptoms of disease. Also, therapeutic intraluminal metronidazole levels are only achieved in the setting of diarrhea that is not evinced by asymptomatic carriers [31,63].

Other anti–Clostridium difficile therapies

Nonabsorbable anion-exchange–binding resins, such as cholestyramine and colestipol, have been given in cases of relapsing, recurrent, or refractory C difficile disease. Cholestyramine has been associated with a better overall response rate than colestipol [69]. Both of these medications also bind with other substances, such as vancomycin. Therefore, it is important to space the times at which the medicines are taken by at least 2 to 3 hours. These medications should not be used for longer than a couple of weeks and should not be prescribed for patients who have a hard time keeping track of their dosing times. Tolevamer is a newly developed resin that binds C difficile toxins and may help to protect against antibiotic-associated diarrhea [70]. There is an ongoing randomized study to evaluate the efficacy of this agent compared with oral vancomycin or metronidazole [63]. In some case reports, intravenous methylprednisolone was used successfully for CDAD treatment [71]. Rifampin also has been used in combination with vancomycin and was effective in treating multiple relapses of CDAD [72].

Nitazoxamide is an antihelminthic and antiprotozoal drug that has been used with success in treating parasitic infections globally as well as within the United States. It possesses anti–C difficile activity in vitro as well. In one study involving 22 patients who had failed therapy for CDAD, 17 (76%) displayed a vigorous response to therapy with nitazoxamide. In total,

14 (64%) patients were cured, with complete resolution of their symptoms from *C difficile*, after taking nitazoxamide [73]. In one double-blind, prospective study, nitazoxamide and metronidazole possessed equal efficacy [73]. Another medication, bacitracin, was used successfully to treat *C difficile* colitis [74]; it had similar efficacy to vancomycin and metronidazole in previous trials, and it may be tried as an alternative for the treatment of CDAD worldwide because of its low cost and better availability [75,76].

Other medications with activity against *C difficile* include teicoplanin and fusidic acid, neither of which is available in the United States. Both of these medications displayed efficacies comparable to those of metronidazole and oral vancomycin. One prospective European study evaluated cure rates among 119 patients afflicted with *C difficile* colitis; each received antimicrobial therapy in the form of teicoplanin, metronidazole, fusidic acid, or oral vancomycin. Clinical cure rates ranged from 93% to 96% [77].

Other pharmaceutical products are undergoing evaluation in phase II and III trials, including tiacumicin B (possesses 8 to 10 times the activity of vancomycin with respect to action against *C difficile*), ramoplanin, rifaximin (nonabsorbable antibiotic approved for the treatment of traveler's diarrhea), and rifalazil (a type of rifamycin).

Probiotics

The theory behind the development of probiotic therapy involves the use of live microorganisms to repopulate the colon with normal colonic flora in the hopes of preventing the colonization or infection with *C difficile*. Two such probiotics are *Lactobacillus* and *Bifidobacterium*. Another such organism is the nonpathogenic yeast *Saccharomyces boulardii*, which is used throughout Europe to prevent antibiotic-associated diarrhea [78]. It is available in the United States as an over-the-counter product, Florastor (250 mg capsules). Additionally, it may protect against *C difficile*–induced colitis [79]. Commercial preparations of *S boulardii* are not regulated by the US Food and Drug Administration; therefore, they are not standardized and may lack quality control testing. The administration of *Saccharomyces* to the elderly and the immunocompromised should be used only after careful consideration, especially because fungemia—although rare—has been reported in these populations following its consumption. Baker's yeast, also known as *S cerevisiae*, should not be substituted for *S boulardii* for the same reason [80–82].

Recent meta-analyses of randomized controlled trials showed favorable risk reduction with probiotics use in the prevention of antibiotic-associated diarrhea and treatment efficacy for CDAD [79,83,84]. Encouraging the CD-affected patient to add yogurt to their diet at multiple meals also can help to achieve this objective.

Fecal bacteriotherapy

Bacteriotherapy involves the use of fecal enemas containing fresh feces from a healthy relative of a CDAD-infected patient, as reported in one study, or it can relate to the use of rectal infusions of anaerobic and aerobic bacterial mixtures. This was a successful method for treating relapsing CDAD and pseudomembranous colitis, with resolution of symptoms and disappearance of *C difficile* toxins from the stool [85,86]. *Bacteroides* spp. were able to be isolated from the stool that was lacking *C difficile* toxins. The fact that these bacteria were absent in the presence of *C difficile* may point to the possibility of their presence in normal colonic flora being protective to the development of CDAD [78].

Intravenous immunoglobulin and vaccine

Multiple case reports reveal successful treatment of refractory, severe, or relapsing CDAD with intravenous immunoglobulin, with resolution of symptoms in 1 to 2 weeks [87,88]. The inability to produce an antibody response to toxin exposure has been linked with a 48-fold increased risk for the acquisition of CDAD [23]. Research is ongoing regarding the development of a vaccine against *C difficile* that would stimulate the immune system to develop anti–*C difficile* toxin antibodies against toxins A and B. The vaccine is composed of a partially purified mixture of inactivated *C difficile* toxins A and B. In a trial study of this vaccine preparation, three patients with recurrent CDAD involving multiple episodes received four intramuscular injections of the vaccine every 2 weeks for 8 weeks. None of the patients had further relapses when followed up after 6 months [89]. In another study, a parenteral *C difficile* toxoid vaccine induced high levels of anti–*C difficile* antibodies against toxin A and may protect against *C difficile* infection [90].

Summary

The morbidity and mortality attributable to initial and relapsing episodes of CDAD have been on the rise over the past decade. This is especially true with regard to the geriatric portion of the general population. Several risk factors have been implicated in the development of CDAD. Chief on this list is prior antibiotic use as well as frequency and duration of use, regardless of the particular type of antibiotic, although the most frequently implicated ones are clindamycin, third-generation cephalosporins, and fluoroquinolones. Age greater than 65 years also is considered an independent CDAD-related risk factor as is increased duration of residence in a hospital; long-term, acute-care facility; or nursing home. Severe or persistent CDAD may result in life-threatening complications, such as sepsis, toxic megacolon, intestinal perforation, or death.

Supportive therapy, including discontinuing any antibiotic therapy other than what is absolutely necessary, intravenous fluid rehydration, and electrolyte replacement efforts, should be combined with antimicrobial therapy with metronidazole as the primary drug of choice, especially for an initial case. Oral vancomycin may be considered when dealing with a severe, recurrent, or refractory case. For recalcitrant cases, adjunctive therapy using anion-binding resins to bind *C difficile* toxins, immunotherapy with intravenous immunoglobulin containing high levels of antibodies to *C difficile* toxins, bacteriotherapy, and probiotic therapy have been used with varying degrees of success. There are new drugs in the pipeline, such as tolevamer and rifaximin, as well as the potential for a vaccine directed against the toxins that hopefully will be available in the near future. In the meantime, careful isolation and hand hygiene precautions when dealing with patients who have CDAD, coupled with proper cleaning of environmental surfaces potentially contaminated with *C difficile* with bleach-containing cleaning solutions, will go a long way toward decreasing the incidence and prevalence of CDAD.

Viral gastroenteritis

In the general population, hospitalization due to diarrhea of viral etiology ranges from 13.6% to 27.4% [2,91], mortality due to viral causes is 7.1%, and the mortality due to bacterial causes is 71.7% of the total deaths due to foodborne gastroenteritis [91]. Acute epidemic viral gastroenteritis is self-limiting, lasting 24 to 48 hours, with one or more of the symptom cluster: nausea, vomiting, diarrhea, abdominal cramps, fever, chills, and headache. It can be debilitating in the elderly and has resulted in a death rate of more than 50% in persons aged 75 years and older [3]. Infections with foodborne viruses generally do not confer immunity [92,93]. Viral gastroenteritis usually peaks in the winter in the nursing home setting, a pattern suggestive of the highly contagious nature of the viruses. Stricter infection control measures, such as the restriction of residents and staff to their own units and not allowing staff from affected units to work on other units, had no significant effect on attack rate and duration of outbreak [92]; however, another study showed that rapid response and strict infection control contained a hospital outbreak of Norwalk-like viral gastroenteritis [94].

The traditional agents responsible for common viral diarrhea involve the viruses of four distinct families: caliciviruses (Norwalk, norovirus, Sapporo viruses), rotaviruses, adenoviruses, and astroviruses. Adenovirus was transmitted in a long-term care facility contaminated by vomitus [95]; outbreaks of astrovirus and rotavirus were found in elderly homes, with more severe diarrhea and longer duration of illness occurring in the rotavirus outbreak [96,97]. Furthermore, no specific pathogen was identified in two thirds of the foodborne disease outbreaks. This is due, in the large part, to the failure to collect or submit specimens for testing [98]. In a study in which stool kits were delivered to improve the collection rate, an etiologic pathogen was identified in two thirds of the cases; of those positive results, 76% were identified as norovirus and 24% were of bacterial origin. Twenty-five percent of affected patients did not return kits because of the resolution of symptoms [98].

Norovirus, formerly known as Norwalk-like or small round structured viruses, has been established as a major cause of epidemic viral gastroenteritis outbreaks in nursing homes, hospital wards, and cruise ships; its incidence has been increasing worldwide in recent years [92,94,99–102]. Noroviruses are highly infectious, stable, and cause severe disease in young children, the elderly, and in those with chronic diseases and persistent infection in immunosuppressed patients. It is responsible for approximately 60% of all gastroenteritis with a known enteric pathogen in the United States yearly and accounts for most deaths due to viral causes—6.9% of the total cases [91]. In the nursing home setting, restriction of visitation was used to contain the infection, but it resulted in staff shortages because of transmission to caretakers [103].

Noroviruses are commonly responsible for winter outbreaks of "stomach flu" in nursing homes, with nonbloody diarrhea noted more frequently than vomiting, and fever being less common in the elderly. Transmission modes may be person-to-person, fecal–oral, via vomitus [104], foodborne, and airborne, especially during vomiting or in a closed space [104–107]. A crowded living condition facilitates transmission of the virus, as in a recent outbreak among the 24,000 Hurricane Katrina evacuees from New Orleans. More than 1000 people were affected with gastroenteritis, and the only pathogens isolated were noroviruses [108]. Aerosolization also may occur with cleaning toilets, vomitus, vacuuming, changing bed linens, or doing soiled, contaminated laundry. Appropriate contact precautions, including gowns, masks, and gloves, should be taken when caring for the elderly with disease, [107]. Restricting and controlling visitors, separation of affected individuals 2 to 3 days after their last symptoms because of prolonged viral shedding, and controlled staff interactions between outbreak ward and unaffected ward are recommended in times of outbreak [107]. A fresh 10% bleach solution is recommended for use instead of the usual quaternary ammonia disinfectants, because the quaternary ammonia does not inactivate the virus adequately [107,109]. Alcohol gels do not provide optimal antiviral protection; however, soap and good handwashing techniques do [109]. Cleaning commonly used areas, such as doorknobs, light switches, faucet handles, and physical therapy equipment, is recommended. Practitioners and medical directors are advised to contact the local public health department during suspected outbreaks for questions and assistance on infection control and diagnostic testing.

Other infectious causes

Bacterial agents that cause significant foodborne gastroenteritis include *Shigella, Salmonella, Campylobacter jejuni*, and less frequently, *Escherichia coli* O157:H7. Older patients are at increased risk for these infections because of multiple comorbidities, achlorhydria, frequent and chronic use of proton pump inhibitors, decreased intestinal motility, and more frequent antibiotic use. These conditions alter the normal protective gastrointestinal flora, and in the setting of impaired cell-mediated immunity in the elderly, increase the rate of invasive infection and colonization by pathogenic agents. Residents of long-term care facilities, institutions, hospitals, and daycare facilities are at increased risk for outbreaks from gastrointestinal diseases. This is due to crowded communal living conditions; common delivery of medical care, food, and water; and medical personnel. These risk factors facilitate transmission by way of various routes, including fecal–oral, person-to-person, and foodborne. In reported outbreaks of foodborne gastrointestinal diseases between 1975 and 1987, nursing home outbreaks accounted for 2% of cases but almost 20% of deaths [110].

The incidence of salmonellosis in the United States has decreased in recent years, but it still carries a high fatality rate in persons aged 65 years and older [111]. For reported cases in California (1990–1999), mortality for persons older than 65 years was 59%, with *Salmonella* septicemia and gastroenteritis as the major causes of death [112]. Of the reported outbreaks of gastroenteritis with a known cause in nursing homes, *Salmonella* was the most reported pathogen, accounting for 52% of cases and 81% of deaths; staphylococcal foodborne disease was the next common cause and accounted for 23% of outbreaks [110].

Previous epidemic outbreaks of *E coli* O157:H7 infections in nursing homes in Scotland, Canada, and in the United States were reviewed. Elderly patients had similar or higher hospitalization rates compared with children aged younger than 10 years. Older patients also had a higher rate of developing postdiarrhea sequelae of thrombotic thrombocytopenic purpura (TTP) and hemolytic uremic syndrome (HUS) and carried a much higher mortality from these complications compared with the general population [113]. Bloody diarrhea was reported in 65% to 75% of patients, whereas others experienced nonspecific symptoms, such as bloating, nausea, watery diarrhea, and distension [113]. *E coli* O157:H7 is the agent most commonly isolated from visibly bloody specimens of bacterial causes of diarrhea [114]. Most elderly patients did not mount a fever response, and with a report of some bleeding per rectum and other nonspecific symptoms, most patients initially were misdiagnosed and had other unnecessary diagnostic tests performed before a suspicion for infectious diarrhea arose. This was the case in San Mateo County, California [113], where a delay in diagnosis led to excessive diagnostic tests and delay in supportive care for the elderly, who are at higher risk for dehydration and possibly higher risk for progression to HUS/TTP.

An outbreak of *E coli* in Missouri in 1990 was due to an unchlorinated water supply. This outbreak was responsible for the largest number of affected people, 243, with four deaths, all occurring in the elderly [115]. The most recent outbreak of *E coli* O157:H7 spans several states, with a common contaminated source of raw spinach that could be traced back to a single manufacturing facility on a particular day. The general population affected included 199 persons in 26 states; of those, 14% were 60 years or older. Two elderly women and a 2-year-old child died [116].

Other responsible agents for gastroenteritis outbreaks include *Cryptosporidium* in the 1993 Milwaukee outbreak of contaminated drinking water. Elderly persons had an increased risk for contracting the disease and had a more severe disease than did other adults. They also had a shorter incubation period and higher risk for secondary transmission [117].

In a retrospective chart review of a hospital in Rhode Island, chronically ill elderly patients accounted for 36% of affected cases—and in almost half of the affected elderly—coinfection with *Cryptosporidium* and *C difficile* was identified [118]. Traveler's diarrhea often is self-limiting, is more common in young travelers, and has the lowest incidence in people older than 55 years of age [119]; however, giardiasis and amebiasis need to be considered in traveling elderly retirees, in elder immigrants at risk for exposure to unsanitary conditions, and in those presenting with persistent diarrhea. Giardiasis was detected on small bowel biopsy of two elderly patients who presented with anorexia, weight loss, and diarrhea, and in one elderly person with a history of dyspepsia, hematemesis, and malabsorption [120]. Amebiasis also should be considered in the elderly with watery diarrhea, abdominal bloating, and pruritus, especially in the traveling retired elderly, in the elderly working abroad, or in an elderly immigrant from a developing country.

Noninfectious acute diarrhea

Although diarrhea in an elderly person may get early recognition by nurses or a caregiver, treatment with antidiarrheal agents may exacerbate an underlying problem of fecal impaction. Diarrhea may represent the initial sign of fecal impaction, which is a potentially life-threatening condition if not treated appropriately and timely. In the setting of fecal impaction, this initial diarrhea is termed "overflow diarrhea." In a retrospective investigation of institutionalized elderly, fecal impaction was the most common cause of diarrhea (55% of cases), laxative-induced diarrhea occurred in 20% of cases, and gastrointestinal infections resulted in 5% of cases [121]. Absent or hypoactive bowel sounds and abdominal distension, with or without a change in mental status, in the setting of diarrhea should prompt the physician and staff to look for underlying fecal impaction [122]. This can be diagnosed easily and readily with a rectal examination and plain abdominal radiograph. Sometimes a routine problem requires more than a routine solution; it requires close observation and examination of the patient. An "as-needed" medication, such as an antidiarrheal, could make fecal impaction worse, and the patient may end up in a hypoactive delirious state.

Diarrhea is a common side effect of many drugs. The mechanism is poorly understood; however, for many drugs, diarrhea is caused by interaction of the drug with intestinal receptors. Other drug reactions include mucosal cell toxicity commonly induced by anticancer drugs, bacterial overgrowth, and changes in normal colonic flora due to antibiotics and osmotic laxatives [123]. Several classes of drugs commonly cause diarrhea in the elderly; the most commonly encountered are digitalis (a specific splanchnic vasoconstrictor), β-blockers, angiotensin-converting enzyme inhibitors, antiarrhythmics, diuretics, cholesterol lowering drugs, and anti–Parkinson disease drugs, such as levodopa [123]. Other drugs prescribed commonly in the elderly population include antiulcer agents, lactulose, and histamine receptor blockers. Withdrawal of one medication at a time, as a therapeutic measure in the case of diarrhea of unknown cause, may be needed to evaluate the possibility of the diarrhea being related to an adverse drug reaction.

Although antibiotic-induced diarrhea is common in hospitalized patients, tube feeding can result in a significant number of patients developing diarrhea [124]. This occurred in up to 39% of patients on general medical floors [125–128] and in up to 63% of patients in critical care units [129,130]. In those patients whose enteral formula was supplemented with fiber, stool frequency was lower, and stool consistency was significantly higher [131]. It is believed that the composition of the enteral formula may have an adverse effect on the colonic microflora, which normally produces short-chain fatty acids (SCFAs) [132]. SCFAs are believed to be trophic to the colonic flora, are used as fuel, and normally are absorbed in the colon. Their absorption enhances water and electrolyte absorption [133]. Fecal SCFAs are low in acute diarrhea, and colonic water and sodium absorption is restored with increasing level of luminal SCFAs [133,134].

Chronic diarrhea

Other diarrheal diseases need to be considered in the elderly population, including celiac disease and inflammatory bowel diseases, such as Crohn's disease and ulcerative colitis. Although celiac disease traditionally has been described as a disease of childhood, more than 80% of cases have been diagnosed in adulthood [135,136]. For those elderly with a delay in diagnosis, duration of symptoms lasted 11 ± 19 years and most were incorrectly diagnosed with irritable bowel syndrome [137]. Several case reports established that celiac disease is underdiagnosed in the elderly population [138–141]. Older patients with celiac disease frequently present with diarrhea, weight loss, abdominal pain and discomfort, and malabsorption syndromes that can result in anemia, electrolyte disturbances, and osteoporosis; however, they can present with atypical findings of hyperimmunoglobulin A [141] or neurologic and psychiatric symptoms [142]. In another case report, celiac disease was confirmed only after a second work-up with positive duodenal biopsy and antibody titers with worsening symptoms over a 3-month period, including anorexia, rapid weight loss, and gastrointestinal symptoms [143]. Histologically, intestinal biopsy shows villous atrophy in celiac disease. It was believed that the changes in the mucosa are patchy and skipped; a repeat biopsy may be required when the first biopsy is negative or inconclusive and symptoms persist. Although antigliadin and antiendomysial antibodies are highly sensitive and specific in cases of celiac disease, there have been cases of negative titers in lesser grades of villous atrophy. Although uncommon, seronegative celiac disease has been reported [144–146]. The only effective treatment is a gluten-free diet. There is an increased association with malignant intestinal lymphoma in patients who have celiac disease, with a prevalence of up to 22% in elderly who had celiac disease in one study [147]. Early recognition and diagnosis would improve outcome and reverse the associated morbidities significantly.

Inflammatory bowel disease (IBD) is another malady that is commonly thought of as a disease of the youth, with peak incidences occurring in the second to fourth decades of life; however, some studies showed a bimodal distribution, with a second, small peak in the sixth through eighth decades of life that was responsible for 10% to 15% of diagnosed cases [148,149]. Symptoms of IBD in elderly patients are similar to those in young adults; however, the elderly group seems to requires less surgical intervention than the younger group, but may have more postoperative complications as a result of preexisting comorbidities [150,151] and a longer hospital stay [150]. Crohn's disease in the elderly usually is confined to the colon. Left-sided Crohn's disease often is misdiagnosed as diverticular disease in the elderly [151]. Ulcerative colitis is more severe in the elderly and often presents as distal disease. Mortality may be increased in the elderly, probably because of other comorbid conditions. Treatment of IBD in the elderly is the same as that in younger adults, but extra caution needs to be taken when steroids are used. This is due to the multiple adverse effects of corticosteroids on the elderly, including poor glycemic control, cataract formation, steroid-induced psychosis, and an increased risk for osteoporosis. Steroid-sparing drugs, such as mercaptopurine and mesalamine, are tolerated better and should be maximized before starting steroids. When indicated, calcium supplementation and bisphosphonate prophylaxis and treatment are advised to prevent further bone loss.

Microscopic colitis, an entity including collagenous colitis and lymphocytic colitis, has emerged as a new common cause of chronic diarrhea in the general population. Microscopic colitis has a peak incidence at around 65 years of age and is more prevalent in women, with a female to male ratio of 7:1 in collagenous colitis and 2.4:1 in lymphocytic colitis [152]. The classic clinical presentation is that of a 65-year-old woman with chronic, recurrent nonbloody watery diarrhea, often nocturnal, abdominal pain, and weight loss. Dehydration and severe complications requiring medical attention are rare. The onset may mimic acute infectious diarrhea but the course is benign, chronic, and relapsing. No associated increased risk for colorectal cancer was reported, but an association with other autoimmune diseases was reported in up to 40% to 50% of cases [152]. The most common associated diseases are diabetes, thyroid disease, celiac disease, and rheumatoid arthritis. Colonoscopy commonly shows normal mucosa; occasionally, mucosal irritation or redness may be seen. Diagnosis is confirmed by proximal colonic biopsies showing classic histopathologic changes. Treatment is supportive with loperamide and cholestyramine in mild cases. Budesonide, a corticosteroid, is effective compared with placebo but has a high relapse rate upon drug discontinuation [152]. Immunomodulators, such as mesalamine and sulfasalazine, have been used; however, they have not been evaluated in randomized, controlled trials.

Special considerations

Carcinoid tumor of the intestines frequently present with diarrhea, abdominal pain, weight loss, and, in some cases, intractable nausea and vomiting. The disease course can be complicated by recurrent intestinal obstruction and seems to mimic other diseases radiographically, such as Crohn's ileitis [153]. The diagnosis often is delayed until specific diagnostic tests are ordered or until a postoperative histopathologic diagnosis is made. With common usage of selective serotonin-reuptake inhibitors in the elderly to treat depression, diarrhea can be exacerbated in patients who have undiagnosed carcinoid tumor.

For the elderly who have predisposed conditions of atherosclerosis, peripheral vascular disease, heart failure, and treatment with diuretics, digitalis, or antihypertensives, ischemic colitis occurs as a result of treatment because of hypovolemia and hypoperfusion to the intestines, especially the large intestine. The patient typically presents with acute, crampy abdominal pain and bloody diarrhea or a pink mucous bowel movement. The course of the disease is frequently reversible; however, in severe cases it can progress to ulceration, stricture formation, gangrene, and perforation. This condition is especially common after abdominal aortic aneurysm surgery. Management includes early recognition and diagnostic studies with abdominal roentgenogram and colonoscopy studies. Intravenous fluids, antibiotics, and bowel rest normally resolve the symptoms in 24 to 48 hours; however, stool studies should be sent to exclude other causes, because *C difficile* colitis and bacterial enteritis have similar presentations to that of ischemic colitis.

Summary

Diarrhea in the elderly population is one disease that needs special attention in treatment and management, especially in acute and long-term care residents because of their multiple comorbidities, immunosenescence, frailty, and poor nutritional status. Close follow-up to ensure adequate hydration and electrolyte replacement and infection control measures to contain outbreaks should be emphasized to caregivers and nursing staff in acute- and long-term–care facilities. Although *C difficile* colitis causes significant morbidity and mortality in this population, the judicious use of antibiotics is important to decrease the incidence and recurrence of the disease. When the diarrhea is chronic and all stool testings and serologies have been performed, the patient may benefit from endoscopy and colonoscopy for biopsy. An attentive and vigilant nursing staff is critical to the timely diagnosis and treatment of diarrheal diseases to improve quality of life and reduce mortality.

References

[1] Sahyoun N, Lentzner H, Hoyert D, et al. Trends in causes of death among the elderly. Centers for Disease Control and Prevention. Aging Trends 2001;1–10.
[2] Mounts AW, Holman RC, Clarke MJ, et al. Trends in hospitalizations associated with gastroenteritis among adults in the United States, 1979–1995. Epidemiol Infect 1999; 123(1):1–8.
[3] Lew JF. Diarrheal deaths in the United States, 1979 through 1987. A special problem for the elderly. JAMA 1991;265(24):3280–4.
[4] Guerant RL, Van Gilder T, Steriner TS, et al. Practice guidelines for the management of infectious diarrhea. Clin Infect Dis 2001;132(3):331–51.
[5] AGA guideline: evaluation and management of chronic diarrhea. Gastroenterology 1999; 116:1461–3.
[6] Feldman M, Friedman LS, Brandt LJ. Sleisenger & Fordtran's gastrointestinal and liver disease. 8th edition. Chapter 9 online. Philadelphia, PA: W.B. Saunders; 2006.
[7] Gangarosa RE, Glass RI, Lew JF, et al. Hospitalizations involving gastroenteritis in the United States, 1985: the special burden of the disease among the elderly. Am J Epidemiol 1992;135(3):281–90.
[8] Dryden MS, Gabb RJ, Wright SK. Empirical treatment of severe acute community-acquired gastroenteritis with ciprofloxacin. Clin Infect Dis 1996;22(6):1019–25.
[9] Musher DM, Musher BL. Contagious acute gastrointestinal infections. N Engl J Med 2004; 351:2417–27.
[10] Simor AE, Bradley SF, Strausbaugh LJ, et al. Clostridium difficile in long-term care facilities for the elderly. Infect Control Hosp Epidemiol 2002;23(11):696–703.
[11] Kuijper EJ, Coignard B, Tull P, et al. Emergence of Clostridium difficile-associated disease in North America and Europe. Clin Microbiol Infect 2006;12(Suppl 6):2–18.
[12] Buchner AM, Sonnenberg A. Epidemiology of Clostridium difficile infection in a large population of hospitalized US military veterans. Dig Dis Sci 2002;47(1):201–7.
[13] McDonald LC, Owings M, Jernigan DB. Clostridium difficile infection in patients discharged from US short-stay hospitals, 1996–2003. Emerg Infect Dis 2006;12(3):409–15.
[14] Pepin J, Valiquette L, Alary ME, et al. Clostridium difficile-associated diarrhea in a region of Quebec from 1991 to 2003: a changing pattern of disease severity. CMAJ 2004;171: 466–72.
[15] Dallal RM, Harbrecht BG, Boujoukas AJ, et al. Fulminant Clostridium difficile: an underappreciated and increasing cause of death and complications. Ann Surg 2002; 235(3):363–72.
[16] Morris AM, Jobe BA, Stoney M, et al. Clostridium difficile colitis: an increasingly aggressive iatrogenic disease? Arch Surg 2002;137(10):1096–100.
[17] Jobe BA, Grasley A, Deveney KE, et al. Clostridium difficile colitis: an increasing hospital-acquired illness. Am J Surg 1995;169(5):480–3.
[18] Wren SM, Ahmed N, Jamal A, et al. Preoperative oral antibiotics in colorectal surgery increase the rate of Clostridium difficile colitis. Arch Surg 2005;140(8):752–6.

[19] Bulstrode NW, Bradbury AW, Barrett S, et al. *Clostridium difficile* colitis after aortic surgery. Eur J Vasc Endovasc Surg 1997;14(3):217–20.

[20] Synnott K, Mealy K, Merry C, et al. Timing of surgery for fulminating pseudomembranous colitis. Br J Surg 1998;85(2):229–31.

[21] Olson M, Shanholtzer CJ, Lee TJ Jr, et al. Ten years of prospective *Clostridium difficile*-associated disease surveillance and treatment at the Minneapolis VA Medical Center, 1982–1991. Infect Control Hosp Epidemiol 1994;15:371–81.

[22] Moshkowitz M, Ben Baruch E, Kline Z, et al. Clinical manifestations and outcome of pseudomembranous colitis in an elderly population in Israel. Isr Med Assoc J 2004;6:201–4.

[23] Kyne L, Warny M, Qamar A, et al. Association between antibody response to toxin A and protection against recurrent *Clostridium difficile* diarrhoea. Lancet 2001;357(9251):189–93.

[24] Musher DM, Aslam S, Logan N, et al. Relatively poor outcome after treatment of *Clostridium difficile* colitis with metronidazole. Clin Infect Dis 2005;40:1586–90.

[25] Loo VG, Poirier L, Miller MA, et al. A predominantly clonal multi-institutional outbreak of *Clostridium difficile*-associated diarrhea with high morbidity and mortality. N Engl J Med 2005;353:2442–9.

[26] Hirschhorn LR, Trnka Y, Onderdonk A, et al. Epidemiology of community-acquired *Clostridium difficile*-associated diarrhea. J Infect Dis 1994;169:127–33.

[27] Levy DG, Stergachis A, McFarland LV, et al. Antibiotics and *Clostridium difficile* diarrhea in the ambulatory care setting. Clin Ther 2000;22:91–102.

[28] Kim KH, Fekety R, Batts DH, et al. Isolation of *Clostridium difficile* from the environment and contacts of patients with antibiotic-associated colitis. J Infect Dis 1981;143:42–50.

[29] McFarland LV, Mulligan ME, Kwok RY, et al. Nosocomial acquisition of *Clostridium difficile* infection. N Engl J Med 1989;320:204–10.

[30] Gerding DN, Johnson S, Peterson LR, et al. *Clostridium difficile*-associated diarrhea and colitis. Infect Control Hosp Epidemiol 1995;16(8):459–77.

[31] Sunenshine RH, McDonald LC. *Clostridium difficile*-associated disease: new challenges from an established pathogen. Cleve Clin J Med 2006;71(2):187–97.

[32] Wanahita A, Goldsmith EA, Marino BJ, et al. *Clostridium difficile* infection in patients with unexplained leukocytosis. Am J Med 2003;115(7):543–6.

[33] Raveh D, Rabinowitz B, Breuer GS, et al. Risk factors for *Clostridium difficile* toxin-positive nosocomial diarrhoea. Int J Antimicrob Agents 2006;28(3):231–7.

[34] Bingley PJ, Harding GM. *Clostridium difficile* colitis following treatment with metronidazole and vancomycin. Postgrad Med J 1987;63:993–4.

[35] Tedesco FJ, Barton RW, Alpers DH. Clindamycin-associated colitis. A prospective study. Ann Intern Med 1974;81(4):429–33.

[36] Gaynes R, Rimland D, Killum E, et al. Outbreak of *Clostridium difficile* infection in a long-term care facility: association with gatifloxacin use. Clin Infect Dis 2004;38(5):640–5.

[37] Yip C, Loeb M, Salama S, et al. Quinolone use as a risk factor for nosocomial *Clostridium difficile*-associated diarrhea. Infect Control Hosp Epidemiol 2001;22(9):572–5.

[38] McCusker ME, Harris AD, Perencevich E, et al. Fluoroquinolone use and *Clostridium difficile*-associated diarrhea. Emerg Infect Dis 2003;9(6):730–3.

[39] Muto CA, Pokrywka M, Shutt K, et al. A large outbreak of *Clostridium difficile*-associated disease with an unexpected proportion of deaths and colectomies at a teaching hospital following increased fluoroquinolone use. Infect Control Hosp Epidemiol 2005;26(3):273–80.

[40] Palmore TN, Sohn S, Malak SF, et al. Risk factors for acquisition of *Clostridium difficile*-associated diarrhea among outpatients at a cancer hospital. Infect Control Hosp Epidemiol 2005;26(8):680–4.

[41] Brown E, Talbot GH, Axelrod P, et al. Risk factors for *Clostridium difficile* toxin-associated diarrhea. Infect Control Hosp Epidemiol 1990;11(6):283–90.

[42] Dial S, Alrasadi K, Manoukian C, et al. Risk of *Clostridium difficile* diarrhea among hospital inpatients prescribed proton pump inhibitors: cohort and case control studies. CMAJ 2004;171(1):33–8.

[43] Dial S, Delaney JA, Barkun AN, et al. Use of gastric acid-suppressive agents and the risk of community-acquired *Clostridium difficile*-associated disease. JAMA 2005;294(23):2989–95.

[44] Al-Tureihi FI, Hassoun A, Wolf-Klein G, et al. Albumin, length of stay, and proton pump inhibitors: key factors in *Clostridium difficile*-associated disease in nursing home patients. J Am Med Dir Assoc 2005;6(2):105–8.

[45] Cunningham R, Dale B, Undy B, et al. Proton pump inhibitors as a risk factor for *Clostridium difficile* diarrhoea. J Hosp Infect 2003;54(3):243–5.

[46] Thibault A, Miller MA, Gaese C. Risk factors for the development of *Clostridium difficile*-associated diarrhea during a hospital outbreak. Infect Control Hosp Epidemiol 1991;12(6):345–8.

[47] Kyne L, Sougioultzis S, McFarland LV, et al. Underlying disease severity as a major risk factor for nosocomial *Clostridium difficile* diarrhea. Infect Control Hosp Epidemiol 2002; 23(11):653–9.

[48] Modena S, Bearelly D, Swartz K, et al. *Clostridium difficile* among hospitalized patients receiving antibiotics: a case-control study. Infect Control Hosp Epidemiol 2005;26(8): 685–90.

[49] Bliss DZ, Johnson S, Savik K, et al. Acquisition of *Clostridium difficile* and *Clostridium difficile*-associated diarrhea in hospitalized patients receiving tube feeding. Ann Intern Med 1998;129(12):1012–9.

[50] Jiang ZD, DuPont HL, Garey K, et al. A common polymorphism in the interleukin 8 gene promoter is associated with *Clostridium difficile* diarrhea. Am J Gastroenterol 2006;101(5): 1112–6.

[51] Kyne L, Warny M, Qamar A, et al. Asymptomatic carriage of *Clostridium difficile* and serum levels of IgG antibody against toxin A. N Engl J Med 2000;342(6):390–7.

[52] Barbut F, Kajzer C, Planas N, et al. Comparison of three enzyme immunoassays, a cytotoxicity assay, and toxigenic culture for diagnosis of *Clostridium difficile*-associated diarrhea. J Clin Microbiol 1993;31(4):963–7.

[53] Lyerly DM, Neville LM, Evans DT, et al. Multicenter evaluation of the *Clostridium difficile* TOX A/B test. J Clin Microbiol 1998;36(1):184–90.

[54] Aldeen WE, Bingham M, Aiderzada A, et al. Comparison of the TOX A/B test to a cell culture cytotoxicity assay for the detection of *Clostridium difficile* in stools. Diagn Microbiol Infect Dis 2000;36(4):211–3.

[55] Malnick SD, Zimhony O. Treatment of *Clostridium difficile*-associated diarrhea. Ann Pharmacother 2002;36(11):1767–75.

[56] Nair S, Yadav D, Corpuz M, et al. *Clostridium difficile* colitis: factors influencing treatment failure and relapse – a prospective evaluation. Am J Gastroenterol 1998;93(10):1873–6.

[57] Barbut F, Richard A, Hamadi K, et al. Epidemiology of recurrences or reinfections of *Clostridium difficile*-associated diarrhea. J Clin Microbiol 2000;38(6):2386–8.

[58] Gerding DN. Metronidazole for *Clostridium difficile*-associated disease: is it ok for mom? Clin Infect Dis 2005;40(11):1598–600.

[59] Fekety R. Guidelines for the diagnosis and management of *Clostridium difficile*-associated diarrhea and colitis. American College of Gastroenterology, Practice Parameters Committee. Am J Gastroenterol 1997;92(5):739–50.

[60] Surowiec D, Kuyumjian AG, Wynd MA, et al. Past, present and future therapies for *Clostridium difficile*-associated disease. Ann Pharmacother 2006;40(12):2155–63.

[61] Koss K, Clark MA, Sanders DS, et al. The outcome of surgery in fulminant *Clostridium difficile* colitis. Colorectal Dis 2006;8(2):149–54.

[62] Longo WE, Mazuski JE, Virgo KS, et al. Outcome after colectomy for *Clostridium difficile* colitis. Dis Colon Rectum 2004;47(10):1620–6.

[63] Aslam S, Musher DM. An update on diagnosis, treatment, and prevention of *Clostridium difficile*-associated disease. Gastroenterol Clin North Am 2006;35(2):315–35.

[64] Tedesco FJ, Gordon D, Fortson WC. Approach to patients with multiple relapses of antibiotic-associated pseudomembranous colitis. Am J Gastroenterol 1985;80(11):867–8.

[65] Bartlett JG, Tedesco FJ, Shull S, et al. Symptomatic relapse after oral vancomycin therapy of antibiotic-associated pseudomembranous colitis. Gastroenterology 1980;78(3):431–4.

[66] McFarland LV, Surawicz CM, Greenberg RN, et al. A randomized placebo-controlled trial of Saccharomyces boulardii in combination with standard antibiotics for Clostridium difficile disease. JAMA 1994;271(24):1913–8.

[67] Hubert B, Loo VG, Bourgault AM, et al. A portrait of the geographic dissemination of the Clostridium difficile North American pulsed-field type I strain and the epidemiology of C. difficile-associated in Quebec. Clin Infect Dis 2007;44(2):238–44.

[68] McFarland LV, Elmer GW, Surawicz CM. Breaking the cycle: treatment strategies for 163 cases of recurrent Clostridium difficile disease. Am J Gastroenterol 2002;97(7):1769–75.

[69] Kreutzer EW, Milligan FD. Treatment of antibiotic-associated pseudomembranous colitis with cholestyramine resin. Johns Hopkins Med J 1978;143(3):67–72.

[70] Braunlin W, Xu Q, Hook P, et al. Toxin binding of tolevamer, a polyanionic drug that protects against antibiotic-associated diarrhea. Biophys J 2004;87(1):534–9.

[71] Cavagnaro C, Berezin S, Medow MS. Corticosteroid treatment of severe, non-responsive Clostridium difficile induced colitis. Arch Dis Child 2003;88(4):342–4.

[72] Buggy BP, Fekety R, Silva J Jr. Therapy of relapsing Clostridium difficile-associated diarrhea and colitis with the combination of vancomycin and rifampin. J Clin Gastroenterol 1987;9(2):155–9.

[73] Musher DM, Logan N, Hamill RJ, et al. Nitazoxanide for the treatment of Clostridium difficile colitis. Clin Infect Dis 2006;43(4):421–7.

[74] Chang TW, Gorbach SL, Bartlett JG, et al. Bacitracin treatment of antibiotic-associated colitis and diarrhea caused by Clostridium difficile toxin. Gastroenterology 1980;78:1584–6.

[75] Young GP, Ward PB, Bayley N, et al. Antibiotic-associated colitis due to Clostridium difficile: double-blind comparison of vancomycin with bacitracin. Gastroenterology 1985; 89:1038–45.

[76] Dudley MN, McLaughlin JC, Carrington G, et al. Oral bacitracin vs vancomycin therapy for Clostridium difficile-induced diarrhea. A randomized double-blind trial. Arch Intern Med 1986;146:1101–4.

[77] Wenisch C, Parschalk B, Hasenhundl M, et al. Comparison of vancomycin, teicoplanin, metronidazole, and fusidic acid for the treatment of Clostridium difficile-associated diarrhea. Clin Infect Dis 1996;22:813–8.

[78] Elmer GW, Surawicz CM, McFarland LV. Biotherapeutic agents. A neglected modality for the treatment and prevention of selected intestinal and vaginal infections. JAMA 1996;275: 870–6.

[79] McFarland LV. Meta-analysis of probiotics for the prevention of antibiotic associated diarrhea and the treatment of Clostridium difficile disease. Am J Gastroenterol 2006;101: 812–22.

[80] Cherifi S, Robberecht J, Miendje Y. Saccharomyces cerevisiae fungemia in an elderly patient with Clostridium difficile colitis. Acta Clin Belg 2004;59(4):223–4.

[81] Munoz P, Bouza E, Cuenca-Estrella M, et al. Saccharomyces cerevisiae fungemia: an emerging infectious disease. Clin Infect Dis 2005;40(11):1625–34.

[82] Lestin F, Pertschy A, Rimek D. Fungemia after oral treatment with Saccharomyces boulardii in a patient with multiple comorbidities [English abstract]. Dtsch Med Wochenschr 2003;128(48):2531–3 [in German].

[83] Sazawal S, Hiremath G, Dhingra U, et al. Efficacy of probiotics in prevention of acute diarrhea: a meta-analysis of masked, randomized, placebo-controlled trials. Lancet Infect Dis 2006;6(6):374–82.

[84] Cremonini F, Di Caro S, Nista EC, et al. Meta-analysis: the effect of probiotic administration on antibiotic-associated diarrhoea. Aliment Pharmacol Ther 2002;16(8): 1461–7.

[85] Borody TJ, Warren EF, Leis SM, et al. Bacteriotherapy using fecal flora: toying with human motions. J Clin Gastroenterol 2004;38:475–83.

854   TRINH & PRABHAKAR

[86] Tvede M, Rask-Madsen J. Bacteriotherapy for chronic relapsing *Clostridium difficile* diarrhoea in six patients. Lancet 1989;1(8648):1156–60.

[87] Salcedo J, Keates S, Pothoulakis C, et al. Intravenous immunoglobulin therapy for severe *Clostridium difficile* colitis. Gut 1997;41(3):366–70.

[88] McPherson S, Rees CJ, Ellis R, et al. Intravenous immunoglobulin for the treatment of severe, refractory, and recurrent *Clostridium difficile* diarrhea. Dis Colon Rectum 2006; 49(5):640–5.

[89] Sougioltzis S, Kyne L, Drudy D, et al. *Clostridium difficile* toxoid vaccine in recurrent *C. difficile*-associated diarrhea. Gastroenterology 2005;128(3):764–70.

[90] Aboudola S, Kotloff KL, Kyne L, et al. *Clostridium difficile* vaccine and serum immunoglobulin G antibody response to toxin A. Infect Immun 2003;71(3):1608–10.

[91] Mead PS, Slutsker L, Dietz V, et al. Food-related illness and death in the United States. Emerg Infect Dis 1999;5(5):607–25.

[92] Augustin AK, Simor AE, Shorrock C, et al. Outbreaks of gastroenteritis due to Norwalk-like virus in two long-term care facilities for the elderly. Can J Infect Control 1995;10(4): 111–3.

[93] Parashar U, Quiroz ES, Mounts AW, et al. "Norwalk-like viruses": public health consequences and outbreak management. MMWR Recomm Rep 2001;50(RR-9):1–17.

[94] McCall J, Smithson R. Rapid response and strict control measures can contain a hospital outbreak of Norwalk-like virus. Commun Dis Public Health 2002;5(3):243–6.

[95] Reid JA, Breckon D, Hunter PR. Infection of staff during an outbreak of viral gastroenteritis in an elderly persons' home. J Hosp Infect 1990;16(1):81–5.

[96] Lewis DC, Lightfoot NF, Cubitt WD, et al. Outbreaks of astrovirus type 1 and rotavirus gastroenteritis in a geriatric inpatient population. J Hosp Infect 1989;14(1):9–14.

[97] Feeney SA, Mitchell SJ, Mitchell F, et al. Association of the G4 rotavirus genotype with gastroenteritis in adults. J Med Virol 2006;78(8):1119–23.

[98] Jones TF, Bulens SN, Gettner S, et al. Use of stool collection kits delivered to patients can improve confirmation of etiology in foodborne disease outbreaks. Clin Infect Dis 2004;39: 1454–9.

[99] Green KY, Belliot G, Taylor JL, et al. A predominant role for Norwalk-like viruses as agents of epidemic gastroenteritis in Maryland nursing homes for the elderly. J Infect Dis 2002;185:133–46.

[100] Calderon-Margalit R, Sheffer R, Halperin T, et al. A large-scale gastroenteritis outbreak associated with Norovirus in nursing homes. Epidemiol Infect 2004;133:35–40.

[101] Odelin MF, Ruel N, Berthelot P, et al. Investigation of an outbreak of norovirus gastroenteritis in a geriatric hospital. Ann Biol Clin (Paris) 2006;64(2):141–7 [in French].

[102] Jiang X, Turf E, Hu J, et al. Outbreaks of gastroenteritis in elderly nursing homes and retirement facilities associated with human caliciviruses. J Med Virol 1996;50(4):335–41.

[103] Drinka PJ. Norovirus outbreaks in nursing homes. J Am Geriatr Soc 2005;53:1839–40.

[104] Chadwick PR, McCann R. Transmission of a small round structured virus by vomiting during a hospital outbreak of gastroenteritis. J Hosp Infect 1994;26:251–9.

[105] Marks PJ, Vipond IB, Carlisle D, et al. Evidence for airborne transmission of Norwalk-like virus (NLV) in a hotel restaurant. Epidemiol Infect 2000;124:481–7.

[106] Ho MS, Monroe SS, Stine S, et al. Viral gastroenteritis aboard a cruise ship. Lancet 1989; 2:961–5.

[107] Virginia Department of Health. Guidelines for the control of a suspected or confirmed outbreak of viral gastroenteritis in a nursing home-updated 2/13/04. Available at: www.vhd.state.va.us/epi/noro_outbreak_guidelines.pdf.

[108] Palacio H, Shah U, Kilborn C, et al. Norovirus outbreak among evacuees from hurricane Katrina: Houston, Texas, September 2005. MMWR Morb Mortal Wkly Rep 2005;54: 1016–8.

[109] Doultree JC, Druce JD, Birch CJ, et al. Inactivation of feline calicivirus. A Norwalk virus surrogate. J Hosp Infect 1999;41:51–7.

[110] Levine WC, Smart JF, Archer DL, et al. Foodborne disease outbreaks in nursing homes, 1975 through 1987. JAMA 1991;266:2105–9.

[111] Summary of notifiable diseases, United States, 1998. MMWR Morb Mortal Wkly Rep 1999;47(53):1–93.

[112] Trevejo RT, Courtney JG, Starr M, et al. Epidemiology of salmonellosis in California, 1990–1999: morbidity, mortality, and hospitalization costs. Am J Epidemiol 2003;157(1): 48–57.

[113] Reiss G, Kunz P, Koin D, et al. Escherichia coli O157:H7 infection in nursing homes: review of literature and report of recent outbreak. J Am Geriatr Soc 2006;54:680–4.

[114] Slutsker L, Ries AA, Greene KD, et al. Escherichia coli O157:H7 diarrhea in the United States: clinical and epidemiologic features. Ann Intern Med 1997;126(7):505–13.

[115] Swerdlow DL, Woodruff BA, Brady RC, et al. A waterborne outbreak in Missouri of Escherichia coli O157:H7 associated with bloody diarrhea and death. Ann Intern Med 1992;117(10):812–9.

[116] Centers for Disease Control and Prevention. Update on multi-state outbreak of E. coli O157:H7 infections from fresh spinach October 6, 2006. National Center for Infectious Diseases. Available at: http://www.cdc.gov/ecoli/2006/september/. Accessed January 8, 2007.

[117] Naumova EN, Egorov AI, Morris RD, et al. The elderly and waterborne Cryptosporidium infection: gastroenteritis hospitalizations before and during the 1993 Milwaukee outbreak. Emerg Infect Dis 2003;9(4):418–26.

[118] Neill MA, Rice SK, Ahmad NV, et al. Cryptosporidiosis: an unrecognized cause of diarrhea in elderly hospitalized patients. Clin Infect Dis 1996;22(1):168–70.

[119] Steffen R. Epidemiologic studies of travelers' diarrhea, severe gastrointestinal infections, and cholera. Rev Infect Dis 1986;8(Suppl 2):S122–30.

[120] Beaumont DM, James OFW. Unsuspected giardiasis as a cause of malnutrition and diarrhea in the elderly. Br Med J (Clin Res Ed) 1986;293(6546):554–5.

[121] Kinnunen O, Jauhonen P, Salokannel J, et al. Diarrhea and fecal impaction in elderly long-stay patients. Z Gerontol 1989;22(6):321–3.

[122] Hahn K. Think twice about diarrhea. Nursing 1987;17(9):78–80.

[123] Holt PR. Diarrhea and malabsorption in the elderly. Gastroenterol Clin North Am 2001; 30(2):427–44.

[124] McErlean A, Kelly O, Bergin S, et al. The importance of microbiological investigations, medications and artificial feeding in diarrhoea evaluation. Ir J Med Sci 2005;174(1): 21–5.

[125] Heymsfield SB, Bethel RA, Ansley JD, et al. Enteral hyperalimentation: an alternative to central venous hyperalimentation. Ann Intern Med 1979;90:63–71.

[126] Heibert JM, Brown A, Anderson RG, et al. Comparison of continuous vs intermittent tube feedings in adult burn patients. JPEN J Parenter Enteral Nutr 1981;5:73–5.

[127] Cataldi-Betcher EL, Seltzer MH, Slocum BA, et al. Complications occurring during enteral nutrition support: a prospective study. JPEN J Parenter Enteral Nutr 1983;7:546–52.

[128] Whelan K, Hill L, Preedy VR, et al. Formula delivery in patients receiving enteral tube feeding on general hospital wards: the impact of nasogastric extubation and diarrhea. Nutrition 2006;22(10):1025–31.

[129] Keohane PP, Attrill H, Love M, et al. Relation between osmolality and gastrointestinal side effects in enteral nutrition. Br Med J (Clin Res Ed) 1984;288:678–80.

[130] Kelly TW, Patrick MR, Hillman KM. Study of diarrhoea in critically ill patients. Crit Care Med 1983;11:7–9.

[131] Vandewoude MF, Paridaens KM, Suy RA, et al. Fibre-supplemented tube feeding in the hospitalised elderly. Age Ageing 2005;34(2):120–4.

[132] Whelan K, Judd PA, Preedy VR, et al. Enteral feeding: the effect on faecal output, the faecal microflora and SCFA concentrations. Proc Nutr Soc 2004;63(1):105–13.

[133] Bowling TE, Raimundo AH, Grimble GK, et al. Reversal by short-chain fatty acids of colonic fluid secretion induced by enteral feeding. Lancet 1993;342(8882):1266–8.

[134] Ramakrishna BS, Mathan VI. Colonic dysfunction in acute diarrhoea: the role of luminal short chain fatty acids. Gut 1993;34(9):1215–8.

[135] Zipser RD, Patel S, Yahya KZ, et al. Presentations of adult celiac disease in a nationwide patient support group. Dig Dis Sci 2003;48:761–4.

[136] Green PHR, Stavros SN, Panagi SG, et al. Characteristics of adult celiac disease in the USA: results of a national survey. Am J Gastroenterol 2001;96:126–31.

[137] Patel D, Kalkat P, Baisch D, et al. Celiac disease in the elderly. Gerontology 2005;51(3): 213–4.

[138] Koutroutsos K, Tsiachris D, Papatheodoridis GV, et al. Simultaneous diagnosis of ulcerative jejunoileitis and coeliac disease in an elderly man. Digestion 2006;73(1):20–4.

[139] Cankurtaran M, Ulger Z, Doan S, et al. Complications due to late diagnosis of celiac disease with co-existing plasma cell dyscrasia in an elderly patient. Aging Clin Exp Res 2006;18(1):75–7.

[140] Baroni F, Ghisla MK, Ritchie Leonardi, et al. Celiac disease in the elderly: a case report. Ann Ital Med Int 2005;20(4):253–7 [in Italian].

[141] Menardo G, Bertolotti MG, Minetti F, et al. Hyperimmunoglobulin A and celiac disease in the elderly. J Am Geriatr Soc 2005;53(6):1074–5.

[142] Dseplat-Jego S, Bernard D, Bagneres D, et al. Neuropsychiatric symptoms in the elderly: let us not forget celiac disease. J Am Geriatr Soc 2003;51(6):884–5.

[143] Sanders DS, Hurlstone DP, McAlindon ME, et al. Antibody negative coeliac disease presenting in elderly people–an easily missed diagnosis. BMJ 2005;330(7494):775–6.

[144] Thomas PD, Forbes A, Green J, et al. Guidelines for the investigation of chronic diarrhoea, 2nd edition. Gut 2003;52(Suppl 5):v1–v15.

[145] Fasano A, Catassi C. Current approaches to diagnosis and treatment of celiac disease: an evolving spectrum. Gastroenterology 2001;120:636–51.

[146] Rostami K, Kerckhaert J, Tiemessen R, et al. Sensitivity of antiendomysium and antigliadin antibodies in untreated celiac disease: disappointing in clinical practice. Am J Gastroenterol 1999;94:888–94.

[147] Freeman HJ. Lymphoproliferative and intestinal malignancies in 214 patients with biopsy-defined celiac disease. J Clin Gastroenterol 2004;38(5):429–34.

[148] Robertson DJ, Grimm IS. Inflammatory bowel disease in the elderly. Gastroenterol Clin North Am 2001;30:409–26.

[149] Russel M, Stockbrugger RW. Epidemiology of inflammatory bowel disease: an update. Scand J Gastroenterol 1996;31:417–27.

[150] Page MJ, Poritz LS, Kunselman SJ, et al. Factors affecting surgical risk in elderly patients with inflammatory bowel disease. J Gastrointest Surg 2002;6(4):606–13.

[151] Pardi DS, Loftus EV Jr, Camilleri M. Treatment of inflammatory bowel disease in the elderly. Drugs Aging 2002;19(5):355–63.

[152] Nyhlin N, Bohr J, Eriksson S, et al. Systemic review: microscopic colitis. Aliment Pharmacol Ther 2006;23:1525–34.

[153] Bassi A, Loughran C, Foster P. Carcinoid tumor of the terminal ileum simulating Crohn disease. Scand J Gastroenterol 2003;9:1004–6.

ELSEVIER
SAUNDERS

CLINICS IN
GERIATRIC
MEDICINE

Clin Geriatr Med 23 (2007) 857–869

Fecal Incontinence in Older Adults

Syed H. Tariq, MD, FACP

*Department of Internal Medicine, Divisions of Geriatric Medicine, Saint Louis University
School of Medicine, 1402 South Grand Avenue, M-238, Saint Louis, MO 63104, USA*

Fecal incontinence is usually defined as the involuntary loss of bowel control, which normally allows the passage of gas or stool at a socially acceptable norm. Normal continence results from an integrated activity of the anal sphincters, pelvic floor muscles, and adequate neural input. It is also influenced by stool consistency, rectal capacity and compliance, the anorectal sampling reflex, normal resting anal tone, and normal anorectal sensation. Failure in any of the mechanisms that are responsible for maintaining continence results in fecal incontinence. Fecal incontinence is underreported because it is not socially acceptable, which places the onus on physicians to ask about anorectal problems and encourage patients to seek effective treatment options.

Prevalence and impact of fecal incontinence

The prevalence of fecal incontinence is 2.2% in the general population and up to 21% in community-dwelling older adults [1–4]. The frequency of fecal incontinence increases with age from 3.7% to 27% (Table 1). The prevalence of fecal incontinence in geriatric hospital wards is reported to be between 20% and 32% and up to 56% in geriatric psychiatry [5,6]. The prevalence of fecal incontinence in long-term care is approximately 50% [7,8]. Approximately 80% of elderly patients who are hospitalized and have dementia have experienced fecal incontinence [9].

Double incontinence (ie, fecal incontinence and urinary incontinence) occurs 12 times more commonly than fecal incontinence alone, with 50% to 70% of patients experiencing both [4,6,14]. This fact is not surprising, as the combination of urinary and fecal incontinence is the second most common cause of nursing home placement [15,16].

E-mail address: tariqsh@slu.edu

Table 1
Prevalence of fecal incontinence

Location	Prevalence age > 65 years (%)
Europe	
New Zealand [1]	3.1
Netherlands [2]	4.2–16.9
England [10][a]	21
France [9][a]	58
Asia	
Japan [11]	8.7 M; 6.6 F
United States	
Boston [12]	17
Minnesota [13]	17 M; 27 F[b]
Minnesota [3]	3.7
Wisconsin [14][a]	47

[a] Studies reporting prevalence in long-term care.
[b] Age older than 50 years.
Abbreviations: F, female; M, male.

Fecal incontinence results in anxiety, embarrassment, social demoraliza-
tion, silent suffering, isolation, and depression [17]. Fecal incontinence is
also a marker for poorer overall health and is associated with increased mortality [7,11]. Incontinent nursing home residents experience more urinary
tract infections and pressure ulcers [18]. The total health care cost attributable to fecal incontinence is unknown. The nursing home–related costs for
incontinence reported in 1987 were $3.26 billion and the yearly cost of adult
diapers alone is $400 million [19,20]. The additional health expenditures
exceed $9000 per patient year of incontinence [18].

Causes of fecal incontinence and risk factors

Clinically fecal incontinence could be classified into three subgroups:
overflow, reservoir, and rectosphincteric. The causes of incontinence of
these subgroups are shown in Box 1. Some of the risk factors for fecal incontinence include a history of urinary incontinence, the presence of neurologic
or psychiatric disease, poor mobility, age older than 70 years, and dementia
[21,22].

Possibly the most common predisposing condition to fecal incontinence
is fecal impaction, which is reported in 42% of older adults [23]. Some
risk factors that contribute to fecal impaction are outlined in Box 2. These
patients are often chronically constipated and receive large doses of laxatives, causing incontinence from seepage of stools around the obstruction.
Fecal incontinence is also seen in individuals who have diabetes resulting
from autonomic neuropathy and is exacerbated in the presence of diabetic
diarrhea [24]. Fecal incontinence can be caused by surgical procedures (eg,

---

Box 1. Classification of fecal incontinence and its causes

Overflow
Cognitively impaired
Bedridden individuals in a nursing home

Reservoir dysfunction (diminished colonic or rectal capacity)
Radiation proctopathy
Chronic rectal ischemia
Idiopathic inflammatory bowel disease
Proctocolectomy with ileoanal anastomosis

Rectosphincteric
Structural damage to one or both anal sphincters
Pudendal neuropathy
Degenerative
Myogenic disorders affecting internal or external anal sphincter

---

hemorrhoidectomy, anal fissure repair, and anal dilatation may disrupt the anal sphincter muscles) or trauma (eg, sphincter damage, pudendal neuropathy) [25–27]. Fecal incontinence is seen in 40% of patients who undergo total internal sphincterotomy and 8% to 15% who undergo partial sphincterotomy [28–30].

Box 2. Risk factors for overflow incontinence

Medication
Narcotics
Antipsychotics
Antidepressants
Calcium channel blockers
Diuretics

Metabolic abnormalities
Hypothyroidism
Hypercalcemia
Hypokalemia

Inadequate fiber and water intake

Immobility and inadequate toileting facilities

Delirium

Evaluation of fecal incontinence

The goal in evaluating fecal incontinence includes establishing the severity of incontinence and providing appropriate therapy. This goal is accomplished through history, physical examination, and investigations targeted to determining the cause of fecal incontinence. Questioning the patient or caregiver about bowel habits and continence is very helpful. Clinicians should try to determine when the symptoms first occurred and if the patient has any sensation, such as the passage of stool or gas, fullness in the rectum, or warning symptoms such as abdominal cramps and urgency.

In evaluating fecal incontinence, several components of the neurologic history deserve attention. A cerebrovascular accident may limit a patient's physical ability to use the toilet. The new onset of fecal incontinence may also indicate the presence of cord compression, especially when associated with other neurologic symptoms.

A review of medication, including over-the-counter medicine and supplements, may reveal an underlying cause for the altered bowel habit. Some commonly used products causing diarrhea include magnesium-containing antacids and poorly absorbed sugars, such as sorbitol and mannitol (used in dietetic products). Sorbitol is also frequently used as a base in elixirs (eg, theophylline elixir). The intentional or inadvertent use of cathartics may contribute to diarrhea and incontinence.

Physical examination helps identify the pathophysiology of fecal incontinence and can guide the ordering of appropriate tests for further evaluation [31]. The usual physical examination may be supplemented with a Mini Mental Status Examination (MMSE) or Saint Louis University Mental Status (SLUMS) examination, which helps identify patients who have cognitive impairment [32,33]. The neurologic examination includes assessment of general patient mobility, motor strength, and sensory testing. The perineum should be inspected for dermatitis, hemorrhoids, fistula, surgical scars, skin tags, rectal prolapse, anal winking, soiling, and ballooning of the perineum (suggesting weakness of the pelvic floor). Digital rectal examination is the next step, with a positive predictive value of 67% for detecting decreased anal tone compared with anal manometry [34]. Patients who have high or normal sphincter tone can also be incontinent, especially in the setting of large rectal volumes or altered rectal sensation.

Excluding fecal impaction is most important in the elderly population. If impaction is suspected, the patients should undergo a digital rectal examination and plain abdominal radiograph to exclude anal and higher impaction, respectively. A flexible sigmoidoscopy or colonoscopy examines the colorectal mucosa for evidence of colitis, neoplasia, inflammatory bowel disease, colonic and rectal ischemia, laxative abuse, and other structural abnormalities. Anorectal manometry provides comprehensive information about anorectal function, because it quantifies anal sphincter tone and assesses anorectal sensory responses, the rectoanal inhibitory reflex, and rectal compliance [35]. A finding of lower rectal compliance may indicate fecal incontinence from increased stress on the continence mechanism as the stool is received in the rectum [36]. Electromyography measures the neuromuscular integrity between the distal portion of pudendal nerve and the anal sphincter muscle [37]. Electromyography correlates well with anorectal manometry, but its use in the routine assessment of fecal incontinence is controversial [38,39]. Anal ultrasound defines the internal and external anal sphincters [40]. Anal ultrasound can be used to identify isolated sphincter defects, present in approximately two thirds of patients who are incontinent [41,42]. Ultrasonographic findings correlate with surgical and electromyographic findings [43,44]. MRI has also been used to evaluate the sphincter defects, with definition superior to anal ultrasound, because it provides higher spatial resolution and better contrast for lesion characterization [45].

Treatment

The treatment of fecal incontinence depends on the underlying cause and severity of the incontinence. Minor degrees of fecal incontinence can be treated conservatively, where patients experiencing severe fecal incontinence require more aggressive treatment [46,47]. The subjective complaints and symptoms of fecal incontinence must be made more objective, which can be accomplished using the widely used and validated Cleveland Clinic Florida score [48]. This scale measures the frequency of incontinence to gas, liquid, and solid stool; the degree of alteration in lifestyle; and the use of protective devices (0 = total control, 20 = complete incontinence). A score of greater than 9 is associated with a significant alteration in quality of life and can be used as an indication for surgical intervention in appropriately selected patients [49].

Conservative therapy

Patients who have cognitive impairment, such as those with dementia, may simply need to be directed to the toilet or reminded. Physical limitations and environment obstacles must be addressed if they contribute to incontinence, because they can often be overcome through simple measures. Habit training involves a regular schedule of defecation, usually after breakfast. Habit training is particularly effective for patients experiencing overflow incontinence. Prompted voiding increases the number of continent bowel movements and reduces the number of incontinent bowel movements. This study was designed primarily for urine incontinence [50].

Diarrhea is one of its most common aggravating factors. The mainstay of the medical management of fecal incontinence is the control of diarrhea through dietary modifications and a wide variety of antidiarrheal medications. Of course, infectious causes should be ruled out before using antidiarrheal agents. When gut dysmotility is suspected, especially in patients who have diabetes, clonidine may be used, with the topical preparation preferred because of fewer side effects. A trial of cholestyramine may also be helpful when bile acid malabsorption is suspected. Antidiarrheal agents are helpful when the stool is loose [51]. In a 4-week, double-blind crossover trial of 30 patients receiving loperamide, codeine, or diphenoxylate with atropine, all agents reduced the stool frequency, but loperamide and codeine were more effective in reducing fecal incontinence than diphenoxylate [52]. Diphenoxylate and codeine had more central nervous system side effects than loperamide and are generally best to avoid in elderly patients in this setting.

Sphincter training exercises (*Kegel exercises*) alone do not increase the number of continent episodes but are effective in treating urinary incontinence [53]. Biofeedback is an operant conditioning first described by Engel and colleagues [54]. Biofeedback is a nonsurgical, noninvasive, inexpensive outpatient method of treating fecal incontinence [55]. Biofeedback for fecal incontinence involves improving external sphincter strength and anorectal sensation [53]. Biofeedback provides immediate and long-term improvements and is described in Table 2 [56–72]. Better results are achieved when treating motivated, mentally capable patients. Patients should also have some degree of rectal sensation and be able to contract the external anal sphincter [73,74]. Miner and colleagues [75] compared active sensory biofeedback with sham retraining. Although the control group showed no improvement, biofeedback training reduced incontinent episodes by 80% per week in the active group. This improvement lasted more than 2 years in 73% patients available for follow-up. One study involving 13 geriatric patients who continued to be incontinent with conservative treatment [53] showed that biofeedback improved sphincter strength and reduced incontinence episodes by more than 75%. In a review of biofeedback, Enck and colleagues [76] showed improved continence in 13 of 14 studies. Improved continence occurred in at least one half of 1364 female patients treated with biofeedback. No specific details regarding age-related differences were noted [77].

Surgical therapy

Surgical intervention is generally considered when more conservative measures have failed in patients who have severe incontinence and identifiable anatomic defects. Although surgery is more commonly recommended in younger patients, appropriately selected elderly patients will respond fairly well to surgical intervention [78].

Some available surgical procedures include sphincter repair, neosphincter operations, and alternative therapies. Repair of an isolated sphincter defect, especially anterior sphincteroplasty, is very successful [55,79]. Improvement in anal function shown with anal manometry before and after anterior

Table 2
Results of biofeedback therapy

Reference	N	Age range (mean)	Improved	Follow-up duration months (mean)
[76]	25	17–76 y	77% biofeedback	24
			42% sham	
[53]	18	65–92 y (73 y)	77%	Post-biofeedback
			50%	6
			42%	12
[56]	24	39–72 y (60 y)	75%	6
		16 biofeedback	19%	24–36 (30)
		8 control		
[57]	17	35–84 y (64 y)	50%[a]	3
		8 biofeedback	38%[a]	12
		9 medical therapy		
[58]	50	25–76 y (55 y)	72%	12
[59]	22	15–78 y (50 y)	≥75% = 53%	12
			≥50% = 100%	
[60]	12	12–78 y	83%	3–24
[61]	17	10–79 y (48 y)	71%	2–38 (15)
[62]	28	30–74 y (52.9 y)	75%	4–47 (21)
[63]	26	32–82 y (61 median)	64%	12–48 (21)
[64]	14	24–75 y (49 y)	75%	3–21 (15)
[65]	50	5–97 y (46 y)	72%	4–108 (32)
[66]	21	14–84 y (60 y)	86%	1.5 or 3
[67]	72	34–87 y (70 y)	85%	Not stated
[26]	30	29–85 y (68 median)	27%	1.5
[68]	37	22–82 y (61 median)	9%	12–59 (44)
[69]	13	13–66 y	92%	16–30
[70]	100	14–82 y (49 median)	43% (cure)	Not specified
			24% (improved)	
[71]	25	31–82 y (63 y)	92%	7
[72]	27	29–74 y (53 y)	30%	Not reported

[a] Unchanged from controls.

sphincter repair has been reported [80,81]. A 96% improvement was seen in anal function compared with preoperative symptoms (all women aged 22–75 years, mean age, 37.8 years). The outcome of surgical repair is variable, because some patients may continue to experience incontinence and others develop new bowel problems postoperatively [79,80].

Muscle transposition may be considered for severe fecal incontinence when standard therapy fails. Techniques include graciloplasty, dynamic graciloplasty, and gluteus maximus transposition. The result of graciloplasty varies significantly [82–84]. The results of graciloplasty are improved through electrical stimulation after electrical electrodes and a pulse generator are implanted [85]. Electrical stimulation provides the gracilis muscle with the properties to function as a sphincter [86]. In a prospective multicenter trial, 66% of patients who underwent graciloplasty achieved continence at 2-year follow-up [87]. The performance of graciloplasty specifically in elderly patients has not been reported.

Some new techniques have been developed to treat fecal incontinence, but these are described predominantly in younger age groups. In a multicenter prospective trial of 12 patients who did not experience response to conventional management for severe fecal incontinence and had an artificial anal sphincter implanted, 75% of the patients (mean age, 33 years) experienced successful outcome [88]. This surgical technique has not been specifically studied in the geriatric population.

Injections of glutaraldehyde cross-linked collagen are simple and well tolerated for patients who do not experience response to conservative therapy and have a surgically uncorrectable problem (internal sphincter dysfunction). In a study of 17 patients (mean age, 53 years), 65% experienced symptomatic improvement, 12% experienced minimal improvement, and 18% showed no improvement [89]. However, the long-term results are less encouraging than the initial results of the small pilot trials. The slow deterioration in fecal continence after the initial improvement was attributed to migration or flattening of the bulking material, sometimes necessitating additional injections.

Durasphere FI is a gel consisting of approximately 97% water and 3% β-glucan and is injected in the submucosal space. Weiss and colleagues [90] presented their experience with Durasphere FI in a prospective, open-label pilot trial of 10 patients (7 women) who had severe fecal incontinence, showing that 8 of the patients experienced symptomatic improvement. Davis and colleagues [91] used Durasphere FI in a slightly different manner. They treated 18 incontinent patients who had internal anal sphincter defects and injected the compound submucosally only adjacently to the area of the disrupted sphincter until the regularity of the anal canal was restored. A strong correlation was seen between the number of sites that were injected and the degree of improvement in the incontinence. A significant improvement occurred in Fecal Incontinence Quality-of-Life (FIQOL) scores in addition to the symptomatic improvement. Durasphere FI achieves its effect through several potential mechanisms: (1) the bulk provides additional resistance to the passage of stool and allows for improved sensation and discrimination, (2) the physical filling of sphincter defects restores the normal contour of the anal canal, and (3) the continuous fibrosis adds further volume to the sphincter muscles. This procedure has proven to be safe, simple, inexpensive, and effective for treating moderate to severe fecal incontinence.

Sacral nerve stimulation (SNS) for fecal incontinence has been shown to improve fecal incontinence along with quality of life in selected patients [92]. A recent systematic review of SNS for treating fecal incontinence evaluated six studies in which 266 patients underwent percutaneous nerve evaluation, of whom 149 (56%) had a permanent stimulator implanted and underwent follow-up for 1 to 99 months. Complete continence was reported in approximately 55% of patients, with 90% having more than 50% improvement in incontinence; no deterioration of the effect of SNS occurred over time [93].

A colostomy offers definitive treatment for individuals with fecal incontinence when all other options have failed. Patients and physicians remain apprehensive about this option because quality of life with a colostomy is presumably worse than living with fecal incontinence. A cross-sectional postal survey of patients who had fecal incontinence and underwent colostomy used the Short Form 36 (SF-36) and the FIQOL score to determine patient satisfaction. The SF-36 showed a higher social function score in the colostomy group compared with the fecal incontinence group. The FIQOL scores on the coping, embarrassment, lifestyle scales, and depression scales were higher in the colostomy group than the fecal incontinence group. This study suggests that colostomy is a viable option for patients who experience fecal incontinence and offers improved quality of life as an alternative to other ineffective treatments [94].

Summary

Fecal incontinence is a common problem in the elderly population. Fecal incontinence causes inconvenience to the patient and caregivers, is a marker of poorer health, and is associated with increased mortality. All patients experiencing fecal incontinence warrant medical evaluation, including the exclusion of fecal impaction through rectal examination and radiograph of the abdomen. Cognitively impaired patients benefit most from habit training and redirection. Minor cases of fecal incontinence could be treated conservatively and severe cases could be referred for possible surgical intervention in selected cases.

References

[1] Campbell AJ, Reinken J, McCosh L. Incontinence in the elderly: prevalence and prognosis. Age Ageing 1985;14:65–70.
[2] Kok AL, Voorhorst FJ, Burger CW, et al. Urinary and faecal incontinence in community-residing elderly women. Age Ageing 1992;21:211–5.
[3] Talley NJ, O'Keefe EA, Zinsmeister AR, et al. Prevalence of gastrointestinal symptoms in the elderly: a population-based study. Gastroenterology 1992;102:895–901.
[4] Nelson R, Norton N, Cautley E, et al. Community-based prevalence of anal incontinence. JAMA 1995;274:559–61.
[5] Thomas TM, Ruff C, Karran O, et al. Study of the prevalence and management of patients with faecal incontinence in old people's homes. Community Med 1987;9:232–7.
[6] Issac B, Walkley FA. A survey of incontinence in elderly hospital patients. Gerontol Clin 1964;6:367–76.
[7] Chassagne P, Landrin I, Neveu C, et al. Fecal incontinence in the institutionalized elderly: incidence, risk factors, and prognosis. Am J Med 1999;106:185–90.
[8] Prather CM, Tariq SH, Walker D, et al. Biofeedback for fecal incontinence in elderly nursing home residents: a pilot study. Gastroenterology 2001;120:5S:A747.
[9] Taylor BM, Beart RW, Phillips SF. Longitudinal and radial variations of pressure in the human anal sphincter. Gastroenterology 1984;86:693–7.
[10] Peet SM, Castleton CM, McGrother CW. Prevalence or urinary and fecal incontinence in hospitals and residential nursing homes for older people. Br Med J 1995;311:1063–4.

[11] Nakanishi N, Tatara K, Shinsho F, et al. Mortality in relation to urinary and faecal incontinence in elderly people living at home. Age Ageing 1999;28:301–6.

[12] Resnick M, Beckett LA, Branch LG. Short term variability of self reported incontinence in older persons. J Am Geriatr Soc 1994;42:202–7.

[13] Robert RO, Jacobson SJ, Reiley WT. Prevalence of combined fecal and urinary incontinence: a community based study. J Am Geriatr Soc 1999;47:895–901.

[14] Ouslander JG, Kane RL, Abrass IB. Urinary incontinence in elderly nursing home patients. JAMA 1982;248:1194–8.

[15] Nelson R, Furner S, Jesudason V. Fecal incontinence in Wisconsin nursing homes: prevalence and associations. Dis Colon Rectum 1998;41:1226–9.

[16] O'Donnell BF, Drachman DA, Barnes HJ, et al. Incontinence and troublesome behaviors predict institutionalization in dementia. J Geriatr Psychiatry Neurol 1992;5:45–52.

[17] Johanson JF, Lafferty J. Epidemiology of fecal incontinence: the silent affliction. Am J Gastroenterol 1996;91:33–6.

[18] Borrie MJ, Davidson HA. Incontinence in institutions: costs and contributing factors. CMAJ 1992;147:322–8.

[19] Hu TW. Impact of urinary incontinence on health-care costs. J Am Geriatr Soc 1990;38: 292–5.

[20] Mandelstam DA. Faecal incontinence: a social and economic factors. In: Henry MM, Swash M, editors. Coloproctology and the pelvic floor: pathophysiology and management. London: Butterworths; 1985. p. 217–22.

[21] Madoff RD, Williams JG, Caushaj PF. Fecal incontinence. N Engl J Med 1992;326:1002–7.

[22] Tobin GW, Brocklehurst JC. Faecal incontinence in residential homes for the elderly: prevalence, aetiology and management. Age Ageing 1986;15:41–6.

[23] Read NW, Abouzekry L. Why do patients with faecal impaction have faecal incontinence. Gut 1986;27:283–7.

[24] Schiller LR, Santa Ana CA, Schmulen AC, et al. Pathogenesis of fecal incontinence in diabetes mellitus: evidence for internal-anal-sphincter dysfunction. N Engl J Med 1982;307: 1666–71.

[25] Sultan AH, Kamm MA, Hudson CN, et al. Third degree obstetric anal sphincter tears: risk factors and outcome of primary repair. BMJ 1994;308:887–91.

[26] Rieger NA, Wattchow DA, Sarre RG, et al. Prospective trial of pelvic floor retraining in patients with fecal incontinence. Dis Colon Rectum 1997;40:821–6.

[27] Read MG, Read NW, Haynes WG, et al. A prospective study of the effect of haemorrhoidectomy on sphincter function and faecal continence. Br J Surg 1982;69:396–8.

[28] Bennet RC, Goligher JC. Results of internal sphincterotomy for anal fissure. Br J Surg 1962; 2:1500–3.

[29] Walker WA, Rothenberger DA, Goldberg SM. Morbidity of internal sphincterotomy for anal fissure and stenosis. Dis Colon Rectum 1985;28:832–5.

[30] Pernikoff BJ, Eisenstat TE, Rubin RJ, et al. Reappraisal of partial lateral internal sphincterotomy. Dis Colon Rectum 1994;37:1291–5.

[31] Rosen L. Physical examination of the anorectum: a systematic technique. Dis Colon Rectum 1990;33:439–40.

[32] Crum RM, Anthony JC, Bassett SS, et al. Population-based norms for the mini-mental state examination by age and educational level. JAMA 1993;269:2386–91.

[33] Tariq SH, Tumosa N, Chibnall JT, et al. The Saint Louis University mental status (*SLUMS*) examination for detecting mild cognitive impairment and dementia is more sensitive than mini mental status examination (MMSE)—a pilot study. Am J Geriatr Psychiatry 2006; 14(11):900–10.

[34] Hill J, Corson RJ, Brandon H, et al. History and examination in the assessment of patients with idiopathic fecal incontinence. Dis Colon Rectum 1994;37:473–7.

[35] Rao SS, Patel RS. How useful are manometric tests of anorectal function in the management of defecation disorders? [see comments]. Am J Gastroenterol 1997;92:469–75.

[36] Rasmussen O, Christensen B, Sorensen M, et al. Rectal compliance in the assessment of patients with fecal incontinence. Dis Colon Rectum 1990;33:650–3.

[37] Rao SS. Manometric evaluation of defecation disorders: part II. Fecal incontinence. Gastroenterologist 1997;5:99–111.

[38] Barnett JL, Hasler WL, Camilleri M. American Gastroenterological Association medical position statement on anorectal testing techniques. American Gastroenterological Association. Gastroenterology 1999;116:732–60.

[39] Wexner SD, Marchetti F, Salanga VD, et al. Neurophysiologic assessment of the anal sphincters. Dis Colon Rectum 1991;34:606–12.

[40] Law PJ, Kamm MA, Bartram CI. Anal endosonography in the investigation of faecal incontinence. Br J Surg 1991;78:312–4.

[41] Chen H, Humphreys MS, Kettlewell MG, et al. Anal ultrasound predicts the response to nonoperative treatment of fecal incontinence in men. Ann Surg 1999;229:739–43 [discussion: 743–4].

[42] Liberman H, Faria J, Ternent CA, et al. A prospective evaluation of the value of anorectal physiology in the management of fecal incontinence. Dis Colon Rectum 2001;44: 1567–74.

[43] Deen KI, Kumar D, Williams JG, et al. Anal sphincter defects. Correlation between endoanal ultrasound and surgery. Ann Surg 1993;218:201–5.

[44] Meyenberger C, Bertschinger P, Zala GF, et al. Anal sphincter defects in fecal incontinence: correlation between endosonography and surgery. Endoscopy 1996;28:217–24.

[45] Beets-Tan RG, Morren GL, Beets GL, et al. Measurement of anal sphincter muscles: endoanal US, endoanal MR imaging, or phased-array MR imaging? A study with healthy volunteers. Radiology 2001;220:81–9.

[46] Tariq SH, Prather CM, Morley JE. Fecal incontinence in the elderly patient. Am J Med 2003; 115:217–26.

[47] Tariq SH. Geriatric fecal incontinence. Clin Geriatr Med 2004;20:571–87.

[48] Jorge JM, Wexner SD. Etiology and management of fecal incontinence. Dis Colon Rectum 1993;36:77–97.

[49] Rothbarth J, Bemelman WA, Meijerink WJ, et al. What is the impact of on fecal incontinence quality of life? Dis Colon Rectum 2001;44:67–71.

[50] Ouslander JG, Simmons S, Schnelle J, et al. Effects of prompted voiding on fecal continence among nursing home residents. J Am Geriatr Soc 1996;44:424–8.

[51] Read M, Read NW, Barber DC, et al. Effects of loperamide on anal sphincter function in patients complaining of chronic diarrhea with fecal incontinence and urgency. Dig Dis Sci 1982;27:807–14.

[52] Palmer KR, Corbett CL, Holdsworth CD. Double-blind cross-over study comparing loperamide, codeine and diphenoxylate in the treatment of chronic diarrhea. Gastroenterology 1980;79:1272–5.

[53] Whitehead WE, Burgio KL, Engel BT. Biofeedback treatment of fecal incontinence in geriatric patients. J Am Geriatr Soc 1985;33:320–4.

[54] Engel BT, Nikoomanesh P, Schuster MM. Operant conditioning of rectosphincteric responses in the treatment of fecal incontinence. N Engl J Med 1974;290:646–9.

[55] Mavrantonis C, Wexner SD. A clinical approach to fecal incontinence. J Clin Gastroenterol 1998;27:108–219.

[56] Guillemot F, Bouche B, Gower-Rousseau C, et al. Biofeedback for the treatment of fecal incontinence. Long-term clinical results. Dis Colon Rectum 1995;38:393–7.

[57] Loening-Baucke V. Efficacy of biofeedback training in improving faecal incontinence and anorectal physiologic function. Gut 1990;31:1395–402.

[58] MacLeod JH. Biofeedback in the management of partial anal incontinence. Dis Colon Rectum 1983;26:244–6.

[59] Rao SS, Welcher KD, Happel J. Can biofeedback therapy improve anorectal function in fecal incontinence? Am J Gastroenterol 1996;91:2360–6.

[60] Goldenberg DA, Hodges K, Hershe T, et al. Biofeedback therapy for fecal incontinence. Am J Gastroenterol 1980;74:342–5.

[61] Wald A. Biofeedback therapy for fecal incontinence. Ann Intern Med 1981;95:146–9.

[62] Sangwan YP, Coller JA, Barrett RC, et al. Can manometric parameters predict response to biofeedback therapy in fecal incontinence? Dis Colon Rectum 1995;38:1021–5.

[63] Glia A, Gylin M, Akerlund JE, et al. Biofeedback training in patients with fecal incontinence. Dis Colon Rectum 1998;41:359–64.

[64] Chiarioni G, Scattolini C, Bonfante F, et al. Liquid stool incontinence with severe urgency: anorectal function and effective biofeedback treatment. Gut 1993;34:1576–80.

[65] Cerulli MA, Nikoomanesh P, Schuster MM. Progress in biofeedback conditioning for fecal incontinence. Gastroenterology 1979;76:742–6.

[66] Berti Riboli E, Frascio M, Pitto G, et al. Biofeedback conditioning for fecal incontinence. Arch Phys Med Rehabil 1988;69:29–31.

[67] Patankar SK, Ferrara A, Larach SW, et al. Electromyographic assessment of biofeedback training for fecal incontinence and chronic constipation. Dis Colon Rectum 1997;40:907–11.

[68] Ryn AK, Morren GL, Hallbook O, et al. Long-term results of electromyographic biofeedback training for fecal incontinence. Dis Colon Rectum 2000;43:1262–6.

[69] Buser WD, Miner PB Jr. Delayed rectal sensation with fecal incontinence. Successful treatment using anorectal manometry. Gastroenterology 1986;91:1186–91.

[70] Norton C, Kamm MA. Outcome of biofeedback for fecal incontinence. Br J Surg 1999;86:1159–63.

[71] Ko CY, Tong J, Lehman RE, et al. Biofeedback is effective therapy for fecal incontinence and constipation. Arch Surg 1997;132(8):829–34.

[72] Leroi AM, Dorival MP, Lecouturier MF, et al. Pudendal neuropathy and severity of incontinence but not presence of an anal sphincter defect may determine the response to biofeedback therapy in fecal incontinence. Dis Colon Rectum 1999;42(6):762–9.

[73] Enck P, Daublin G, Lubke HJ, et al. Long-term efficacy of biofeedback training for fecal incontinence. Dis Colon Rectum 1994;37:997–1001.

[74] Latimer PR, Campbell D, Kasperski J. A components analysis of biofeedback in the treatment of fecal incontinence. Biofeedback Self Regul 1984;9:311–24.

[75] Miner PB, Donnelly TC, Read NW. Investigation of mode of action of biofeedback in treatment of fecal incontinence. Dig Dis Sci 1990;35:1291–8.

[76] Enck P, Daublin G, Lubke H. Long-term efficacy of biofeedback training for fecal incontinence. Dis Colon Rectum 1994;37:997–1001.

[77] Norton C, Kamm MA. Anal sphincter biofeedback and pelvic floor exercises for faecal incontinence in adults–a systematic review. Aliment Pharmacol Ther 2001;15:1147–54.

[78] Simmang C, Birnbaum EH, Kodner IJ, et al. Anal sphincter reconstruction in the elderly: does advancing age affect outcome? Dis Colon Rectum 1994;37:1065–9.

[79] Karoui S, Leroi AM, Koning E, et al. Results of sphincteroplasty in 86 patients with anal incontinence. Dis Colon Rectum 2000;43:813–20.

[80] Fleshman JW, Peters WR, Shemesh EI, et al. Anal sphincter reconstruction: anterior overlapping muscle repair. Dis Colon Rectum 1991;34:739–43.

[81] Yoshioka K, Keighley MR. Critical assessment of the quality of continence after postanal repair for faecal incontinence. Br J Surg 1989;76:1054–7.

[82] Leguit P Jr, van Baal JG, Brummelkamp WH. Gracilis muscle transposition in the treatment of fecal incontinence. Long-term follow-up and evaluation of anal pressure recordings. Dis Colon Rectum 1985;28:1–4.

[83] Corman ML. Gracilis muscle transposition for anal incontinence: late results. Br J Surg 1985;72:S21–2.

[84] Corman ML. Follow-up evaluation of gracilis muscle transposition for fecal incontinence. Dis Colon Rectum 1980;23:552–5.

[85] Baeten CG, Geerdes BP, Adang EM, et al. Anal dynamic graciloplasty in the treatment of intractable fecal incontinence. N Engl J Med 1995;332:1600–5.

[86] George BD, Williams NS, Patel J, et al. Physiological and histochemical adaptation of the electrically stimulated gracilis muscle to neoanal sphincter function. Br J Surg 1993;80: 1342–6.
[87] Madoff RD, Rosen HR, Baeten CG, et al. Safety and efficacy of dynamic muscle plasty for anal incontinence: lessons from a prospective, multicenter trial. Gastroenterology 1999;116: 549–56.
[88] Wong WD, Jensen LL, Bartolo DC, et al. Artificial anal sphincter. Dis Colon Rectum 1996; 39:1345–51.
[89] Kumar D, Benson MJ, Bland JE. Glutaraldehyde cross-linked collagen in the treatment of faecal incontinence. Br J Surg 1998;85:978–9.
[90] Weiss EG, Efron JE, Nogueras JJ, et al. Submucosal injection of carbon coated beads is a successful and safe office based treatment for fecal incontinence. Dis Colon Rectum 2002;45: A46–7.
[91] Davis K, Kumar D, Poloniecki J. Preliminary evaluation of an injectable anal sphincter bulking agent (Durasphere) in the management of faecal incontinence. Aliment Pharmacol Ther 2003;18:237–43.
[92] Vaizey CJ, Kamm MA, Roy AJ, et al. Double-blind crossover study of sacral nerve stimulation for fecal incontinence. Dis Colon Rectum 2000;43:298–302.
[93] Jarrett ME, Mowatt G, Glazener CM, et al. Systematic review of sacral nerve stimulation for fecal incontinence and constipation. Br J Surg 2004;91:1559–69.
[94] Colquhoun P, Kaiser R Jr, Efron J, et al. Wexner SD is the quality of life better in patients with colostomy than patients with fecal incontinence? World J Surg 2006;30(10):1925–8.

ELSEVIER
SAUNDERS

Clin Geriatr Med 23 (2007) 871–887

CLINICS IN
GERIATRIC
MEDICINE

Mesenteric Ischemia in the Elderly

Nuri Ozden, MD[a,b,*], Burak Gurses, MD[c]

[a]Department of Internal Medicine, Meharry Medical College, 1005 Dr. D.B. Todd, Jr.
Boulevard, Nashville, TN 37208-3599, USA
[b]Division of Gastroenterology and Hepatology, Meharry Medical College,
1005 Dr. D.B. Todd, Jr. Boulevard, Nashville, TN 37208-3599, USA
[c]Pulmonary and Critical Care Medicine, Meharry Medical College,
1005 Dr. D.B. Todd, Jr. Boulevard, Nashville, TN 37208-3599, USA

Intestinal ischemia constitutes a number of clinical disorders that limit tissue oxygenation secondary to reduced splanchnic or mesenteric blood flow in the overall territory or region. The spectrum of intestinal ischemia comprises a number of syndromes that include: acute mesenteric ischemia (AMI), as a result of emboli, arterial or venous thrombi; nonocclusive mesenteric ischemia (NOMI), resulting from vasoconstriction secondary to low flow states; and chronic mesenteric ischemia (CMI), caused by transient and recurrent episodes of inadequate intestinal blood flow, causing an inability to sustain metabolic needs or to support increased metabolic demands that are associated with digestion (Box 1) [1].

Acute ischemia

Arterial embolism

Arterial emboli are the most frequent cause of AMI and are responsible of 40% to 50% of cases. Most common causes are myocardial ischemia or infarction, atrial tachyarrhythmia, valvular disorders, cardiomyopathies, ventricular aneurysms, and angiography. One third of all patients with a superior mesenteric artery (SMA) embolus have a history of an embolic incident. Visceral arterial emboli preferentially lodge in the SMA because it emerges from the aorta at an oblique angle. Whereas 15% of arterial emboli occur at the origin of the SMA, 50% lodge distally to the origin of the

---
* Corresponding author. Meharry Medical College, 1005 Dr. D.B. Todd, Jr. Boulevard, Nashville, TN 37208-3599.
E-mail address: nozden@mmc.edu (N. Ozden).

Box 1. Mesenteric ischemia

Acute ischemia (95% of cases)
   Emboli 50%
   Arterial Thrombosis 25% to 30%
   Nonocclusive mesenteric ischemia 20% to 25%
   Venous Thrombosis 5% to 10%
Chronic mesenteric ischemia (5% of cases)
Chronic mesenteric ischemia

---

middle colic artery, which is the first major branch of the SMA. As most SMA emboli lodge distally to the origin of the middle colic artery, by allowing the inferior pancreaticoduodenal branches to be perfused, the proximal jejunum is spared, whereas the rest of the small bowel is ischemic or infracted [2].

The onset of symptoms is dramatic as a result of inadequate collateral circulation. Patients develop abrupt onset of severe abdominal pain associated with nausea, vomiting and diarrhea, which may become bloody. Classically, the severity of abdominal pain is out of proportion to the physical findings. Laboratory findings include metabolic acidosis with elevated anion gap and lactate levels, leuokocytosis, and hemoconcentration.

Arterial thrombosis

Acute mesenteric thrombosis constitutes 25% to 30% of acute mesenteric ischemic events. Arterial thrombosis occurs in the setting of severe atherosclerosis, with the most frequent site near the origin of SMA. Patients usually can tolerate the major visceral obstruction because the slow progressive nature of atherosclerosis allows the development of collateral vessels. The extent of the bowel ischemia or infarction is typically greater than that of an embolism, extending from the duodenum to the transverse colon. Perioperative mortality ranges from 70% to 100%. The increased mortality is caused by the extensive nature of the bowel ischemia-infarction and the need for more complex surgical revascularization.

Patients with SMA thrombosis frequently report a prodromal symptom complex of postprandial pain, nausea, and weight loss associated with chronic intestinal insufficiency. Patients with a subacute onset tend to seek medical care much later than those with arterial emboli. However, when ischemia from mesenteric thrombosis becomes acute, patients present in a similar fashion to those who have acute SMA embolism [3,4].

Nonocclusive mesenteric ischemia

Approximately 20% to 25% of patients with mesenteric ischemia have nonocclusive disease. The pathophysiology of NOMI is poorly understood but involves a low cardiac output state associated with diffuse mesenteric vasoconstriction. The resultant low state causes intestinal hypoxia and necrosis. Vasoactive drugs, especially Digoxin, have been implicated as an etiologic factor. Digitalis preparations induce contraction of splanchnic venous and arterial vascular smooth muscle in vitro and in vivo.

Conditions predisposing to NOMI include an age older than 50 years, myocardial infarction, congestive heart failure, aortic insufficiency, cardiopulmonary bypass, renal or hepatic disease, dialysis, cocaine, excessive physical exercise, vasopressors, and major abdominal or cardiovascular surgery. Infrequently, NOMI has been described in patients who have undergone the stress of surgical procedure or trauma and are receiving enteral nutrition in intensive care units, related most likely to an imbalance between demand and supply. The reported incidence of AMI in these patients is 0.3% to 8.5% and survival is poor (56%). Some patients may not have any underlying risk factors. In comparison to prior decades, mortality rate associated with NOMI has declined with increased use of afterload reducing agents and vasodilators. NOMI occurs most frequently in the elderly, critically ill patients, and in those with severe mesenteric atherosclerosis. These patients develop unexplained worsening in their clinical or physical condition [5].

Mesenteric venous thrombosis

Mesenteric venous thrombosis (MVT) constitutes up to 10% of all patients with mesenteric ischemia. In the past, most cases were secondary related to intra-abdominal pathologic conditions (intra-abdominal infection, malignancy, and pancreatitis). Currently most cases are secondary because of underlying primary clotting disorders, with only 10% of cases now being classified as idiopathic. Mesenteric venous thrombosis is usually segmental, with edema and hemorrhage of the bowel wall and focal exfoliation of the mucosa. Hemorrhagic infarctions occur when the intramural vessels are occluded. Involvement of the inferior mesenteric vein and colon is uncommon. The transition from normal to ischemic intestine is more gradual with venous embolism than with arterial embolism or thrombosis. Except in the most fulminant cases, patients with MVT typically present late (ie, 1 to 2 weeks after onset), complaining of diffuse, nonspecific abdominal pain associated with anorexia, nausea, vomiting, and diarrhea. If the pain is localized, it is most often localized in the lower quadrants. In comparison to arterial thrombosis, MVT generates fewer prodromal symptoms with food intake. Fever, ileus, and heme-positive stools are the most common signs. Bloody ascites and significant third space losses can occur, leading to dehydration and hypotension, causing progression of thrombosis and worsening of the mesenteric ischemia. Mortality depends on the type of MVT (acute or chronic) and the extent of venous involvement. Patients with acute disease, with involvement of the superior mesenteric or portal vein, have a 30-day mortality approaching 30%. Long-term survival is

30% to 40% in patients with acute MVT, as compared with at least 80% in those with the chronic form (Box 2) [6].

Chronic mesenteric ischemia

Chronic mesenteric ischemia (intestinal angina) is characterized by post-prandial pain and marked weight loss, and is caused by repeated, transient episodes of inadequate intestinal blood flow, usually provoked by the increased metabolic demands associated with digestion.

Mesenteric artery stenosis is a common finding in free-living elderly patients (17.5% of age greater than 70 years). At a mean follow-up of 6.5 years, the presence of asymptomatic mesenteric artery stenosis was not associated with death or adverse cardiovascular events. Patients with asymptomatic mesenteric artery stenosis by duplex ultrasonographic criteria did not experience intestinal infarction or develop chronic intestinal ischemia. Superior mesenteric artery stenosis and celiac artery occlusion demonstrated an independent association with weight loss and concurrent renal artery disease [7–9].

Diagnosis

Prompt diagnosis and treatment are of paramount importance for the long-term morbidity or mortality. In a report from Madrid, Spain of 21 patients with superior mesenteric artery embolus, intestinal viability was achieved in 100% of patients if the duration of the symptoms was less than 12 hours, in 56% if duration was between 12 and 24 hours, and in only 18% if symptoms were more than 24 hours in duration before diagnosis [10]. A high index of suspicion within the setting of a compatible history and physical examination should be the main goal to early diagnosis of mesenteric ischemia. Acute mesenteric ischemia should be considered in the differential diagnosis when a patient is older than 50 years, has a history of atrial fibrillation, recent myocardial infarction, congestive heart failure, carotid artery stenosis, atherosclerosis, arterial or venous emboli, postprandial abdominal pain that is out of proportion to that suggested by physical exam, sepsis, bloody diarrhea, unexplained weight loss, hypercoagulable states, or vasculitis.

Unfortunately there is no definitive diagnostic test available, but laboratory abnormalities include hemoconcentration, leukocytosis, increased anion gap metabolic acidosis, lactic acidosis, increased levels of amylase, aspartate aminotransferase, lactate dehydrogenase, creatine phosphokinase, hyperphosphatemia, and hyperkalemia. Serum lactate, an established marker of cell hypoxia, has been shown to have a sensitivity of 96% in patients with mesenteric ischemia that has, unfortunately, found to be a late manifestation [11]. Recently, plasma D-Dimer has been suggested as an earlier marker of acute ischemia but needs confirmation in large scale trials

Box 2. Conditions associated with MVT

Hematological and hypercoagulable states
Sickle cell anemia
Polycythemia vera
Thrombocytosis
Antithrombin III deficiency
Protein C or S deficiency
Factor V Leiden mutation (activated protein C resistance)
Lupus anticoagulant
Factor II 20,210A mutation
Neoplasms or carcinomatosis
Migratory thrombophlebitis
Peripheral deep vein thrombosis
Pregnancy
Local venous congestion and stasis
Hepatic cirrhosis
Congestive splenomegaly
Compression of portal venous system by tumor

Intra-abdominal inflammation and sepsis
Cholangitis
Pancreatitis
Diverticulitis
Appendicitis
Peritonitis
Inflammatory bowel disease
Pelvic or intra-abdominal abscess

Parasitic infection
Ascaris lumbricoides

Blunt abdominal trauma

Decompression sickness

Iatrogenic
Abdominal operations (especially splenectomy
    and pancreatectomy)
Colonoscopy
Sclerotherapy of esophageal varices
Arterial chemoembolization for hepatocellular carcinoma
Estrogens (oral contraceptives)

Adapted from Burns BJ, Brandt LJ. Intestinal ischemia. Gastroenterol Clin North Am 2003;32:1127–43; with permission.

[12,13]. The plain abdominal X-rays are nonspecific. In the early stage of the disease, 25% of patients may have normal findings on abdominal radiography. Characteristic radiographic abnormalities, such as thumbprinting or thickening of bowel loops, occur in less than 40% of patients at presentation. Air in the portal vein is a late finding and is associated with a poor prognosis. Barium enema has no place in the diagnosis of AMI. Duplex sonography (Doppler ultrasonograpy) is highly specific (92%–100%) for identification of occlusions or severe stenosis of the splanchnic, but has a sensitivity of only 70% to 89% for detection of greater than 70% diameter stenoses or occlusions of the celiac and superior mesenteric arteries when performed in highly experienced laboratories. Although the expected increase in intestinal arterial flow that results from food ingestion can be detected and quantified by duplex scanning, this information has not added to the diagnostic accuracy of the test for establishing whether abdominal symptoms that are present are the result of intestinal ischemia.

Duplex scanning of visceral vessels is technically difficult but can be accomplished in more than 85% of subjects in the elective setting. Unfortunately, duplex sonography is of no value in detecting emboli beyond the proximal main vessel or in diagnosing NOMI [14].

Magnetic resonance angiography has shown a specificity of 95% but needs to be confirmed in large cohorts. Li and colleagues [15] used magnetic resonance oximetry to evaluate the percentage of oxygenated hemoglobin in the preprandial and postprandial SMA in patients with chronic ischemic symptoms. In comparison to asymptomatic atherosclerotic patients, this study showed a statistically significant increase in oxygen extraction and a decrease in oxygenated hemoglobin in the mesenteric ischemia group. Oximetry combined with magnetic resonance angiography may hold promise as a diagnostic modality [16]. Multidetector row computer tomography (CT) has emerged as the gold standard for evaluation of mesenteric ischemia. In a prospective series, the positive and negative predictive values in a series of 291 subjects were found to be 90% and 98%, respectively. In another series of 62 subjects evaluated for mesenteric ischemia with multidetector CT and mesenteric angiography, the sensitivity and specificity was found to be 96% and 94%, respectively. CT is more sensitive in diagnosing venous thrombosis [17–20].

In the absence of a clinical indication for emergency laparotomy, mesenteric angiography remains the modality of choice. Early angiography has been shown to improve survival rates. Mesenteric angiography can usually differentiate embolic from thrombotic arterial occlusions. Emboli usually lodge where the artery tapers, which is just after the first branch of the SMA; in contrast, in thrombotic disease the middle colic artery usually involves the origin of the SMA. Mesenteric venous thrombosis is characterized by a generalized slowing of arterial flow in conjunction with lack of opacification of the corresponding mesenteric or portal venous outflow tracts. This is usually segmental in comparison to NOMI, which is diffuse and shows normal venous runoff. In addition, NOMI characteristically shows narrowing and multiple irregularities of the major SMA tributaries, the "string of sausages" sign (Table 1) [21].

Endoscopy has been used to diagnose ischemic colitis; however, it does not visualize much of the small bowel, which is frequently involved in the AMI. In addition, endoscopy may not have adequate sensitivity and specificity in detecting ischemic changes rather than the infarction. A recent study suggests that chronic mesenteric ischemia is detectable during endoscopy by use of visible light spectroscopy, and that successful endovascular treatment results in near normalization of mucosal oxygen saturation but needs to be confirmed in large scale studies [22].

Although many tests have been proposed to establish the presence of CMI, none have proven sensitive and specific as mesenteric angiography that also guides for treatment. In the absence of any specific, reliable diagnostic test, diagnosis must be based on clinical symptoms, arteriographic demonstration of an occlusive process of the splanchnic vessels, and—to a great extent—with exclusion of other gastrointestinal disorders. In most

Table 1
Single institution comparisons of mesenteric angioplasty or stenting versus surgery

First author and procedure	Year	Reference	No. of patients	Successfully revascularized (%)	30-day mortality (%)	Recurrence (%)
Kasirajan[a]	2001	(850)				
Angioplasty			28	93	11	27
Surgery			85	98	8	24
Rose[b]	1995	(850a)				
Angioplasty/ stenting			8	80	13	33
Surgery			9	100	11	22
Bowser[c]	2002	(850b)				
Angioplasty/ stenting			18	88	11	46
Surgery			22	100	9	19

A diagnostic and therapeutic algorithm involving various clinical spectrums of intestinal ischemia is depicted in Figs. 1–5.

[a] Surgical controls were historic; mean postprocedure follow-up was 3 years for both groups.

[b] Mean follow-up for surgery was 3 years; for angioplasty or stenting, 9 months.

[c] Mean follow-up was 14 months.

Data from Hirsch AT, et al. Guidelines for the management of patients with peripheral arterial disease (lower extremity, renal, mesenteric, and abdominal aortic): a collaborative report from the American Associations for Vascular Surgery/Society for Vascular Surgery, Society for Cardiovascular Angiography and Interventions, Society for Vascular Medicine and Biology, Society of Interventional Radiology, and the ACC/AHA Task Force on Practice Guidelines (writing committee to develop guidelines for the management of patients with peripheral arterial disease)—summary of recommendations. J Vasc Interv Radiol 2006;17(9):1383–97.

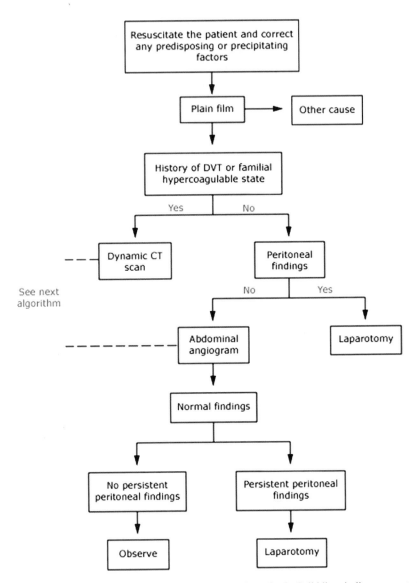

Fig. 1. Diagnosis and treatment of mesenteric venous thrombosis. Solid lines indicate accepted management plan; dashed lines indicate alternate management plan. DVT, deep vein thrombosis. (*Adapted from* American Gastroenterological Association Medical Position Statement: guidelines on intestinal ischemia. Gastroenterology 2000;118:952; with permission.)

patients with CMI, at least two of the three splanchnic vessels are either completely obstructed or severely stenosed. In a comprehensive review of patients with CMI, 91% had occlusion of at least two vessels, and 55% had involvement of all three; 7% and 2% had isolated occlusion of the

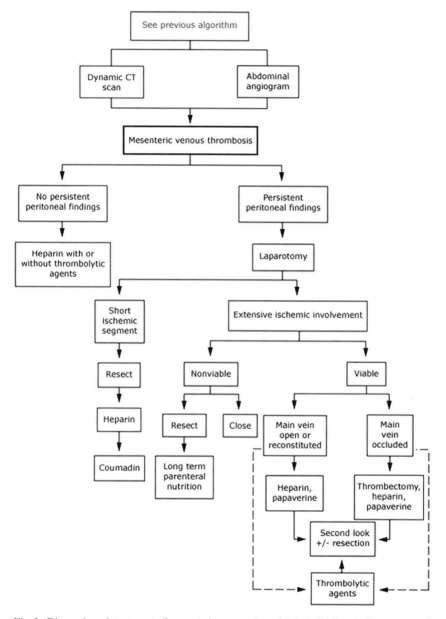

Fig. 2. Diagnosis and treatment of mesenteric venous thrombosis. Solid lines indicate accepted management plan; dashed lines indicate alternate management plan. (*Adapted from* American Gastroenterological Association Medical Position Statement: guidelines on intestinal ischemia. Gastroenterology 2000;118:952; with permission.)

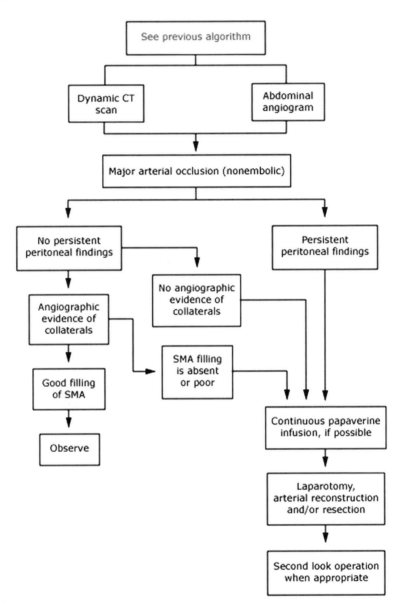

Fig. 3. Diagnosis and treatment of intestinal ischemia. Solid lines indicate accepted manage-ment plan. (*Adapted from* American Gastroenterological Association Medical Position State-ment: guidelines on intestinal ischemia. Gastroenterology 2000;118:952; with permission.)

SMA and celiac axis, respectively. Arteriogram provides definitive diagnosis of intestinal arterial lesions. Lateral aortography is best suited for display of the typical origin lesions, which may not be apparent on frontal projections. The presence of an enlarged "arc of Riolan" (an enlarged collateral vessel

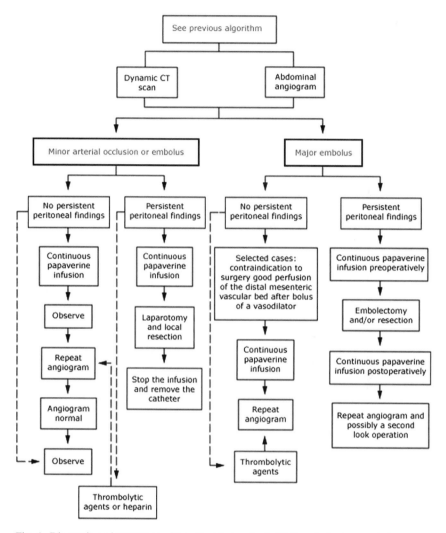

Fig. 4. Diagnosis and treatment of intestinal ischemia. Solid lines indicate accepted management plan; dashed lines indicate alternate management plan. (*Adapted from* American Gastroenterological Association Medical Position Statement: guidelines on intestinal ischemia. Gastroenterology 2000;118:952; with permission.)

connecting the left colic branch of the inferior mesenteric artery with the superior mesenteric artery) is an arteriographic sign of proximal mesenteric arterial obstruction that is visible on anteroposterior aortograms. Selective arteriography of the intestinal vessels may fail to visualize the typical atherosclerotic origin lesions because the selective catheter may be positioned beyond them in the affected vessel [23].

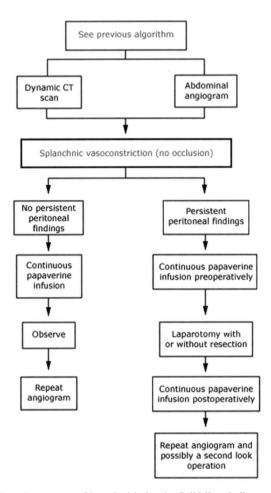

Fig. 5. Diagnosis and treatment of intestinal ischemia. Solid lines indicate accepted management plan. (*Adapted from* American Gastroenterological Association Medical Position Statement: guidelines on intestinal ischemia. Gastroenterology 2000;118:952; with permission.)

Treatment

As soon as diagnosis of the AMI is made, treatment should be initiated
without delay. This should include resuscitation and treatment of the underlying condition, reducing the associated vasospasm, preventing propagation
of the intravascular clotting process, and minimizing the reperfusion injury.
Ideally, fluid resuscitation should begin before angiography. Supranormal-
ization of hemodynamic values has been attempted, with equivocal results;
it remains to be proven whether such an approach offers an advantage to
patients with AMI. Broad-spectrum antibiotics should be given as early as
possible [24].

If there are no contraindications to anticoagulation, therapeutic intravenous heparin sodium should be administered to maintain the activated partial thromboplastin at least twice the normal value. After hemodynamic status stabilization and anticoagulation, therapy efforts should aim at reducing the mesenteric vasospasm. If the diagnosis of AMI is made without the use of the mesenteric angiography, intravenous glucagon infused initially at 1 μg/kg per minute and titrated up to 10 μg/kg per minute as tolerated may help reduce the associated vasospasm. When angiography is used to establish the diagnosis, the angiographic catheter has been placed in the SMA for infusions of papaverine or other vasodilators. Papavarine, a phosphodiesterase inhibitor, increases mesenteric blood flow to marginally perfused tissues and may considerably improve bowel salvage. The usual dosage is 30 mg per hour to 60 mg per hour. Papaverine use is recommended by some investigators in cases of arterial emboli or nonocclusive disease, because in both conditions the arterial vasospasm persists even after successful treatment of the precipitating event.

Signs of peritonitis indicate bowel infarction rather than ischemia alone and mandate emergency laparotomy. Even in the absence of bowel necrosis, surgical procedures are generally required. Visceral revascularization (embolectomy, thrombectomy, endarterectomy, or bypass) should precede bowel resection in almost all patients with occlusive AMI.

For AMI from arterial thrombosis caused by atherosclerotic disease, a vascular bypass graft is usually necessary, with subsequent resection of clearly nonviable bowel. This allows preservation of the potentially viable gut and reduces the possibility of creating the "short-gut syndrome." Visual examination of the exterior of the bowel is unreliable, especially in cases of NOMI, in which the serosa may appear viable despite the presence of infarcted mucosa. The use of intravenous fluorescein and inspection under a Wood lamp has shown to be more sensitive and specific, but this method is not widely accepted. Uniform uptake suggests bowel viability, in comparison to patchy uptake that is suggestive for questionable viability; these segments are better left in situ with a second-look laparototomy possible. Doppler ultrasonography is an alternative and may be used intraoperatively, but studies have not demonstrated any advantage over clinical judgment in assessment of bowel viability.

Even after the primary operation is successful, the intraoperative assessment of bowel viability is often inaccurate, and few reliable signs are available to detect persistent ischemia or developing infarction in the postoperative period. For this reason, a second-look laparotomy after 24 to 48 hours is usually recommended. The rationale behind this second look is based on the frequent occurrence of the vasospasm after revascularization. Second look laparoscopy has been advocated as a substitute for second look laparotomy, but the reliability of this approach remains unproved. Persistent acidosis, especially in the absence of renal failure, should raise concerns about ongoing uncorrected bowel ischemia or infarction. Adequate volume resuscitation is essential to avoid persistent mesenteric hypoperfusion. The mesenteric capillary leak after mesenteric revascularization is well recognized.

After successful revascularization, efforts should be directed toward limiting any reperfusion injury that may cause progressive mesenteric ischemia or infarction. If the patient's hemodynamic condition allows, infusion of vasodilators should be considered (intravenous glucagon or intra-arterial papaverine). The use of allopurinol, angiotensin converting enzyme inhibitors, activated Protein C, and other free oxygen scavengers may help reduce the reperfusion syndrome [25].

Sepsis and multiple organ dysfunction syndromes occur in many patients with AMI. The presentation and management of such complications are similar to those of complications from other causes; however, the use of vasopressors may worsen ischemia in marginally viable bowel and exacerbate the condition. Vasopressor options include dopamine (3 µg/kg–8 µg/kg per minute) and epinephrine (0.05 µg/kg–0.10 µg/kg per minute); pure α-adrenergic agents should be avoided, if possible. Drotrecogin alfa (activated) has been used safely in patients with sepsis secondary to mesenteric ischemia.

Since early 1980s, endovascular therapy for acute mesenteric ischemia has exponentially expanded. Symptom relief with implantation of stents in the proximal celiac artery has been reported. In addition, the thrombosis rate of mesenteric prostheses has been reduced from 18% to 1% with the addition of antiplatelet therapy. Because thrombolytic therapy in the management of intestinal ischemia was conducted in 1979, in those patients with ostial or short segment occlusion of the SMA and celiac artery, recanalization with or without concomitant fibrinolysis has been shown to have promising initial results. In many centers, intracatheter fibrinolysis with or without embolus retrieval is the initial treatment for SMA thromboembolism. Hallisey and colleagues [26] reported a 75% primary patency rate at a median follow-up of 2.3 years. When the results of open surgery are compared with those of percutaneous angioplasty and stenting, there is a higher incidence of recurrent symptoms after percutaenous angioplasty. A retrospective review conducted by the Dartmouth group noted an increased rate of restenosis and reintervention in the stent group versus an historical surgical group [27]. Clearly, there may be a role for minimally invasive therapy in high-risk patients, but this still requires large-scale randomized trials with long term symptom follow-up.

Effective treatment of NOMI should focus at removing the offending stimulus and correcting the underlying etiology. Vasodilators, anticoagulation, and mesenteric regional blockade have been used in cases which infarction has not yet occurred. Intra-arterial vasodilator therapy has been largely responsible for the decrease in the mortality from 70% in the 1980s, to 50% to 55% during the beginning of the 21st century. Unless the original insult is reversed, mortality in NOMI is similar to that in other forms of AMI. Papaverine is a nonaddictive opium derivative that functions as a phoshodiesterase inhibitor and is usually infused directly into the SMA at a rate of

30 mg per hour to 60 mg per hour. The resultant accumulation of cyclic adenosine monophosphate acts to relax vascular smooth muscle [28]. Treatment of MVT depends on the extent of the intestinal ischemia. Patients without evidence of bowel infarction often recover spontaneously without operative intervention, and many are treated with anticoagulation alone. The presence of peritoneal signs necessitates emergent laparotomy. Intravenous heparin has been shown to reduce the recurrence of thrombosis from 26% to 14%, and mortality from 59% to 22%. For acute main superior mesenteric vein or portal vein thrombosis, thrombectomy may be beneficial. Cases of successful treatment with intravascular thrombolytic agents have also been reported. Thrombolysis is contraindicated when bowel infarction is suspected. After initial treatment of the acute event, the possibility of thrombophilia should be investigated. If a prothrombotic condition is detected, long-term warfarin therapy may be necessary [29,30].

Surgical revascularization has been the method of therapy for most patients with CMI. Since the early 1980s, percutaneous transluminal mesenteric angioplasty (PTMA), alone or with stent insertion, has been offered as alternative therapy. Based on currently available medical literature, patients with CMI who are otherwise appropriate surgical candidates should be treated by surgical revascularization; patients at higher surgical risk should probably have an initial attempt at PTMA with or without stenting to relieve symptoms. Long term studies have shown that patients who survive surgical revascularization have cumulative 5-year survival rates of 81% to 86% (see Table 1) [31–33]. A diagnostic and therapeutic algorithm involving various clinical spectrums of intestinal ischemia is depicted in Figs. 1 to 5.

Summary

Intestinal ischemia is a relatively common disorder in the elderly, and if not treated promptly still carries a high morbidity and mortality rate. High degree of clinical suspicion is of paramount importance in diagnosis because there is no specific laboratory test available and physical examination findings may be subtle. Once the diagnosis is made, management relies on early resuscitation, identification, and treatment of the predisposing conditions, along with careful planning of the therapeutic invasive interventions which, altogether, may help reduce the mortality and morbidity associated with this condition.

References

[1] Brandt LJ, Boley SJ. AGA technical review on intestinal ischemia. American Gastrointestinal Association. Gastroenterology 2000;118(5):954–68 [Review].

[2] Oldenburg WA, et al. Acute mesenteric ischemia: a clinical review. Arch Intern Med 2004; 164(10):1054–62 [Review].

[3] Pique JM. Management of gut ischemia. Indian J Gastroenterol 2006;25(Suppl):S39–42.

[4] Yasuhara H. Acute mesenteric ischemia: the challenge of gastroenterology. Surg Today 2005;35(3):185–95 [Review].

[5] Kozuch PL, Brandt LJ. Review article: diagnosis and management of mesenteric ischaemia with an emphasis on pharmacotherapy. Aliment Pharmacol Ther 2005;21(3):201–15 [Review].

[6] Burns BJ, Brandt LJ. Intestinal ischemia. Gastroenterol Clin North Am 2003;32:1127–43.

[7] Sreenarasimhaiah J. Chronic mesenteric ischemia. Curr Treat Options Gastroenterol 2007; 10(1):3–9.

[8] Hansen KJ, et al. Mesenteric artery disease in the elderly. J Vasc Surg 2004;40(1):45–52.

[9] Wilson DB, et al. Clinical course of mesenteric artery stenosis in elderly Americans. Arch Intern Med 2006;166(19):2095–100.

[10] Lobo Martinez E, et al. Embolectomy in mesenteric ischemia. Rev Esp Enferm Dig 1993; 83(5):351–4.

[11] Murray MJ, et al. Serum D(-)-lactate levels as an aid to diagnosing acute intestinal ischemia. Am J Surg 1994;167(6):575–8.

[12] Acosta S, et al. Preliminary study of D-dimer as a possible marker of acute bowel ischaemia. Br J Surg 2001;88(3):385–8.

[13] Antinyollar H, et al. D-dimer as a marker for early diagnosis of acute mesenteric ischemia. Thromb Res 2006;117(4):463–7.

[14] Mitchell EL, Moneta GL. Mesenteric duplex scanning. Perspect Vasc Surg Endovasc Ther 2006;18(2):175–83 [Review].

[15] Li KC, et al. In vivo flow-independent T2 measurements of superior mesenteric vein blood in diagnosis of chronic mesenteric ischemia: a preliminary evaluation. Acad Radiol 1999;6(9): 530–4.

[16] Lauenstein TC, et al. MR imaging of apparent small-bowel perfusion for diagnosing mesenteric ischemia: feasibility study. Radiology 2005;234(2):569–75.

[17] Horton KM, Fishman EK. Mesenteric ischemia: can it be done? Radiographics 2001;21(6): 1463–73 [Review].

[18] Cademartiri F, Krestin GP, et al. Multi-detector row CT angiography in patients with abdominal angina. Radiographics 2004;24(4):969–84 [Review].

[19] Shih MC, Hagspiel KD. CTA and MRA in mesenteric ischemia: Part 1, Role in diagnosis and differential diagnosis. AJR Am J Roentgenol 2007;188(2):452–61 [Review].

[20] Shih MC, Hagspiel KD, et al. TA and MRA in mesenteric ischemia: Part 2, Normal findings and complications after surgical and endovascular treatment. AJR Am J Roentgenol 2007; 188(2):462–71 [Review].

[21] Hirsch AT, et al. Guidelines for the management of patients with peripheral arterial disease (lower extremity, renal, mesenteric, and abdominal aortic): a collaborative report from the American Associations for Vascular Surgery/Society for Vascular Surgery, Society for Cardiovascular Angiography and Interventions, Society for Vascular Medicine and Biology, Society of Interventional Radiology, and the ACC/AHA Task Force on Practice Guidelines (writing committee to develop guidelines for the management of patients with peripheral arterial disease)—summary of recommendations. J Vasc Interv Radiol 2006;17(9):1383–97.

[22] Friedland S, Soetikno R, et al. Diagnosis of chronic mesenteric ischemia by visible light spectroscopy during endoscopy. Gastrointest Endosc 2007;65(2):294–300.

[23] Landis MS, Sniderman KW. Percutaneous management of chronic mesenteric ischemia: outcomes after intervention. J Vasc Interv Radiol 2005;16(10):1319–25.

[24] Chang RW, Chang JB, Longo WE. Update in management of mesenteric ischemia. World J Gastroenterol 2006;12(20):3243–7 [Review].

[25] Mallick IH, Seifalian AM, et al. Ischemia-reperfusion injury of the intestine and protective strategies against injury. Dig Dis Sci 2004;49(9):1359–77 [Review].

[26] Sheeran SR, Hallisey MJ, et al. Stent placement for treatment of mesenteric artery stenoses or occlusions. J Vasc Interv Radiol 1999;10(7):861–7.

[27] Brown DJ, Cronenwett JL, et al. Mesenteric stenting for chronic mesenteric ischemia. J Vasc Surg 2005;42(2):268–74.

[28] Trompeter M, Reimer P, et al. Non-occlusive mesenteric ischemia: etiology, diagnosis, and interventional therapy. Eur Radiol 2002;12(5):1179–87.

[29] Bayraktar Y, Harmanci O. Etiology and consequences of thrombosis in abdominal vessels. World J Gastroenterol 2006;12(8):1165–74 [Review].

[30] Kumar S, Sarr MG, Kamath PS. Mesenteric venous thrombosis. N Engl J Med 2001; 345(23):1683–8 [Review].

[31] Kasirajan, et al. Chronic mesenteric ischemia: open surgery versus percutaneous angioplasty and stenting. J Vasc Surg 2001;33(1):63–71.

[32] Rose SC, et al. Revascularization for chronic mesenteric ischemia: comparison of operative arterial bypass grafting and percutaneous transluminal angioplasty. J Vasc Interv Radiol 1995;6(3):339–49 [Review].

[33] Sivamurthy N, Davies MG, et al. Endovascular versus open mesenteric revascularization: immediate benefits do not equate with short-term functional outcomes. J Am Coll Surg 2006;202(6):859–67.

CLINICS IN
GERIATRIC
MEDICINE

ELSEVIER
SAUNDERS

Clin Geriatr Med 23 (2007) 889–903

Aging Liver and Hepatitis

Omer Junaidi, MD[a],*, Adrian M. Di Bisceglie, MD[a,b]

[a]Department of Internal Medicine, Saint Louis University School of Medicine,
3635 Vista Avenue, Saint Louis, MO 63110, USA
[b]Division of Gastroenterology and Hepatology, Saint Louis University School of Medicine,
3635 Vista Avenue, Saint Louis, MO 63110, USA

Chronic liver disease and cirrhosis are the tenth leading causes of death in the United States and results in approximately 25,000 deaths annually [1]. The economic burden associated with liver disease is also substantial, with approximately 1% of the total national health care expenditure devoted to the care of patients who have liver disease [2]. The incidence of newly diagnosed chronic liver disease seen in gastroenterologists' offices is 72.3 per 100,000 population. As life expectancy in developed countries has increased, so has the number of elderly patients who have liver disease. The most common cause of chronic liver disease is hepatitis C (57%), followed by alcohol (24%), nonalcoholic fatty liver disease (9.1%), and hepatitis B (4.4%). Other causes, such as primary sclerosing cholangitis, primary biliary cirrhosis, hereditary hemochromatosis, autoimmune hepatitis, alpha 1-antitrypsin deficiency, and liver cancer, account for less than 2% of all newly diagnosed cases of chronic liver disease seen by gastrointestinal specialists [1]. With an aging population and chronic liver disease becoming an increasingly significant cause of morbidity and mortality, the various causes for hepatitis will need to be evaluated and available treatments considered, even in the elderly population. This article reviews the likely causes of hepatitis in elderly individuals (which account for more than 60% of all newly diagnosed chronic liver disease) and discusses evidence for treating this population.

Age-related changes in liver function

Studies examining the changes that occur with age in the structure and function of the human liver are limited. An inverse correlation between

---

* Corresponding author.
E-mail address: junaidio@slu.edu (O. Junaidi).

0749-0690/07/$ - see front matter © 2007 Elsevier Inc. All rights reserved.
doi:10.1016/j.cger.2007.06.006 *geriatric.theclinics.com*

age and liver volume and hepatic blood flow has been shown [3–5]. Liver weight is reduced by 6.5% in men and 14.3% in women [6]. Studies using postmortem tissue suggest that livers of subjects older than 60 years exhibit increased hepatocyte volume, an increase in binuclear hepatocyte index, decreased hepatic concentration of smooth endoplasmic reticulum, and decreased activity of microsomal enzymes, such as mono-oxygenases and glucose-6-phosphatase [6,7]. Volume of mitochondria in hepatocytes increases and the number of mitochondria per hepatocyte decreases with age [8]. Although these changes are not dramatic, coupled with decreased hepatic blood flow they may be responsible for reduced metabolism of some drugs.

Comparison of in vitro and in vivo studies provides unique insight into a potential mechanism of impaired drug metabolism by the aging liver. In hepatocytes isolated from both young and old people and rats, no differences were seen between the rates of phase I oxidative metabolism and phase II conjugation reactions [9,10]. However, in vivo rates of oxidative phase I drug metabolism in older rats were impaired, whereas glucuronidation was preserved [11]. One hypothesis for this difference between in vitro and in vivo oxidative metabolism is that older animals experience decreased oxygen delivery to the hepatocytes because of a diffusion barrier created by pseudocapillarization of hepatic sinusoids. Older rats have sinusoids with fewer fenestrae, thicker endothelium, and some deposition of type IV collagen in the space of Disse. This process of pseudocapillarization is believed to be different from the capillarization of hepatic sinusoids that occurs during cirrhosis, because the formation of a complete basal membrane does not occur (usually absent in sinusoids but present in cirrhotic livers). Therefore pseudocapillarization leads to relative hypoxia of hepatocytes in older rats and may be reflected by lower ATP/ADP ratios in older versus younger rats [12]. This process could be important for drug therapy in old age, because the clearance of drugs undergoing oxidative metabolism, such as theophylline and propranolol, has been shown to be impaired [11].

Toxic injury in older rats has been shown to result in slower regeneration of the liver compared with younger rats [13–15], which may explain the length of time needed for an elderly liver to recover from an acute toxic or viral injury. One possible mechanism may be an age-related decrease in mitogen-activated protein kinase activity seen in rat hepatocytes [16]. However, because the overall capability for regeneration is unchanged, hepatic resections for hepatocellular carcinoma can be performed in elderly patients.

A factor that may be overlooked while drawing inferences from animal studies is the difference between frail and healthy robust elderly patients. Studies on the metabolism of some drugs, such as metoclopramide and acetaminophen, have shown impairment in only elderly patients who are frail [17,18].

These changes in the liver with aging are minor compared with other organ systems. They affect the ability of the liver to metabolize certain drugs and decrease its capacity to rapidly recover from severe hepatic injury. They do not result in age-related changes in liver blood tests, and abnormalities in serum bilirubin, aminotransferases, and alkaline phosphatase must be further evaluated just as in younger persons.

Viral hepatitis

Hepatitis A

Hepatitis A virus (HAV) is an RNA virus from the Picornaviridae family, which is highly contagious and spread through the fecal–oral route. Acute hepatitis A infection is usually a mild disease in children; however, middle-aged and older patients are more susceptible to severe HAV infections and experience serious complications. Older patients have been shown to have a higher incidence of acute liver failure and a higher mortality rate compared with younger individuals [19–22]. Case-fatality rates have been estimated to be less than 1% for children and young adults, rising to approximately 2.5% in individuals older than 50 years. The reason for this may be multifactorial and the ability to recover may be impaired by a higher prevalence of other comorbid conditions, decline in immune function, and slower regeneration capacity of the liver. However, studies have shown that the prevalence of anti-HAV antibody is high among the older population; as high as 80% in an American nursing home, according to Chien and colleagues [23], which may be why acute HAV infection remains rare in patients older than 65 years.

Recent recommendations by the Advisory Committee on Immunization Practices (ACIP) to begin immunizing all children against HAV at age 12 to 23 months will help eradicate this infection. However, US Centers for Disease Control and Prevention (CDC) recommendations for adults only support vaccination of individuals within high-risk groups, such as international travelers, homosexual men, and intravenous drug users. Increased mobility of elderly persons, including travel to endemic areas, may lead to increased exposure to HAV. Vaccination at least 4 weeks before traveling to developing countries is recommended for all elderly individuals. Individuals who have been vaccinated are protected 4 weeks from the first dose, although a second dose 6 to 12 months later is necessary for long-term protection. Because protection might not be complete until 4 weeks after vaccination, persons traveling to a high-risk area less than 4 weeks after receiving the initial dose should also be administered immunoglobulin. Persons who have chronic liver disease are not at increased risk for HAV infection because of their liver disease alone; however, they are at increased risk for fulminant hepatitis A if they become infected. Elderly patients who have chronic liver disease should be vaccinated, including those who are awaiting or have undergone liver transplantation [24].

Hepatitis B

Hepatitis B virus (HBV) is a double-shelled, enveloped DNA virus in the Hepadnaviridae family. HBV is spread predominantly through the parenteral route or sexual contact, and because high-risk sexual behavior and intravenous drug use are uncommon in the elderly population, acute hepatitis B is rare after 65 years of age. However, the cases that occur seem to have a higher risk for progressing to chronic infection. In a nursing home in Japan, as many as 59% of patients aged 77.4 ± 9.3 years developed chronic HBV infection after an outbreak, whereas only 2% to 7% of immunocompetent adults who have acute HBV infection usually do so [25].

In the geriatric population, the most prevalent form of HBV is likely to be chronic hepatitis B, because it affects approximately 0.5% of the United States population. Physicians caring for elderly people of Asian origin must be aware that the prevalence of chronic hepatitis B will be higher in this group. According to Chien and colleagues [23], the prevalence of the hepatitis B surface antigen (HBsAg) in an American nursing home was 0%, whereas it was 5% in a Japanese nursing home [26]. HBV causes liver injury through an immune response against the virus-infected liver cells and is usually not directly cytotoxic. The four drugs approved by the U.S. Food and Drug Administration for treating HBV are interferon alpha, lamivudine, adefovir, and entecavir. They effectively decrease replication of the virus and reduce inflammation and fibrosis. The decision to treat must be individualized and the clinical condition of the patient, viral load, aminotransferase levels, coexisting liver disease, family history of hepatocellular cancer, and liver biopsy findings must be taken into account [27–29]. In general, those who have active liver disease, as evidenced through elevated aminotransferases and viral titers exceeding 1 million copies per milliliter, are considered to require treatment. No studies evaluate the advantages of hepatitis B treatment in the elderly, and therefore decisions must be made on an individual basis.

Patients who have chronic hepatitis B are at higher risk for developing hepatocellular carcinoma, even without the presence of cirrhosis, and should be appropriately screened. Resolution of chronic hepatitis B significantly diminishes the risk for subsequent hepatocellular carcinoma, as does seroconversion to hepatitis B e antigen (HBeAg) negativity. Additionally, patients who have active or inactive chronic HBV infection while undergoing chemotherapy or after bone marrow transplantation may experience reactivation, leading to severe hepatitis during or after chemotherapy [30]. Lamivudine seems effective as prophylaxis or for treating HBV reactivation in these patients.

The ACIP has recommended a comprehensive strategy to eliminate HBV transmission, including prevention of perinatal HBV transmission; universal vaccination of infants; catch-up vaccination of unvaccinated children and adolescents; and vaccination of unvaccinated adults at increased risk for infection [31]. Box 1 lists the adults for whom routine hepatitis B vaccination is recommended.

Hepatitis C

Hepatitis C virus (HCV) is a small RNA virus in the Flaviviridae family. Nearly 4 million people are estimated to be infected with HCV in the United States [32] and the worldwide total approaches 170 million [33]. Alter and colleagues [34], in their United States survey, showed that the seroprevalence of anti-HCV was 0.9% between ages 60 and 69 years and 1.0% for individuals 70 years and older. These rates are significantly lower than the average prevalence of 1.8% in the United States and 3.0% to 3.9% for persons between ages 30 and 49 years. As the middle-aged population grows older in the next 2 to 3 decades, the prevalence of HCV infection in the older population is expected to increase. Prolonged infection in these patients may

---

Box 1. Adults for whom routine hepatitis B vaccination is recommended

All persons who wish to be protected from HBV infection; the CDC states that patients do not need to disclose a risk factor to receive hepatitis B vaccine
Persons who are at risk for sexual exposure
Sexually active persons who are not in long-term mutually monogamous relationships
Sex partners of persons who are HBsAg-positive
Persons seeking evaluation or treatment for a sexually transmitted disease
Men who have sex with men
Persons at risk for infection by percutaneous or mucosal exposure to blood
Current or recent injection-drug users
Household contacts of persons who are HBsAg-positive
Residents and staff of facilities for developmentally challenged persons
Health care and public safety workers with reasonably anticipated risk for exposure to blood or blood-contaminated body fluids
Persons with end-stage renal disease and those receiving dialysis
Travelers to areas with moderate or high rates of HBV infection
Persons who have chronic liver disease
Persons who have HIV infection

lead to higher rates of advanced liver disease, which would result in increased economic pressure on health care systems worldwide.

HCV is spread through the parenteral route, and transfusion of blood and blood products was an important source of transmission before 1990. Currently, intravenous drug use is the major risk factor [34]. Most elderly patients who have hepatitis C today probably acquired it from prior injection drug therapy that used nondisposable instruments and inadequate methods to sterilize needles and syringes [35,36]. According to the 2004 guideline of the American Association for the Study of Liver Diseases (AASLD), persons who received transfusion of blood or blood products before July 1992 should be checked for HCV infection [37].

The major risk factors associated with the progression of chronic HCV infection are older age at infection, male gender, and daily alcohol ingestion [38,39]. Poynard and colleagues [40] showed that age at infection was a main risk factor for fibrosis in 2235 infected patients. The rate at which fibrosis progressed was low in individuals infected when younger than 20 years, intermediate in those infected at age 21 to 40 years, increased in those infected at age 40 to 50 years, and highest in those infected at 50 years of age or older. Roudot-Thoraval and colleagues [41] reported comparable results in 2500 patients who had chronic HCV, showing that the risk for cirrhosis was independently related to the age at HCV exposure and reached a peak of 46.8% in patients who acquired HCV infection at age 60 years or older. In these studies and others, the severity of liver disease was greater in older patients than younger patients, with the same duration of infection [42]. The reason for more rapid progression of liver fibrosis in older patients who have chronic hepatitis C is unknown but may relate to the decline in immune function with age.

Treatment of HCV infection in the elderly population remains a controversial issue and evidence is limited. Current recommendations for treatment of the general population are based on large, multicenter, randomized, controlled studies [43,44]. However, these studies excluded patients older than 65 years [45] and those who had diseases common in elderly persons, such as dementia, depression, renal, coronary, or cerebral vascular diseases, which poses problems for applying the results to the elderly population.

Currently, standard care for HCV infection is pegylated interferon (IFN)-alpha and oral ribavirin [37]. The rate of sustained virologic response (defined as the absence of serum HCV RNA at and 6 months after the end of treatment) reported for younger populations treated with pegylated IFN and ribavirin averages 55% [43,44]. In these large, multicenter, randomized trials with pegylated IFN and ribavirin involving cohorts with a mean age of 42 to 43 years, older age was associated with poorer response to treatment. According to Fried and colleagues [44], age older than 40 years was an independent predictor of poor response (odds ratio, 2.60 for sustained response of those aged younger than 40 years).

   Studies on treatment of HCV infection in older patients are few, and
early ones did not assess the rate of sustained virologic response [46,47].
Later studies, although assessing sustained virologic response, used treatments such as IFN monotherapy or IFN with amantadine [48–50], which
are now considered obsolete. However, in these studies the rate of sustained
virologic response for patients older than 60 years (mean age, 64 years) was
similar to that for younger patients (mean age, 48 years; 18% [9/50] versus
20% [21/104]) [49]. IFN monotherapy has been shown to reduce liver-
related mortality among patients older than 60 years (mean age, 63 years)
who had chronic hepatitis C [50]. Furthermore, patients (median age, 57
years) who had cirrhotic hepatitis C treated with IFN had a reduced risk
for hepatocellular carcinoma and an improved survival rate compared
with patients who underwent no treatment [51]. Even one of the most recent
studies reporting the efficacy of therapy had relatively small numbers of
older adults who were treated with the current standard treatment, pegylated IFN and ribavirin. In this study, Thabut and colleagues [52] reported
a 45% (9 of 20 patients) sustained virologic response to pegylated IFN and
ribavirin in patients aged 65 years and older. However, treatment was
stopped in 25% (5/20) of patients because of poor tolerance and doses
were lowered in 30% (6/20) of patients. Nudo and colleagues [53], comparing 30 patients older than 60 years (mean age, 65.13 ± 4.2 years) with 41
control patients younger than 60 years (mean age, 44.5 ± 8.7 years), report
no significant difference in sustained virologic response after treatment with
either interferon, interferon and ribavirin, or pegylated interferon and
ribavirin. However, they noted that patients older than 60 years were
more likely to develop anemia, neutropenia, and thrombocytopenia while
on treatment. Nevertheless, the AASLD guideline does not stipulate an
upper age limit for antiviral therapy [37], although in practice, elderly
patients are less often considered and referred for treatment. Therapy
should be considered for male and female patients up to 75 years of age,
because in the United States they have an average life expectancy of 10.3
and 12.4 years, respectively [54].

Autoimmune hepatitis

   Autoimmune hepatitis (AIH) is a chronic disease of the hepatic paren-
chyma characterized by hypergammaglobulinemia, circulating autoantibodies, and morphologic changes of interface hepatitis. AIH was first
described in jaundiced peripubertal girls in the 1950s by Waldenstrom [55]
and Kunkel and colleagues [56], and subsequently described as a separated
disease entity called *lupoid hepatitis* [57]. Since then, its clinical description
has been expanded to include both men and women and has a bimodal
incidence. Patients may not only present with AIH between 10 and 30 years
of age, but recent studies have shown that another peak in presentation
occurs between 50 and 70 years of age [58–61].

AIH is not diagnosed with a single sensitive and specific diagnostic test, and often may be a diagnosis of exclusion. Serologic clues are hypergamma-globulinemia (ie, immunoglobulin G) and autoantibodies, but these are usually diverse. Antinuclear (ANA), antismooth muscle (SMA), anti–liver kidney microsomal (LKM), and antisoluble liver/pancreas antigen (SLA/LP) autoantibodies may all be detected in these patients [62]. Except for SLA/LP, none of these autoantibodies is specific for AIH and can be seen in other conditions such as rheumatologic diseases, drug reactions, and virus-associated autoimmunity. AIH may be classified into two types based on the presence of certain serum autoantibodies. Type I (classic) charac-terized by presence of ANA and SMA antibodies is more common in older patients [61]. Type II AIH is characterized by the presence of anti–LKM 1 and anti–liver cytosol antibodies and the absence of ANA and SMA and is more prevalent in younger patients. These antibodies should be present in a titer of at least 1:80 in adults to meet criteria for diagnosis.

As a treatable chronic liver disease, AIH has an excellent prognosis if remission can be induced; a timely diagnosis must be made and therapy initiated immediately. However, until recently, studies of AIH in elderly patients have been limited perhaps partly because of the belief that these patients have a tendency to have milder disease [63]. Controversy has also existed over whether elderly patients benefit from treatment [64]. In 1985, Lebovics and colleagues [65] concluded that elderly patients received less benefit from treatment and experienced more adverse side effects, whereas in 1986, Selby and colleagues [66] reported good responses to treatment and few adverse side effects. More recent studies note that elderly patients can present with severe disease and suggest that this may be partly because of delays in diagnosis and initiation of therapy [60,67]. All of these studies involved small numbers and heterogeneous populations of patients, includ-ing those who had probable and definite AIH and some who also had fea-tures of primary sclerosing cholangitis or primary biliary cirrhosis (so-called "overlap syndromes"). Additionally, the earlier reports (before the discov-ery of the HCV) may have included patients who had chronic HCV infec-tion. Most recently, Al-Chalabi and colleagues [68] presented data from a cohort of 164 patients in the United Kingdom, including 43 individuals aged 60 years and older who had definite AIH according to the revised In-ternational Autoimmune Hepatitis Group (IAIHG) scoring system. Sub-stratification of patients younger and older than 40 years showed that older patients had more fibrosis. Rates of complete, partial, and failed re-sponse were similar, and the median number of relapses was lower in older patients. However, this did not lead to differences in liver-related deaths in both groups (12% versus 15%).

Older patients present with AIH with an increased prevalence after 40 years of age and require treatment, which has a favorable outcome. Whether this represents new-onset AIH or presentation of previously ongoing asymptomatic AIH remains unresolved. Clinicians should remain vigilant about the possibility of AIH in older individuals and be aware that these patients are more likely to present with extrahepatic immune-mediated disease manifestations, such as thyroiditis, rheumatoid arthritis, hyperparathyroidism, ulcerative colitis, and vitiligo [68]. Standard therapy in AIH consists of steroids alone or in combination with azathioprine. For maintenance, azathioprine monotherapy may be used, but induction with azathioprine alone is not effective. Caution should be used when administering steroids to elderly patients, especially in women who may have osteopenia or diabetes. Cushingoid facies development occurs at a higher frequency among older individuals but disappeared in all patients who were switched to azathioprine monotherapy. Apart from this, drug-related adverse events were not significantly among elderly and younger patients [66]. Recommendations for the treatment of AIH suggest that the steroidal side effects be weighed against the potential benefit of therapy and, depending on comorbidities, that not all elderly patients who have AIH are good candidates for steroid treatment.

Drug-induced hepatitis

A marked disparity in medication use exists between elderly and younger patients, Elderly patients have higher rates of polypharmacy, and their risk for drug-induced hepatotoxicity is correspondingly elevated. Drugs are the causative agents for one third of suspected acute hepatitis cases and responsible for liver dysfunction in 0.8% of outpatients [69]. Presentation of drug-induced liver disease is usually nonspecific. Mild serum aminotransferase or alkaline phosphatase elevation are most commonly seen, which may be incidentally noted and typically do not cause symptoms. At the other extreme, patients may experience fulminant hepatic failure leading to the need for liver transplantation or death. However, most clinical presentation lies between the two extremes, and therefore distinguishing drug-induced liver disease from other liver diseases, such as viral hepatitis and cholestatic disorders, can be challenging.

The diagnosis of drug-induced hepatic injury is often based on circumstantial evidence [70,71] and is usually a diagnosis of exclusion. Physicians should be aware that the onset of liver injury may be related to the introduction of certain medications, and resolution of manifestations after drug withdrawal may provide the strongest supporting evidence. Acute drug-induced liver disease may be variously defined but falls broadly into three injury patterns: hepatocellular (cytotoxic), cholestatic (bile duct injury), or mixed. Certain drug categories merit special attention, such as antibiotics, antiepileptics, and nonsteroidal anti-inflammatory drugs. Some widely prescribed medications that result in abnormalities of liver function tests are discussed in the following sections.

Acetaminophen

Acetaminophen is the leading cause of acute hepatic failure in the United States and is responsible for 42% of cases, according to the Acute Liver Failure Study Group [72]. Although 44% of the cases were caused by an intentional overdose, 42% of cases were caused by an unintentional overdose, which is the group that elderly patients are at higher risk for falling into. Because acetaminophen is found in numerous prescription and over-the-counter products, including cold remedies and pain medications, elderly patients should be counseled about the risk for accidental overdose. Acetaminophen has a dose-related hepatotoxicity and, in chronic alcohol users, may cause liver injury at lower doses. N-acetylcysteine should be used in a timely manner for suspected overdose to minimize injury.

Isoniazid

Isoniazid (INH) has been the mainstay therapeutic agent for treating tuberculosis for more than 50 years and often leads to elevations of aminotransferases and occasionally overt liver disease [73]. Elevations of aminotransferase levels from INH usually appear within several weeks after treatment initiation and are found in 10% to 20% of patients. Usually these elevations are modest and not associated with signs or symptoms suggesting liver disease. In many patients, continued use of INH is well tolerated and often the aminotransferases levels return to or near normal. If INH is discontinued when the elevations are noted, the aminotransferase levels generally return to normal within 1 to 4 weeks. However, a few patients develop significant clinical hepatitis, and drug-induced hepatic failure may occur (0.1%–2.0%). Patients older than 50 years are at an increased risk for developing clinically evident hepatitis from INH [74]. Fountain and colleagues [75] confirmed this in a more recent study showing that patients older than 49 years were almost five times more likely to experience a hepatotoxic event while on INH therapy compared with those aged 25 to 34 years.

Other drugs of interest

HMG-CoA reductase inhibitors and currently available second-generation thiazolidinediones are rarely responsible for hepatotoxicity, and a higher risk amongst the elderly has not been reported. However, because of their widespread use, especially in the elderly population, their effects on the liver are reviewed.

HMG-CoA reductase inhibitors (statins)
Hepatotoxicity has been a concern since statins arrived on the market in 1987 (lovastatin) [76]. Asymptomatic increases in aminotransferase levels develop frequently, but more significant elevations (greater than three times

upper limit of normal) occur in 1% to 3% of patients. A study reviewing the tolerability of atorvastatin in patients older than 65 years found no difference compared with placebo in rates of elevation of transaminases greater than three times upper limit of normal until a dose of 40 mg/d (0.2%) [77]. However, the prevalence of elevated transaminases was higher in the group receiving 80 mg/d (3.2% versus $\leq 0.9\%$ in groups receiving ≤ 40 mg/d). No evidence shows that patients who have elevated baseline alanine aminotransferase levels associated with diabetes, steatohepatitis, or chronic hepatitis C are at increased risk [78,79]. Few well-documented cases exist of statin-induced severe hepatotoxicity. Therefore, present evidence supports the view that statins are safe agents for the liver despite the frequent elevations of alanine aminotransferase.

Thiazolidinediones

Thiazolidinedione agents are peroxisome proliferator–activated receptor gamma agonists used to treat diabetes. They were implicated in hepatotoxicity when troglitazone use caused several instances of acute liver failure leading to death or the need for liver transplantation [80]. Subsequently, troglitazone was withdrawn from the market in 2000. Fewer and less severe cases of hepatotoxicity are associated with second-generation thiazolidinediones (rosiglitazone and pioglitazone) compared with troglitazone [81]. Despite the limited case reports in the literature, second-generation thiazolidinediones are believed safe for the liver, although current labeling requires baseline and serial measurements of liver enzymes in patients taking pioglitazone or rosiglitazone.

Summary

Although the liver is not unscathed by the process of aging, the changes it undergoes are minor compared with other organ systems. Acute viral hepatitis is uncommon in the elderly population but, because it may have grave consequences, vaccination against hepatitis A and B is recommended for patients at risk. Prevalence of chronic hepatitis B and C in elderly individuals is expected to increase as the middle-aged population grows older in the next 2 to 3 decades, and treatment must be considered on an individual basis. Further studies are needed to evaluate the benefits of treatment of chronic hepatitis B and C in the elderly. AIH may present in individuals aged 50 to 70 years and carries an excellent prognosis if prompt diagnosis and treatment lead to remission. Drug-induced hepatitis is a significant cause of acute hepatitis in the elderly, with antibiotics, antiepileptics, and nonsteroidal anti-inflammatory drugs common agents.

References

[1] Murphy SDeaths: final data for 1998. National vital statistics reports, vol. 48. Hyattsville (MD): National Center for Health Statistics; 2000.

[2] Kim WR, Brown RS Jr, Terrault NA, et al. Burden of liver disease in the United States: summary of a workshop. Hepatology 2002;36(1):227–42.

[3] Wynne HA, Cope LH, Much E, et al. The effect of age upon liver volume and apparent liver blood flow in healthy man. Hepatology 1989;9:297–301.

[4] Zoli M, Magalotti D, Bianchi G, et al. Total and functional hepatic blood flow decrease in parallel with ageing. Age Ageing 1999;28(1):29–33.

[5] Marchesisi G, Bua V, Brunori A, et al. Galactose elimination capacity and liver volume in aging man. Hepatology 1988;8(5):1079–83.

[6] Popper H. Aging and the liver. In: Popper H, Schaffner F, editors. Progress in liver diseases, vol. 8. New York: Grune & Stratton; 1986. p. 659–83.

[7] Schmucker DL. Hepatocyte fine structure during maturation and senescence. J Electron Microsc Tech 1990;14(2):106–25.

[8] Tauchi H, Sato T. Age changes in size and number of mitochondria of human hepatic cells. J Gerontol 1968;23(4):454–61.

[9] Williams D, Woodhouse K. Age related changes in O-deethylase and aldrin epoxidase activity in mouse skin and liver microsomes. Age Aging 1996;25:377–80.

[10] Wynne H, Mutch E, James OF, et al. The effect of age on mono-oxygenase enzyme kinetics in rat liver microsomes. Age Aging 1987;16:153–8.

[11] Le Couteur DG, McLean AJ. The aging liver. Drug clearance and an oxygen diffusion barrier hypothesis. Clin Pharmacokinet 1998;34:359–73.

[12] Le Couteur DG, Cogger VC, Markus AM, et al. Pseudocapillarization and associated energy limitation in the aged rat liver. Hepatology 2001;33:537–43.

[13] Sanz N, Diez-Fernandez C, Alvarez AM, et al. Age related changes on parameters of experimentally-induced liver injury and regeneration. Toxicol Appl Pharmacol 1999;154:40–9.

[14] Schmucker DL. Aging and the liver: an update. J Gerontol A Biol Sci Med Sci 1998;53: B315–20.

[15] Tsukamoto I, Nakata R, Kojo S. Effect of aging on rat liver regeneration after partial hepatectomy. Biochem Mol Biol Int 1993;30:773–8.

[16] Liu Y, Guyton KZ, Gorospe M, et al. Age-related decline in mitogen-activated protein kinase activity in epidermal growth factor-stimulated rat hepatocytes. J Biol Chem 1996; 271:3604–7.

[17] Wynne HA, Yelland C, Cope LH, et al. The association of age and frailty with the pharmacokinetics and pharmacodynamics of metoclopramide. Age Aging 1993;22:354–9.

[18] Wynne HA, Cope LH, Herd B, et al. The association of age and frailty with paracetamol conjugation in man. Age Aging 1990;19:419–24.

[19] Forbes A, Williams R. Changing epidemiology and clinical aspects of hepatitis A. Br Med Bull 1990;46:303–18.

[20] Forbes A, Williams R. Increasing age–an important adverse prognostic factor in hepatitis A virus infection. J R Coll Physicians Lond 1988;22:237–9.

[21] Brown GR, Persley K. Hepatitis A epidemic in the elderly. South Med J 2002;95:826–33.

[22] Willner IR, Howard SC, Williams EQ, et al. Serious hepatitis A: an analysis of patients hospitalized during an urban epidemic in the United States. Ann Intern Med 1998;128: 111–4.

[23] Chien NT, Dundoo G, Horani MH, et al. Seroprevalence of viral hepatitis in an older nursing home population. J Am Geriatr Soc 1999;47:1110–3.

[24] CDC. Prevention of hepatitis A through active or passive immunization: recommendations of the Advisory Committee on Immunization Practices (ACIP). Morbidity and Mortality Weekly Report 1999;48(No. RR-12):1–37.

[25] Kondo Y, Tsukada K, Takeuchi T, et al. High carrier rate after hepatitis B virus infection in the elderly. Hepatology 1993;18:768.

[26] Sugauchi F, Mizokami M, Orito E, et al. Hepatitis B virus infection among residents of a nursing home for the elderly: seroepidemiological study and molecular evolutionary analysis. J Med Virol 2000;62:456–62.

[27] Liaw YF, Leung N, Guan R, et al. Asian-Pacific consensus statement on the management of chronic hepatitis B: an update. J Gastroenterol Hepatol 2003;18:239–45.

[28] Franchis R, Hadengue A, Lau GK, et al. EASL Jury. EASL International Consensus Conference on Hepatitis B. J Hepatol 2003;39:S3–25.

[29] Lok AS, McMahon BJ. Chronic hepatitis B. Update of recommendations. Hepatology 2004; 39:857–61.

[30] Li YH, He YF, Jiang WQ, et al. Lamivudine prophylaxis reduces the incidence and severity of hepatitis in hepatitis B virus carriers who receive chemotherapy for lymphoma. Cancer 2006;106(6):1320–5.

[31] CDC. A comprehensive immunization strategy to eliminate transmission of hepatitis B virus infection in the United States. Recommendations of the Advisory Committee on Immunization Practices (ACIP) Part 1: immunization of infants, children, and adolescents. Morbidity and Mortality Weekly Report 2005;54(No. RR-16):1–33.

[32] Alter MJ, Kruszon-Moran D, Nainan OV, et al. The prevalence of hepatitis C virus infection in the United States, 1988 through 1994. N Engl J Med 1999;341:556–62.

[33] WHO. Hepatitis C: global prevalence. Wkly Epidemiol Rec 1997;72:341–4.

[34] Alter MJ. Epidemiology of hepatitis C. Hepatology 1997;26(Suppl 1):62S–5S.

[35] Brind AM, Watson JP, James OFW, et al. Hepatitis C virus infection in the elderly. QJM 1996;89:291–6.

[36] Monica F, Lirussi F, Nassuato G, et al. Hepatitis C virus infection and related chronic liver disease in a resident elderly population: The Silea study. J Viral Hepat 1998;5:345–51.

[37] Strader DB, Wright T, Thomas DL, et al. Diagnosis, management, and treatment of hepatitis C. American Association for the Study of Liver Diseases. Hepatology 2004;39: 1147–71.

[38] Gordon SC, Elloway RS, Long JC, et al. The pathology of hepatitis C as a function of mode of transmission: blood transfusion vs. intravenous drug use. Hepatology 1993;18:1338–43.

[39] Yano M, Yatsuhashi H, Inokuchi K, et al. Epidemiology and long term prognosis off hepatitis C virus infection in Japan. Gut 1993;34(Suppl 1):S13–6.

[40] Poynard T, Bedossa P, Opolon P. Natural history of liver fibrosis progression in patients with chronic hepatitis C. Lancet 1997;349:825–32.

[41] Roudot-Thoraval F, Bastie A, Pawlotsky JM, et al. Epidemiological factors affecting the severity of hepatitis C virus-related liver disease: a French survey of 6,664 patients. The Study Group for the Prevalence and the Epidemiology of Hepatitis C Virus. Hepatology 1997;26: 485–90.

[42] Floreani A, Bertin T, Soffiati G, et al. Anti-hepatitis C virus in the elderly: a seroepidemiological study in a home for the aged. Gerontology 1992;38:214–6.

[43] Manns MP, McHutchison JG, Gordon SC, et al. Peginterferon a-2b plus ribavirin compared with interferon a-2b plus ribavirin for initial treatment of chronic hepatitis C: a randomized trial. Lancet 2001;358:958–65.

[44] Fried MW, Shiffman ML, Reddy KR, et al. Peginterferon a-2a plus ribavirin for chronic hepatitis C virus infection. N Engl J Med 2002;347:975–82.

[45] Strader DB. Understudied populations with hepatitis C. Hepatology 2002;36(Suppl 1): S226–36.

[46] Horiike N, Masumoto T, Nakanishi K, et al. Interferon therapy for patients more than 60 years of age with chronic hepatitis C. J Gastroenterol Hepatol 1995;10:246–9.

[47] Marcus EL, Tur-Kaspa R. Viral hepatitis in older adults. J Am Geriatr Soc 1997;45:755–63.

[48] Bacosi M, Russo F, D'innocenzo S, et al. Amantadine and interferon in the combined treatment of hepatitis C virus in elderly patients. Hepatol Res 2002;22:231–9.

[49] Alessi N, Freni MA, Spadaro A, et al. Efficacy of interferon treatment (IFN) in elderly patients with chronic hepatitis C. Infez Med 2003;11:208–12.

[50] Imai Y, Kasahara A, Tanaka H, et al. Interferon therapy for aged patients with chronic hepatitis C: improved survival in patients exhibiting a biochemical response. J Gastroenterol 2004;39:1069–77.

[51] Shiratori Y, Ito Y, Yokosuka O, et al. Antiviral therapy for cirrhotic hepatitis C: association with reduced hepatocellular carcinoma development and improved survival. Ann Intern Med 2005;142:105–14.

[52] Thabut D, Le Calvez S, Thibault V, et al. Hepatitis C in 6,865 patients 65 yr or older: a severe and neglected curable disease? Am J Gastroenterol 2006;101(6):1260–7.

[53] Nudo CG, Wong P, Hilzenrat N, et al. Elderly patients are at greater risk of cytopenia during antiviral therapy for hepatitis C. Can J Gastroenterol 2006;20(9):589–92.

[54] Arias E. United States life tables, 2002. Natl Vital Stat Rep 2004;53:1–38.

[55] Waldenstrom JL. Blutproteine und Nahrungseiweisse [German]. Dtsch Gesellsch Verd Stoffw 1950;15:113–9.

[56] Kunkel HG, Ahrens EHJ, Eisenmenger WJ. Extreme hypergammaglobulinemia in young women with liver disease of unknown etiology. J Clin Invest 1951;30:654.

[57] Mackay IR, Taft LI, Cowling DC. Lupoid hepatitis. Lancet 1956;2:1323–6.

[58] McFarlane IG. The relationship between autoimmune markers and different clinical syndromes in autoimmune hepatitis. Gut 1998;42:599–602.

[59] Toda G, Zeniya M, Watanabe F, et al. Present status of autoimmune hepatitis in Japan, correlating the characteristics with international criteria in an area with a high rate of HCV infection. Japanese National Study Group of Autoimmune Hepatitis. J Hepatol 1997;26:1207–12.

[60] Schramm C, Kanzler S, Meyer zum Buschenfelde KH, et al. Autoimmune hepatitis in the elderly. Am J Gastroenterol 2001;96:1587–91.

[61] Parker DR, Kingham JG. Type 1 autoimmune hepatitis is primarily a disease of later life. QJM 1997;90:289–96.

[62] Strassburg CP, Manns MP. Autoantibodies and autoantigens in autoimmune hepatitis. Semin Liver Dis 2002;22:339–52.

[63] Donaldson PT, Doherty DG, Hayllar KM, et al. Susceptibility to autoimmune chronic active hepatitis: human leukocyte antigens DR4 and A1-B8-DR3 are independent risk factors. Hepatology 1991;13:701–6.

[64] Yarze JC, Meyer zum Buschenfelde K-H, Lohse AW. Autoimmune hepatitis. N Engl J Med 1996;334:923–4.

[65] Lebovics E, Schaffner F, Klion FM, et al. Autoimmune chronic active hepatitis in postmenopausal women. Dig Dis Sci 1985;30:824–8.

[66] Selby CD, Toghill PJ. Chronic active hepatitis in the elderly. Age Ageing 1986;15:350–6.

[67] Newton JL, Burt AD, Park JB, et al. Autoimmune hepatitis in older patients. Age Ageing 1997;26:441–4.

[68] Al-Chalabi T, Boccato S, Portmann BC, et al. Autoimmune hepatitis (AIH) in the elderly: a systematic retrospective analysis of a large group of consecutive patients with definite AIH followed at a tertiary referral centre. J Hepatol 2006;45:575–83.

[69] Galan MV, Potts JA, Siverman AL, et al. The burden of acute nonfulminant drug-induced hepatitis in a United States tertiary referral center. J Clin Gastroenterol 2005;39:64–7.

[70] Maddrey WC. Clinicopathologic patterns of drug-induced liver disease. In: Kaplowitz N, DeLeve LD, editors. Drug-induced liver disease. New York: Marcel Dekker; 2002. p. 227–42.

[71] Kaplowitz N. Causality assessment versus guilt-by-association in drug hepatotoxicity. Hepatology 2001;33:308–10.

[72] Larson AM, Polson J, Fontana RJ, et al. Acetaminophen-induced acute liver failure: results of a United States multicenter, prospective study. Hepatology 2005;42:1364–72.

[73] Maddrey WC. Isoniazid-induced liver disease. Semin Liver Dis 1981;1:77–84.

[74] Kopanoff DE, Snider DE Jr, Caras GJ. Isoniazid related hepatitis. Am Rev Respir Dis 1978;117:991–1001.

[75] Fountain FF, Tolley E, Chrisman CR, et al. Isoniazid hepatotoxicity associated with treatment of latent tuberculosis infection: a 7 year evaluation from a public health tuberculosis clinic. Chest 2005;128:116–23.

[76] Tolman KG. The liver and lovastatin. Am J Cardiol 2002;89:1374–80.
[77] Hey-Hadavi JH, Kuntze E, Luo D, et al. Tolerability of atorvastatin in a population aged > or =65 years: a retrospective pooled analysis of results from fifty randomized clinical trials. Am J Geriatr Pharmacother 2006;4(2):112–22.
[78] Chalasani N, Aljadhey H, Kesterson J, et al. Patients with elevated liver enzymes are not at higher risk for statin hepatotoxicity. Gastroenterology 2004;126:1287–92.
[79] Khorashadi S, Hasson NK, Cheung RC. Incidence of statin hepatotoxicity in patients with hepatitis C. Clin Gastroenterol Hepatol 2006;4(7):902–7.
[80] Graham DJ, Drinkard CR, Shatin D. Incidence of idiopathic acute liver failure and hospitalized liver injury in patients treated with troglitazone. Am J Gastroenterol 2003;98: 175–9.
[81] Nagasaka S, Abe T, Kawakami A, et al. Pioglitazone-induced hepatic injury in a patient previously receiving troglitazone with success. Diabet Med 2002;19:344–8.

CLINICS IN
GERIATRIC
MEDICINE

ELSEVIER
SAUNDERS

Clin Geriatr Med 23 (2007) 905–921

Alcoholic Liver Disease in the Elderly

Helmut K. Seitz, MD[a],*, Felix Stickel, MD[b]

[a]Department of Medicine & Center of Alcohol Research, Liver Disease and Nutrition,
Salem Medical Center, University of Heidelberg, Zeppelinstrasse 11-33,
D - 69121 Heidelberg, Germany
[b]Institute of Clinical Pharmacology, University of Berne, Murtenstrasse 35,
CH- 3010 Berne, Switzerland

The percentage of individuals over 65 years of age is steadily increasing. This increase in life expectancy is also associated with increasing psychosocial problems, such as loss of husbands or wives, loneliness, and depression. All of these factors may explain why alcohol consumption has increased in the elderly, while overall consumption or consumption in younger age groups has decreased in certain geographic regions. Therefore, it seems noteworthy to identify risk factors in the elderly for the development of alcoholic liver disease (ALD). The liver handles alcohol differently with age, and alcohol toxicity increases with age because of increased organ susceptibility. Additional factors increasing the toxicity of ethanol in the elderly are the use of multiple drugs and the presence of other types of liver disease, especially of nonalcoholic fatty liver disease (NAFLD), which may deteriorate under chronic alcohol consumption. This article focuses on these issues.

Epidemiology of alcohol consumption and alcoholic liver disease in the elderly

Epidemiologic studies have shown that alcohol plays a less important role in individuals over 65 years of age when compared with middle-aged adults. A national study from 1986 showed a decrease of regular ethanol use from 70%, in the 20- to 34-year-old age group, to 43% in the 65- to 74-year-old age group, and to 30% in those over 75 years old. More than

Original research was supported by the Volkswagen Foundation, the Dietrich Götze Foundation, Heidelberg, and the Dietmar Hopp Foundation, Heidelberg.

* Corresponding author.
E-mail address: helmut_karl.seitz@urz.uni-heidelberg.de (H.K. Seitz).

two drinks per day were consumed in 8% of the 65- to 74-year-old
individuals, and in 5% of those over 75 years old [1]. Other studies found
approximately 2% of problem drinkers among individuals over 65 years
of age [2,3]. Sulski and coworkers [4] studied 173 men and 317 women in
Boston who were aged 60 to 95 years old. Fifty five percent of the men
and 44% of the women reported weekly alcohol consumption. Heavy
alcohol abuse dropped from 11% to 4% in the 60- to 69-year-old group,
as compared with those over 80 years old. The corresponding data for
women were 8% and 2%, respectively. On the other hand, no alcohol
problems were reported in a British study of more than 500 individuals
with an age of 65 or more [5]. However, in the last decade a tendency toward
an increase in alcohol consumption has been predicted and, finally, also
noted in the elderly [6,7]. In 1996 it was reported that 62% of 60 to 94
year olds in nursing homes drank alcohol regularly. Thirteen percent of
men and 2% of women had more than two drinks per day [8]. Other reports
on individuals over 60 years of age state that 20% of men and 10% of
women had a higher alcohol consumption than what is classified as
"moderate" [9].

According to the 2001 National Household Survey on Drug Abuse, 33%
of adults aged 65 and older consumed alcohol during the preceding month
[10], and a large national cross-sectional survey of community dwelling
elderly reported that 25% of those surveyed consumed alcohol daily (31%
of them men and 19% of them women). Although in general moderate
alcohol consumption prevailed in this group, approximately 10% reported
binge drinking (five or more drinks at one occasion) at least 12 times in
the previous year, and 5% reported weekly binge drinking [11]. Data for
alcohol related hospitalization vary with respect to region and whether it
is a city or countryside analyzed. However it is a fact that older adults are
less likely to receive a primary diagnosis of alcoholism than younger adults
[12]. In a study with 417 subjects, house officers diagnosed alcoholism only
in 37% of older as compared with 60% of younger alcoholics [13]. According to Iber [14] more than 2% (up to 10%) of people over the age of 65 are
alcoholics.

It is important to note that although women are more susceptible to
developing ALD, alcohol consumption in women over 65 was less
pronounced when compared with men of the same age group [15]. However,
more recently alcohol drinking, including heavy alcohol drinking, in women
has been socially more accepted than in earlier years.

Per capita alcohol consumption is a reliable indicator of the proportion
of heavy drinkers in a given population, and alcohol related problems,
such as cirrhosis of the liver, increase as per capita consumption increases
[16]. Recent age period cohort analysis of European trends in liver cirrhosis
mortality clearly documented that alcohol related cirrhosis of the liver is
likely to decrease in Western and Southern European countries, whereas
an increase is predicted for the North and especially the East of Europe

[17]. One has to keep in mind that alcohol may be an additional "cirrhotic" factor in non-ALD and in hepatitis B and C infections. This may be especially relevant in populations over the age 60 and 70 in Northern and Eastern Europe [17].

Although conventional hospital practice suggests that most patients present with severe ALD in their fifth or sixth decade, one study from the United States suggested that the peak incidence of presentation with alcoholic cirrhosis was the seventh decade [18]. In a British study, ALD was found in 28% of subjects over the age of 60, and a French large retrospective study suggested that as many as 20% of subjects with alcoholic cirrhosis were over the age of 70 [18].

Pathophysiology of alcoholic liver disease, with special emphasis on the elderly

The natural course of ALD is given in Fig. 1. Chronic alcohol ingestion results in 90% to 100% of alcoholic fatty liver (AFL), which is reversible. Alcoholic fatty liver is primarily caused by metabolic disturbances following hepatic alcohol metabolism, including an overproduction of a reduced form of nicotinamide adenine dinucleotide (NADH) and thus a change in the hepatic redox state (Fig. 2) [19]. In many cases AFL may remain silent.

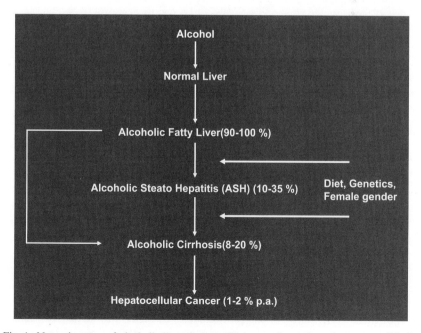

Fig. 1. Natural course of alcoholic liver diseases. Diets, genetics and gender may modify the disease course. p.a., = per annum.

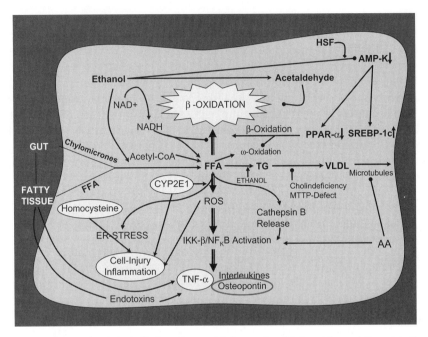

Fig. 2. Pathogenesis of alcoholic fatty liver and inflammation. Fatty acids are delivered to the liver from fat tissue and from the gut as chylomicrones. In addition, the synthesis of free fatty acids (FFA) is enhanced because ethanol metabolism results in the generation of NADH and in a shift of the hepatic redox state, which favors FFA and triglyceride synthesis. Ethanol also inhibits AMP-kinase, leading to a decrease in peroxisome proliferator-activated receptor alpha (PPAR-α) and an increase in SHREB-1c, two nuclear transcription factors, which under normal conditions counteract enhanced fat accumulation by activating gene coding for enzymes involved in fat degradation. Subsequently acetaldehyde, which is also generated from alcohol, injures mitochondria with a decrease in mitochondrial function, such as β oxidation and fat elimination, and also damages the microtubular system, resulting in an inadequate secretion of fat in the form of very low density lipoprotein (VLDL) from the liver to the blood. FFA are hepatotoxic and may be responsible for the release of cathepsine B and induce cytochrome P-4502E1 (CYP2E1). CYP2E1 is also individually induced by chronic alcohol consumption. CYP2E1 produces reactive oxygen species, which result in lipidperoxidation and cell injury. An activation of IKK-β/nuclear factor kappa B occurs, leading to secretion of inteleukines, osteopontin, and especially TNF-α. TNF-α is also released by fat tissue and by hepatic Kupffer cells stimulated via intestinal endotoxins. TNF-α mediates apoptosis and necrosis.

However, only 30% of these patients develop alcoholic fibrosis either with or without inflammation, and only 10% to 20% progress to liver cirrhosis [20]. Because of various pathophysiologic mechanisms, AFL can turn into an alcoholic steatohepatitis (ASH) with a special morphological and clinical entity, or can lead directly to cirrhosis via enhanced fibrogenesis often seen in the elderly. Mechanisms which lead to ASH are summarized in Fig. 2 [21].

An important factor in the pathogenesis of ASH and advanced ALD is the production of reactive oxygen species (ROS) with consecutive lipidperoxidation [21,22]. Several enzymatic systems, including cytochrome

P-4502E1 (CYP2E1), the mitochondrial respiratory chain, and the cytosolic enzymes xanthine oxidase and aldehyde oxidase, have been implicated as sources of ROS in hepatocytes during ethanol oxidation [21,22]. The induction of CYP2E1 is of special importance, as ROS and hydroxylethy radicals are produced through CYP2E1, which leads to lipid peroxidation [23]. These radicals bind covalently to proteins and form neoantigens with a specific antibody response [21–25]. Inhibition of CYP2E1 by specific inhibitors result in an improvement of ALD in animal experiments [26].

Another important pathogenetic factor in ALD is the secretion of cytokines from hepatic Kupffer cells, which is caused by the influx of endotoxins from the gut to the liver [21,27]. Because of alcohol associated injury of the intestinal mucosal barrier, bacteria and bacterial products may enter the portal circulation and are delivered to the liver. Various cytokines, including interleukines 1 and 6 (IL1, IL6), transforming growth factor β1 (TGFβ1), and tumor necrosis factor alpha (TNF-α) are released [28,29]. TNF-α and IL1 have cytotoxic effects against hepatocytes, leading to necrosis. TGFβ1, when liberated, activates hepatic fibrogenesis. The level of TNF-α in the serum correlates inversively and significantly with survival rate [30]. IL6 activates hepatic stellate cells and correlates with the severity of ASH. There is also some evidence that polymorphism of the TNF-α promoter gene and of interleukine 10 may modify the development of ASH [31].

ASH is histomorphologically defined. The histology appearance is indistinguishable from that of nonalcoholic steatohepatitis (NASH). Predominant are hepatocellular degeneration associated with infiltration of neutrophilic granulocytes, ballooning of the hepatocytes, Mallory body formation, and perivenular fibrosis, to name only a few of the most prominant features (Fig. 3) [32].

Effect of age on ethanol metabolism and distribution

In animal experiments, a decrease in ethanol elimination and a decrease in alcohol dehydrogenase (ADH) activity has been shown with age in male but not in female rats [33,34]. The reduction of ethanol elimination in F344 rats is due to an increased body weight to liver weight ratio, a reduced hepatic ADH activity, and a reduced availability of nicotine adenine dinucleotide, a cofactor for ADH [34,35]. Obviously there is a mitochondrial transport defect with age [35]. In addition, age decreases the function of the smooth endoplasmic reticulum, the metabolism of CYP2E1-dependent microsomal ethanol oxidation, and of drug metabolism [36,37]. Studies performed in various animals depend on species, strain, and gender, and may therefore not be conclusive for human beings. However, it is noteworthy that microsomal function, including microsomal CYP2E1-dependent ethanol oxidation, is significantly reduced with age, and that also mitochondrial function including acetaldehyde dehydrogenase activity,

AFL   ASH

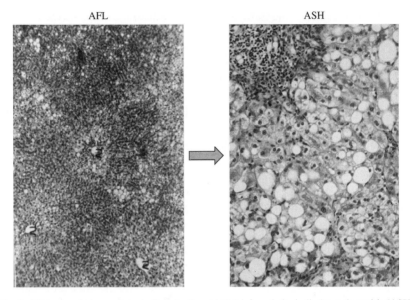

Fig. 3. Histomorphology of alcoholic fatty liver (AFL) left and alcoholic Steatohepatitis (ASH) right. Note that fat deposition is particularly pronounced around the central vein. ASH is characterized by the infiltration of granulocytes, ballooning of hepatocytes, fibrosis, and Mallory bodies.

which is localized intramitochondrial, is also diminished with age [34]. This may lead to increased acetaldehyde levels in the liver with age, and may also explain the enhanced fat accumulation in the elderly following ethanol ingestion, caused by a decrease in mitochondrial fatty acid oxidation (Fig. 4).

In human beings, liver anatomy and physiology changes with age. Liver size is reduced, reflected by a reduction of the number of hepatocytes [38]. In addition, blood flow to the liver also decreases with age [39]. Both factors have an effect on ethanol elimination. Age also affects activity of alcohol metabolizing enzymes. Thus, sigma-ADH, an enzyme which is expressed predominantly in the gastric mucosa and which is predominantly responsible for the gastric first pass metabolism (FPM) of ethanol, is affected by age [40,41]. Younger women already exhibit a lower sigma ADH activity when compared with younger men. However, the higher ADH activity of men decreases when compared with that of women after the age of 60 [40,41]. In this context it is interesting to note that ADH activity in chronic atrophic gastritis is extremely low [40], and that gastric atrophy is a disease which occurs almost exclusively with advanced age. Although it was speculated that the gastric FPM of ethanol is reduced in atrophic gastritis, this could not be demonstrated, most likely because atrophic gastritis delays gastric emptying with a longer exposure of alcohol to the gastric mucosa, which could therefore overcompensate despite the loss of ADH [42]. Thus, the contribution of changes in gastric FPM with age on ethanol uptake and ethanol

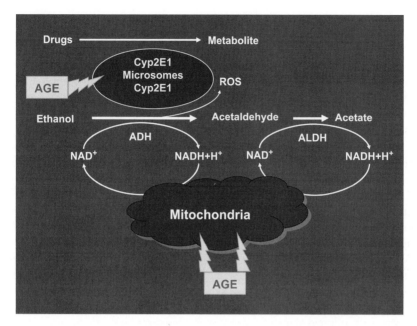

Fig. 4. Aging and ethanol metabolism. Age decreases microsomal and mitochondrial function. Because drugs and ethanol both are metabolized by microsomal cytochrome P-450, an interaction between these compounds may occur more easily with advanced age, resulting in enhanced toxicity. Since mitochondria are important for the reoxidation of NADH, age slows down ADH related ethanol metabolism and decreases fatty acid oxidation, resulting in fatty liver.

blood concentrations is still not completely clear. However, it is unquestionable that age results in elevated blood ethanol concentrations [43,44]. When alcohol is applied to fathers and sons or mothers and daughters in the same dose calculated as gram per kilgoram of body weight, significantly increased blood ethanol concentrations were noted in the parents [44]. This result is primarily explained by the reduced water distribution volume with age, resulting in elevated blood alcohol levels [43,44].

Clinical presentation of alcoholic liver disease in the elderly

The spectrum of presenting symptoms and signs of ALD among elderly patients is very similar to that seen in patients of all ages. A British study has reported that the nonspecific symptoms of general malaise and anorexia are more commonly seen in the elderly [45] than in other age groups. The overall frequency of cirrhosis in those over 60 years old in this study was 79%. In the United States it has been suggested that the peak incidence of presentation of alcoholic cirrhosis is in the seventh decade among white men, and that the proportion of cirrhotics within ALD increases steadily with age [46]. In France, it was found that 22% of the 637 alcoholic cirrhotics studied were over 70 years of age [47]. These data underline the fact that older patients present with more advanced histological disease than younger ones.

ASH is frequently observed in liver biopsies, from alcohol consumers, that are asymptomatic. Seventeen percent of all the biopsies of patients who enter hospital for detoxification also reveal ASH. In addition, 40% of patients with alcoholic cirrhosis of the liver have ASH at the same time. The acute mortality of ASH is between 15% to 25% [48–51].

ASH shows a wide variability of subjective and objective symptoms. Intensity and frequency of these symptoms may divide ASH into mild and severe. A substantial percentage of patients with ASH have an excessive level of liver necrosis with the clinical feature of coma and hepatic encephalopathy. There is no correlation between the severity of the clinical manifestation and the severity of the histology, although presence of ASH cannot be excluded because of an asymptomatic patient. Symptoms include anicteric hepatomegaly, severe jaundice, nausea and vomiting, abdominal pain, and hepatic encephalopathy [48–51]. Frequently, patients with ASH present fever and leucocytosis caused by endotoxemia. Feminization, such as gynecomastia and female body hair type, present in approximately one third of those with ASH without cirrhosis. Because ASH is frequently associated with cirrhosis of the liver, clinical signs of a decompensated liver cirrhosis may occur.

In the laboratory, an increase in gamma glutamyltransferase (GGT) activity and glutamate dehydrogenase (GDH) is seen in all patients with ASH [48–52]. The increased in GGT is an expression of microsomal enzyme induction. The increase in GDH is a sign of mitochondrial damage. The absolute values of transaminase activities do not exceed 300 units per liter. Characteristic is a more pronounced increase in the activity of aspartate aminotransferase (AST) compared with alanine aminotransferase (ALT). An AST/ALT ratio of more than two is the key diagnostic feature for ALD [48–52]. AST is partly of extra hepatic origin, whereas the rather low activity of ALT is primarily caused by a deficiency in vitamin B_6. In addition, an increase in the activity of alkaline phosphatase is noted. The level of serum bilirubin correlates relatively well with the morphological signs of ASH. The concentration of serum proteins are decreased in relation to the severity of the disturbances of liver function. In severe diseases, an increase in beta and gamma globulines is frequently observed. The increase in immunglobulin-A concentrations is especially pronounced. Typical hematological features are macrocytic anemia, low platelets, and leucocytosis with toxic granulations [48–52]. Special laboratory markers may exclude or verify alcohol abuse, such as blood alcohol levels, GGT-activity, mean corpuscular volume, and carbohydrate deficient transferring [52,53].

Natural course and prognostic parameters of alcoholic liver disease

The natural course of ALD is illustrated in Fig. 1. The process of AFL development and fibrogenesis may be accelerated with age, because the aged liver has a lower capacity to handle ethanol and metabolize fat and, therefore, a higher tendency for fat accumulation. Prognosis of ALD depends on the severity at diagnosis. Alcohol abstinence improves ALD at all stages [54]. In patients with severe ASH or cirrhosis a variety of prognostic criteria exists: jaundice, ascites, edema, portal hypertension or esophageal varicel bleeding, as well as hepatic encephalopathy, increase mortality significantly [19,55,56]. Laboratory values with increased mortality include increased bilirubin, decreased serum albumin and prothrombin time, impaired kidney function, as well as anemia and leucocytosis. One-month mortality rate correlates significantly with the extent of protein-calorie malnutrition [57]. Some signs of malnutrition may be present in certain elderly populations.

Histology with poor prognosis includes pervenular fibrosis, cholestasis, the presence of Mallory bodies, and giant mitochondria [19,58]. Fifty percent of patients with ASH who continue to drink develop liver cirrhosis after 10 years. The highest mortality rate for patients with ASH is within one year following diagnosis, regardless of whether cirrhosis is present or not. The most important factors with poor prognosis are severe disease at initial biopsy (Orrego index), continuous alcohol abuse, female gender, presence of cirrhosis, cholestasis, and severe malnutrition [56–59]. The 4-year survival rates in ALD are as follows: AFL 70%, ASH 58%, Cirrhosis 49%, and Cirrhosis with ASH: 35% [56].

For ASH, various severity indices exist:

Discriminate function, according to Maddrey. A value of 32 or more reflects a 1-month mortality of 50% [60].

Combined clinical and laboratory index, according to Orrego and colleagues [59]. This index correlates well with 1-year survival and therefore has prognostic importance.

Mayo Clinic end stage liver disease score, which includes kidney function [61]. A value of 21 or more predicts a 3-month mortality of 20%.

Glasgow score for alcoholic hepatitis [62], which considers age as a significant prognostic factor.

Because individuals with advanced age often also have other diseases and are less resistant to noxae, patients over 60 years of age who have ALD have more severe symptoms and a higher frequency of complications, such as portal hypertension [18]. Prognosis is directly related to age as demonstrated in the Glasgow score for alcoholic hepatitis [62], which characterizes severity and predicts outcome. In a British study, mortality of cirrhosis was 5% at 1 year and 24% at 3 years in patients under 60, compared with 34% and 54%, respectively, in patients over 60 years. Cirrhotics over 70 years had a 75% mortality rate at 1 year. Among the oldest patients, more than half developed hepatocellular carcinoma (HCC) [63]. Indeed, HCC is the number one cause of death in cirrhotics because improvement of treatment, including orthoptic liver transplantation, decreased the other complications, such as hepatorenal syndrome or esophageal varicel bleeding, as causes of death.

Interaction between alcohol and drugs and their importance with respect to liver disease in the elderly

Morbidity increases with age and so does the use of a variety of drugs. Because ethanol and drugs are metabolized through microsomal cytochrome P-45o dependent monooxygenases, it is not surprising that interactions do occur. This is especially relevant for drugs that are predominantly metabolized by CYP2E1. Thus, the liver is the major site for drug and ethanol metabolism and their interactions. Fortunately, it is only the target for the toxic effects of a minority of drugs, such as acetaminophen, phenytoin, and methotrexate [19,64–66]. Chronic ethanol consumption increases hepatic CYP2E1, which leads to an enhanced metabolism of acetaminophen, resulting in the generation of intermediates with hepatotoxic properties. Because ethanol also reduces the hepatic antioxidative defense system, such as glutathione [21], this intermediate can bind to hepatocytes and may initiate severe hepatic damage. Thus, even small doses of acetaminophen (up to 3 g), which may be otherwise harmless, could result in severe hepatic injury, leading to hepatic coma and death in the alcohol consume.

In addition, vitamin use is rather frequent in the elderly, and thus the intake of β-carotene or vitamin A. CYP2E1 also metabolizes retinol and retinoic acid to polar metabolites with apoptotic properties [67,68]. In addition, ethanol activates stellate cells to myofibroblasts with the potency for fibrogenesis [19]. These stellate cells are loaded with vitamin A. Therefore, the combination of chronic alcohol consumption and the intake of β-carotene or vitamin A could lead to hepatic injury and fibrosis [69].

Another drug which is more frequently used with advanced age because of rheumatological disorders, and which interferes with alcohol, is methotrexate. Chronic alcohol consumption, even at a lower dosage, enhances the fibrogenic effect of metothrexat [70]. Therefore, alcohol intake during methotrexat treatment should be avoided. Effects of age and alcohol on hepatic drug metabolism are listed in Table 1.

Alcohol as a cofactor in liver disease of other origin

With advancing age, more than one type of liver disease may occur in one liver. Therefore, chronic alcohol consumption may deteriorate chronic liver disease caused by hepatitis B (HBV) and hepatitis C virus (HCV) infections, as well as lead to NAFLD and hemochromatosis.

HCV infection is common among heavy drinkers. Whether this is caused by a suppressed immune system or a high-risk life style is still not clear.

Table 1
Effect of age and ethanol on drug metabolism

Age effect	Acute ethanol effects	Chronic ethanol effects
Frequently reduced drug oxidation	Inhibition of drug oxidation	Adaptive increase in drug oxidation
Minimal change in glucuronidation of drugs	Slight reduction in glucuronidation of drugs	Possible slight inhibition of conjugation
Reduced distribution volume for water soluble substances, such as ethanol	Elevated serum drug concentrations	Decreased serum drug concentrations. For certain drugs increased concentration of toxic metabolites.

Long-term studies have shown that an increased amount of alcohol also enhances hepatic fibrosis in HCV infection [71,72]. The relative risk for fibrosis with more than 50 g of alcohol per day was calculated as 2.4 [71]. Studies from Europe and the United States have shown that more than 30 g to 50 g of alcohol, per day resulted in an increased fibrosis, cirrhosis, and HCC [72–76]. Most recently, a Swedish study reported data from 78 subjects who had two liver biopsies 6.3 years apart, with less than 40 g of alcohol per day. The authors found more progressive fibrosis with higher alcohol consumption (5.7 g versus 2.6 g per day, $P = .032$), with higher drinking frequency (35 days versus 8 days per year, $P = .006$) and with a higher quantity per occasion (four versus three drinks, which was statistically not significantly different) [76]. These data seem to be especially relevant with respect to age because these alcohol doses are frequently consumed in the elderly. With respect to the development of HCC in HCV infection, the relative risk is 26 if 10 g to 40 g are consumed per day, 63 when 40 g to 80 g are consumed per day, and 126 when more than 80 g are consumed per day [77]. In general, it should be noted that women already had a more severe reaction with lower alcohol dosage.

Data on the interaction between HBV and alcohol are limited. However, a detailed study from Japan showed an earlier occurrence of HCC in patients with HBV who consumed alcohol. In this study, the average occurrence of HCC was at age of 62 years. When less than 25 g of alcohol was consumed daily, the age dropped to 49 years. With 25 g to 75 g per day, age at first diagnosis of HCC was 43 years, and with 75 g to 125 g it was 50 years. Thus, alcohol seems to accelerate carcinogenesis with HBV [78].

Another liver disease with high prevalence in the elderly is NAFLD caused by obesity, metabolic syndrome, and diabetes. The mechanism behind this disease is primarily peripheral insulin resistance with hyperinsulinemia [79]. Although this liver disease can occur at younger age and even in children, the predominant age group is people above 65 years of age. Although there are no evidenced-based data available concerning the effect of ethanol on NAFLD in human beings, indirect data support the theory of an additive damaging effect on the liver [21,80,81]. Fat accumulation is

enhanced by alcohol and more than 95% of overweight (body mass index—
or BMI—greater than 25 kg/m^2) and alcohol consuming (more than 60 g per
day) individuals reveal fatty liver, as compared with 76% of overweight
alone or 46% of drinkers alone [80]. In addition, the major mechanisms
by which NAFLD turns to NASH, namely the involvement of TNF-α
and CYP2E1, are also enhanced by chronic alcohol consumption [21].
A multivariate analysis from a national database on approximately 20,000
patients undergoing liver transplantation showed an increased risk for cry-
progenic cirrhosis (NASH-associated, $P = .02$) and for alcoholic cirrhosis
($P = .002$) in obese (BMI greater than 30 kg/m^2) compared with lean
(BMI less than 25 kg/m^2) individuals [81].

Finally, the risk for HCC in noninsulin dependent diabetes is approximately 4, which increases to almost 10 when alcohol is consumed [82]. All
these data clearly show that alcohol is an important cofactor in other liver
diseases, which results in an acceleration and deterioration of the chronic
liver disease most relevant in the elderly.

Treatment of alcoholic liver disease

Abstinence is the best treatment of ALD regardless of the state and
severity of the disease. While most patients with mild or moderate ASH
respond to abstinence, patients with severe ASH need special attendance.
Patients with a Maddrey index of 32 or more have a poor prognosis, they
must be treated in intensive care units. Hyperalimentation and substitution
with vitamins and minerals are mandatory. In addition, steroids may be
beneficial in a subset of patients. Side effects of steroids are infections and
sepsis. Thus, if steroid therapy (30 mg/d) does not decrease serum
bilirubin within one week, treatment should be stopped. Pentoxyphillin,
a drug which inhibits TNF-α, with almost no side effects, can also be
administered. Finally, TNF antibodies have been tried, but the results
were contradictory. TNF-α antibodies in the elderly seem to be associated
with high risk, because a strong immunsupprossion with advanced age is
risky (for treatment see [48–51,83]).

Summary

Alcoholic liver disease is common in the Western world and its
prevalence increases in elderly individuals because of an increase in alcohol
consumption with age in certain countries. In addition, even moderate
amounts of alcohol may injure the liver in the presence of liver diseases
caused by viruses and metabolic disturbances. The prevalence of obesity
and metabolic syndrome increases in the United States especially, which is
strongly associated with nonalcoholic fatty liver disease, a situation highly
susceptible toward the toxic effect of alcohol. Furthermore, multiple drug

use is frequent in the elderly because of an increased morbidity. Chronic alcohol consumption, even in moderate dosage, may interact with certain drugs and may increase hepatotoxicity of some drugs, such as acetaminophen, phenytoin, and methotrexate. Alcohol is handled differently with age, resulting in a decreased hepatic metabolism caused by a decrease in ethanol metabolizing enzyme activities and a decrease in microsomal and mitochondrial function. This may increase the sensitivity of the liver, leading to more pronounced hepatic fat accumulation and to an enhanced fibrogenesis. In addition, blood ethanol concentrations are higher in the elderly because of a decrease in the water distribution space with age. Although the clinical presentation of alcoholic liver disease with age does not differ from that in younger individuals, prognosis and outcome are significantly worse. Thus, with respect to the liver, regular alcohol consumption is not recommended in the elderly.

Acknowledgments

The authors wish to thank Ms. Marion Schätzle for writing the manuscript.

References

[1] Schoenborn CA, Cohen BH. Trends in smoking, alcohol consumption, and other health practices among US adults 1977–1983. Ulm, Stuttgart, Jena, Lübeck: Fisher Verlag; p. 173–7.

[2] Goodwin JS, Sanchez CJ, Thomas P, et al. Alcohol intake in a healthy elderly population. Am J Public Health 1987;77:173.

[3] Bercsi SJ, Brickner PW, Saha DC. Alcohol use and abuse in the frail, homebound elderly: a clinical analysis of 103 persons. Drug Alcohol depend 1993;33:139–49.

[4] Sulsky SI, Jaques PE, Otradovec CL, et al. Descriptors of alcohol consumption among healthy elderly. J Am Coll Nutr 1990;9(4):326–31.

[5] Livingston G, King M. Alcohol abuse in an inner elderly population: the Gospel Oak survey. Int J Geriatr Psychiatry 1993;8:511–4.

[6] Council on Scientific Affairs, American Medical Association. Alcoholism in the elderly. JAMA 1996;275:797–801.

[7] John W, Culberson MD. Alcohol use in the elderly: beyond the CAGE. Geriatrics 2006; 61(10):23–7.

[8] Mirand AL, Welte JW. Alcohol consumption among the elderly in a general population, Erie Country, New York. Am J Public Health 1996;86:978–84.

[9] Mundle G, Wormstall K, Mann K. Die Alkoholabhängigkeit im Alter [Alcohol dependence and age] [German]. Sucht (Addiction) 1997;43:201–6.

[10] Substance abuse and mental health services administration (office of applied studies). Results from the 2001 National household survey on drug abuse: vol. 1. Summary of National findings. (NHSDA Series H-17, DHHS Publication No. SMA 02-3758) Rockville (MD): Department of Health and Human Services, 2002.

[11] Moore AA, Hays RD, Greendale GA, et al. Drinking habits among older persons: findings from the NHANES I epidemiologic followup study (1982–84), National health and nutrition examination survey. J Am Geriatr Soc 1999;47(4):412–6.

918   SEITZ & STICKEL

[12] Booth BM, Blow FC, Cook CA, et al. Age and ethnicity among hospitalized alcoholics: a nationwide study. Alcohol Clin Exp Res 1992;16(6):1029–34.
[13] Geller G, Levine DM, Mamon JA, et al. Knowledge, attitudes, and reported practices of medical students and house staff regarding the diagnosis and treatment of alcoholism. JAMA 1989;126(21):3115–20.
[14] Iber FL. The elderly alcoholic: experience with Baltimore veterans and private alcoholism patients over age 60. In: Hutchinson ML, Munro HN, editors. Nutrition and aging. Orlando (FL): Academic Press; 1986. p. 169–78.
[15] Barnes GM. Alcohol use among older persons: findings from a western New York State general population survey. J Am Geriatr Soc 1979;27:244–54.
[16] Ledermann S. Alcool, Alcoolisme, Alcoolisation. Donnés scientifiques de caractère physiologique, économique et sociale [Alcohol, Alcoholism, Alcoholization. Psysiological, economic and social scientific data] [French]. Paris: Institute National d'Etudes Démographiques Travaux et Documents, Presses Universitaires de France; 1956;26. p. 124–8.
[17] Corrao G, Ferran P, Zambon A, et al. Trends in liver cirrhosis mortality in Europe, 1970–1989. Int J Epidemiol 1997;26:100–9.
[18] James OFW. Parenchymal liver disease in the elderly. Gut 1997;41:430–2.
[19] Lieber CS. Alcohol and the liver: 1994 update. Gastroenterology 1994;106:1085–105.
[20] Becker U, Dies A, Sorensen TI. Prediction of risk of liver disease by alcohol intake, sex, and age: prospective population study. Hepatology 1996;23:1025–9.
[21] Seitz HK, Stickel F. Risk factors and mechanism of hepatocarcinogenesis with special emphasis on alcohol and oxidative stress. Biol Chem 2006;387:349–60.
[22] Albano E. Free radicals and alcohol-induced liver injury. In: Ethanol and the liver. Sherman CDIN, Preedy VR, Watson RR, editors. London: Taylor and Francis. p. 153–90.
[23] Dupont I, Lucas D, Clot P, et al. Cytochrome P4502E1 inducibility and hydroxyethyl radical formation among alcoholics. J Hepatol 1998;28:564–71.
[24] Clot P, Bellomo G, Tabone M, et al. Detection of antibodies against proteins modified by hydroxyethyl free radicals in patients with alcoholic cirrhosis. Gastroenterology 1995;108: 210–7.
[25] Clot P, Albano E, Elliasson E, et al. Cytochrome P4502E1 hydroxyethyl radical adducts as the major antigenic determinant for autoantibody formation among alcoholics. Gastroenterology 1996;111:206–16.
[26] Gouillon Z, Lucas D, Li J, et al. Inhibition of ethanol-induced liver disease in the intragastric feeding rat model by chlormethiazole. Proc Soc Biol Med 2000;224:302–8.
[27] Thurman RG. Alcoholic liver injury involves activation of Kupffer cells by endotoxins. Am J Physiol 1998;275:G605–11.
[28] McClain C, Barve S, Joshi-Barve S, et al. Dyregulated cytokine metabolism, altered hepatic methionine metabolism and proteasome dysfunction in alcoholic liver disease. Alcohol Clin Exp Res 2005;29(11 Suppl):180S–8S.
[29] Urbaschek R, McCuskey RS, Rudi V, et al. Endotoxin, endotoxin-neutralizing-capacity, sCD14, sICAM-1, and cytokines in patients with various degrees of alcoholic liver disease. Alcohol Clin Exp Res 2001;25:261–8.
[30] Felver ME, Mezey E, McGuire M, et al. Plasma tumor nekrosis factor alpha predicts decreased long-term survival in severe alcoholic hepatitis. Alcohol Clin Exp Res 1990;14: 255–9.
[31] Stickel F, Österreicher CH. Genetic polymorphisms in alcoholic liver disease. Alcohol Alcohol 2006;41(3):209–24.
[32] Hall PM. Alcoholic liver disease. In: MacSween RNM, Alastair DB, Portman BC, et al, editors. Pathology of the liver. 4th edition. London: Churchill Livingstone; 2002. p. 273–312.
[33] Beresford TP, Lucey MR. Ethanol metabolism and intoxication in the elderly. In: Beresford TP, Ganberg E, editors. Alcohol and aging. New York: Oxford University Press; 1995. p. 117–27.

[34] Seitz HK, Meydani M, Ferschke I, et al. Effect of aging on in vivo and in vitro ethanol metabolism and its toxicity in F344 rats. Gastroenterology 1989;97:446–56.

[35] Seitz HK, Yu Y, Simanowski UA, et al. Effect of age and gender on in vivo ethanol elimination, hepatic alcohol dehydrogenase activity, and NAD+ availability in F344 rats. Res Exp Med 1992;192:205–12.

[36] Schmucker DL, Wang RK. Age-related changes in liver drug-metabolizing enzymes. Exp Gerontol 1980;15:423–31.

[37] Schmucker DL. Age-related changes in drug disposition. Pharmacol Rev 1979;30: 455–6.

[38] Thompson EN, Williams R. Effect of age on liver function with particular reference to bromsulphalein excretion. Gut 1965;6:266–9.

[39] Vestal RE, Wood AJJ, Branch RA, et al. Effects of age and cigarette smoking on propanolol disposition. Clin Pharmacol Ther 1979;26:8–15.

[40] Seitz HK, Egerer G, Simanowski UA, et al. Human gastric alcohol dehydrogenase activity: effect of age, gender and alcoholism. Gut 1993;34:1433–7.

[41] Seitz HK, Egerer G, Simanowski UA. High blood alcohol levels in women. N Engl J Med 1990;323:58–62.

[42] Pedrosa MC, Russel RM, Saltzman JS, et al. Gastric emptying and first pass metabolism of ethanol in elderly subjects with and without atrophic gastritis. Scand J Gastroenterol 1996; 31:671–7.

[43] Vestal RE, McGuire EA, Tobin JT, et al. Aging and ethanol metabolism. Clin Pharmacol Ther 1977;21:343–54.

[44] Gärtner U, Schmier M, Bogusz M, et al. Blutalkoholkonzentrationen nach oraler Alkoholgabe – Einfluß von Alter und Geschlecht [Blood alcohol concentrations after oral alcohol administration-effect of sex and age] [German]. Z Gastroenterol 1996;34: 675–9.

[45] Woodhouse KW, James OFW. Alcoholic liver disease in the elderly: presentation and outcome. Age Aging 1985;24:113–8.

[46] Garagliano CF, Lilienfeld AM, Mendeloff AI. Incidence rates of liver cirrhosis and related diseases in Baltimore and selected areas of the United States. J Chron Dis 1979; 32:543–54.

[47] Aron E, Duin M, Jobard P. Les cirrhoses du troisième âge [Cirrhosis and old age] [French]. Ann Gastoenterol Hepatol 1979;15:558–63.

[48] Maher JJ. Alcoholic liver disease. In: Feldman M, Friedman LS, Sleisenger MH, editors. Gastrointestinal and liver disease. 7th edition. St. Loius: Saunders; 2002. p. 1375–87.

[49] Bode JC. Klinik und Therapie alkoholischer Leberschäden [Clinics and therapy of alcoholic liver damage]. In: Seitz, Lieber, Simanowski, editors. Handbuch Alkohol, Alkoholismus, alkoholbedingte Organschäden, 2. [Manual Alcohol, Alcoholism, Alcohol-Associated Organ Damage.] Heidelberg: Johann Ambrosius Barth Verlag; 2000. p. 275–98.

[50] Agarwal K, Kontorinis N, Dieterich D. Alcoholic hepatitis. Curr Treat Options Gastroenterol 2004;7:451–8.

[51] Levitsky J, Mailliard ME. Diagnosis and therapy of alcoholic liver disease. Sem Liver Dis 2004;24:233–47.

[52] Helander A. Biological markers in alcoholism. J Neural Transm Suppl 2003;66:15–32.

[53] Thabut D, Naveau S, Charlotte F, et al. The diagnostic value of biomarkers (AshTest) for the prediction of alcoholic steatohepatitis in patients with chronic alcoholic liver disease. J Hepatol 2006;44:1175–85.

[54] Schenker S. Alcoholic liver disease: evaluation of natural history and prognostic factors. Hepatology 1984;4:36–43.

[55] Teli MR, Day CP, Burt AD, et al. Determinants of progression to cirrhosis or fibrosis in pure alcoholic fatty liver. Lancet 1995;346:987–90.

[56] Chedid A, Mendenhall CL, Gartside P, et al. Prognostic factors in alcoholic liver disease. Am J Gastroenterol 1991;86:210–6.

[57] Mendenhall C, Roselle GA, Gartside P, et al. Relationship of proteins caloric malnutrition to alcoholic liver disease: a re-examination of data from two Veterans Administration Cooperative Studies. Alcohol Clin Exp Res 1995;19(3):635–41.

[58] Nissenbaum M, Chedid A, Mendenhall C, et al. Prognostic significance of cholestatic alcoholic hepatitis. Dig Dis Sci 1990;35:891–6.

[59] Orrego H, Israel Y, Blake YE, et al. Assessment of prognostic factors in alcoholic liver disease: towards a global quantitative expression of severity. Hepatology 1983;3:896–905.

[60] Maddrey WC, Boitnott JK, Bediene MS. Corticosteroid therapy of alcoholic hepatitis. Gastroenterology 1978;75:193–200.

[61] Dunn W, Jamil LH, Brown LS, et al. MELD accurately predicts mortality in patients with alcoholic hepatitis. Hepatology 2005;41:353–8.

[62] Forrest EH, Evans CDJ, Stewart S, et al. Analysis of factors predictive of mortality in alcoholic hepatitis and derivation and validation of the Glasgow alcoholic hepatitis score. Gut 2005;54:1174–9.

[63] Potter JR, James OFW. Clinical features and prognosis of alcoholic liver disease in respect of advancing age. Gerontology 1987;33:380–7.

[64] Seitz HK, Homann N. Effects of alcohol on the oro-gastrointestinal tract, the pancreas, and the liver. In: Heather N, Peters TG, Stockwell T, editors. International handbook of alcohol dependence and problems. West Sussex, UK: John Wiley & sons Ltd; 2001. p. 149–68.

[65] Slattery JT, Nelson SD, Thummel KE. The complex interaction between ethanol and acetaminophen. Clin Pharmacol Ther 1996;60:241–6.

[66] Collins C, Starmer GA. A review of the hepatotoxicity of paracetamol at therapeutic or near-therapeutic dose levels, with particular reference to alcohol abusers. Drug Alcohol Rev 1995;14:63–79.

[67] Liu C, Rassel RM, Seitz HK, et al. Ethanol enhances retinoic acid metabolism into polar metabolites in rat liver via induction of cytochrome P4502E1. Gastroenterology 2001;120: 179–89.

[68] Dan Z, Popov Y, Patsenker E, et al. Alcohol-induced polar retinol metabolites trigger hepatocyte apoptosis via loss of mitochondrial membrane potential. FASEB J 2005;19:1–4.

[69] Ahmed S, Leo MA, Lieber CS. Interactions between alcohol and beta-carotene in patients with alcoholic liver disease. Am J Clin Nutr 1994;60(3):430–6.

[70] Lock G, Schölmerich J. Arzneimittelnebenwirkungen an der Leber [Side effects of drugs on the liver.] [German]. Arzneimitteltherapie 2000;18:275–80.

[71] Polynard T, Bedossa P, Opolon P. Natural history of liver fibrosis progression in patients with chronic hepatitis C. Lancet 1997;349:825–32.

[72] Wiley TE, McCarthy M, Breidi L, et al. Impact of alcohol on the histological and clinical progression of hepatitis C infection. Hepatology 1998;28:805–9.

[73] Corrao G, Aricò S. Independent and combined action of hepatitis C virus infection and alcohol consumption on the risk of symptomatic liver cirrhosis. Hepatology 1998;27:914–9.

[74] Bellentani S, Pozzato G, Saccoccio G, et al. Clinical course and risk factors of hepatitis C virus related liver disease in the general population: report from the Dionysos study. Gut 1999;44:874–80.

[75] Kim WR, Gross JB, Poterucha JJ Jr, et al. Outcome of hospital care of liver disease associated with hepatitis C in the United States. Hepatology 2001;33:201–6.

[76] Westin J, Lagging LM, Spak F, et al. Moderate alcohol intake increases fibrosis progression in untreated patients with hepatitis C virus infection. J Viral Hepat 2002;9:235–41.

[77] Tragger A, Donato F, Ribero ML, et al. Case control study on hepatitis C virus (HCV) as a risk factor for hepatocellular carcinoma: the role of HCV genotypes and the synergism with hepatitis B virus and alcohol. Brescia HCC study. Int J Cancer 1999;81:695–9.

[78] Onishi K. Alcohol and hepatocellular cancer. In: Watson RR, editor. Alcohol and Cancer. Boca Raton (FL): CRC Press; 1992. p. 179–202.

[79] Falck-Ytter Y, Jounossi ZM, Marchesini G, et al. Clinical features and natural history of non-alcoholic steatosis syndroms. Semin Liver Dis 2001;21:17–26.

[80] Bellentani S, Tiribelli C. The spectrum of liver disease in the general population: lesson from the Dionysos study. J Hepatol 2001;35:531–7.
[81] Nair S, Macon A, Eason J, et al. Is obesity an independent risk factor for hepatocellular carcinoma in cirrhosis? Hepatology 2002;36:150–5.
[82] Hassan MH, Hwang LY, Hatten CJ, et al. Risk factors for hepatocellular carcinoma: synergism of alcohol with viral hepatitis and diabetes mellitus. Hepatology 2002;36:1206–13.
[83] Stickel F, Hoehn B, Schuppan D, et al. Review article: nutritional therapy in alcoholic liver disease. Aliment Pharmacol Ther 2003;18:357–73.

ELSEVIER
SAUNDERS

Clin Geriatr Med 23 (2007) 923–926

CLINICS IN
GERIATRIC
MEDICINE

Index

Note: Page numbers of article titles are in **boldface** type.

Gastrointestinal bleeding, causes of,
  770–771
  clinical course of, 771–773
  clinical presentation of, 771–773
  economic impact of, 770
  evaluation and management of, 769
  history taking in, 774–775
  in older adults, **769–784**
  incidence of, 769
  medical therapy in, 776–777
  mortality for, 770
  nonulcer acute, 777–778
  physical examination in, 775–776
  radionuclide scintigraphy in, 778–781
  upper, 773–774

Gastrointestinal motility, in aging, 760

Gastrointestinal peptides, 762

Gastrointestinal symptoms, chronic, in
  elderly, **721–734**

Gastroparesis, diabetic, management of,
  798

Ghrelin, effect of healthy aging on, 747

Glucagon-like peptide-1, satiating effects of,
  746

Glucose intolerance, age-related, factors
  contributing to, 793

Glutaraldehyde, in fecal incontinence, 864

Gut, aging, 743–744
  physiology of, **737–767**

H

Heartburn, and reflux symptoms, 722–724

Hepatitis, and aging liver, **889–903**
  autoimmune, 895–897
  drug-induced, 897–899
  viral, 891–895

Hepatitis A, 891

Hepatitis B, 892–893

Hepatitis C, 893–895

HMG-CoA reductase inhibitors, hepatitis
  induced by, 898–899

Homeostasis, age-related impairment of,
  741–742

Hormones, age-related changes in, 744–749
  peripheral, effects of aging on, 745–748

Hyperglycemia, impaired cognition caused
  by, 794

Hypocretins, and anorexia of aging, 745

Hypotension, postprandial, 758–759

I

Immunoglobulin, intravenous, and vaccine,
  in *Clostridium difficile* infection and
  colitis, 842

Inflammatory bowel diseases, 848
  clinical manifestations of, 810
  colorectal cancer and, 816–817
  differential diagnosis of, 810–811
  epidemiology of, 809
  in elderly, **809–821**
  treatment options in, 811–815

Infliximab, in inflammatory bowel disease,
  815

Insulin, age-associated increases in, 748

Intestinal absorption, with aging, changes
  in, 760–763

Intestinal microflora, 761

Intestines, carcinoid tumor of, diarrhea in,
  849

Irritable bowel syndrome, and constipation,
  in elderly, **823–832**
  clinical features of, 731–732
  definition of, 730
  diagnosis of, 829
  epidemiology of, 730–731

L

Leptin, effects of aging and, 746–747

Liver, aging, and hepatitis, **889–903**
  disease of, in elderly, interaction
    between alcohol and drugs and,
    914
  of nonalcoholic origin, alcohol as
    cofactor in, 914–916
  function of, age-related changes in,
    889–891
  pancreas, and gallbladder, in aging,
    762–763

"Low body weight", in older people, 737

Lubiprostone, 827

M

6-Mercaptopurine, in inflammatory bowel
  disease, 812–813

Mesenteric ischemia, acute, in arterial
  embolism, 871–872
  in arterial thrombosis, 872, 883
  multiple organ dysfunction
    syndromes in, 884
  chronic, diagnosis of, 874–881
  surgical revascularization in, 885
  treatment of, 882–885

United States Postal Service

Statement of Ownership, Management, and Circulation
(All Periodicals Publications Except Requestor Publications)

1. Publication Title
Clinics in Geriatric Medicine

2. Publication Number
0 0 0 - 7 0 4

3. Filing Date
9/14/07

4. Issue Frequency
Feb, May, Aug, Nov

5. Number of Issues Published Annually
4

6. Annual Subscription Price
$178.00

7. Complete Mailing Address of Known Office of Publication (Not printer) (Street, city, county, state, and ZIP+4)

Elsevier Inc.
360 Park Avenue South
New York, NY 10010-1710

Contact Person
Stephen Bushing

Telephone (Include area code)
215-239-3688

8. Complete Mailing Address of Headquarters or General Business Office of Publisher (Not printer)

Elsevier Inc., 360 Park Avenue South, New York, NY 10010-1710

9. Full Names and Complete Mailing Addresses of Publisher, Editor, and Managing Editor (Do not leave blank)

Publisher (Name and complete mailing address)
John Schrefer, Elsevier, Inc., 1600 John F. Kennedy Blvd. Suite 1800, Philadelphia, PA 19103-2899

Editor (Name and complete mailing address)
Lisa Richman, Elsevier, Inc., 1600 John F. Kennedy Blvd. Suite 1800, Philadelphia, PA 19103-2899

Managing Editor (Name and complete mailing address)
Catherine Bewick, Elsevier, Inc., 1600 John F. Kennedy Blvd. Suite 1800, Philadelphia, PA 19103-2899

10. Owner (Do not leave blank. If the publication is owned by a corporation, give the name and address of the corporation immediately followed by the names and addresses of all stockholders owning or holding 1 percent or more of the total amount of stock. If not owned by a corporation, give the names and addresses of the individual owners. If owned by a partnership or other unincorporated firm, give its name and address as well as those of each individual owner. If the publication is published by a nonprofit organization, give its name and address.)

Full Name	Complete Mailing Address
Wholly owned subsidiary of	4520 East-West Highway
Reed/Elsevier, US holdings	Bethesda, MD 20814

11. Known Bondholders, Mortgagees, and Other Security Holders Owning or Holding 1 Percent or More of Total Amount of Bonds, Mortgages, or Other Securities. If none, check box → None

Full Name	Complete Mailing Address
N/A	

12. Tax Status (For completion by nonprofit organizations authorized to mail at nonprofit rates) (Check one)
The purpose, function, and nonprofit status of this organization and the exempt status for federal income tax purposes:
☐ Has Not Changed During Preceding 12 Months
☐ Has Changed During Preceding 12 Months (Publisher must submit explanation of change with this statement)

PS Form 3526, September 2006 (Page 1 of 3 (Instructions Page 3)) PSN 7530-01-000-9931 PRIVACY NOTICE: See our Privacy policy in www.usps.com

---

13. Publication Title
Clinics in Geriatric Medicine

14. Issue Date for Circulation Data Below
August 2007

15. Extent and Nature of Circulation		Average No. Copies Each Issue During Preceding 12 Months	No. Copies of Single Issue Published Nearest to Filing Date
a. Total Number of Copies (Net press run)		1850	1700
b. Paid Circulation (By Mail and Outside the Mail)	(1) Mailed Outside-County Paid Subscriptions Stated on PS Form 3541. (Include paid distribution above nominal rate, advertiser's proof copies, and exchange copies)	858	817
	(2) Mailed In-County Paid Subscriptions Stated on PS Form 3541 (Include paid distribution above nominal rate, advertiser's proof copies, and exchange copies)		
	(3) Paid Distribution Outside the Mails Including Sales Through Dealers and Carriers, Street Vendors, Counter Sales, and Other Paid Distribution Outside USPS®	285	309
	(4) Paid Distribution by Other Classes Mailed Through the USPS (e.g. First-Class Mail®)		
c. Total Paid Distribution (Sum of 15b (1), (2), (3), and (4))	►	1143	1126
d. Free or Nominal Rate Distribution (By Mail and Outside the Mail)	(1) Free or Nominal Rate Outside-County Copies Included on PS Form 3541	97	84
	(2) Free or Nominal Rate In-County Copies Included on PS Form 3541		
	(3) Free or Nominal Rate Copies Mailed at Other Classes Mailed Through the USPS (e.g. First-Class Mail)		
	(4) Free or Nominal Rate Distribution Outside the Mail (Carriers or other means)		
e. Total Free or Nominal Rate Distribution (Sum of 15d (1), (2), (3) and (4))	►	97	84
f. Total Distribution (Sum of 15c and 15e)	►	1240	1210
g. Copies not Distributed (See instructions to publishers #4 (page #3))	►	610	490
h. Total (Sum of 15f and g)	►	1850	1700
i. Percent Paid (15c divided by 15f times 100)		92.18%	93.06%

16. Publication of Statement of Ownership
If the publication is a general publication, publication of this statement is required. Will be printed ☐ Publication not required
in the November 2007 issue of this publication.

17. Signature and Title of Editor, Publisher, Business Manager, or Owner

Stephen Bushing – Executive Director of Subscription Services

Date
September 14, 2007

I certify that all information furnished on this form is true and complete. I understand that anyone who furnishes false or misleading information on this form or who omits material or information requested on the form may be subject to criminal sanctions (including fines and imprisonment) and/or civil sanctions (including civil penalties).

PS Form 3526, September 2006 (Page 2 of 3)

Moving?

Make sure your subscription moves with you!

To notify us of your new address, find your **Clinics Account Number** (located on your mailing label above your name), and contact customer service at:

E-mail: elspcs@elsevier.com

800-654-2452 (subscribers in the U.S. & Canada)
407-345-4000 (subscribers outside of the U.S. & Canada)

Fax number: 407-363-9661

Elsevier Periodicals Customer Service
6277 Sea Harbor Drive
Orlando, FL 32887-4800

*To ensure uninterrupted delivery of your subscription, please notify us at least 4 weeks in advance of move.